AF341605

REVIEWS ON IMMUNOASSAY TECHNOLOGY:
VOLUME 1

Reviews on Immunoassay Technology

Volume 1

Edited by

S. B. Pal

Universität Ulm
Abteilung für Innere Medizin I
7900 Ulm, FR Germany

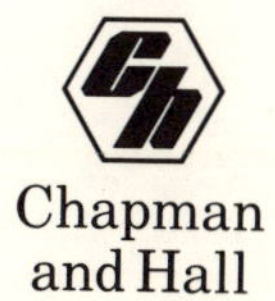

Chapman
and Hall

First published 1988

Published in the USA and Canada by
CHAPMAN & HALL
The Scientific and Technical Division of
Routledge, Chapman and Hall, Inc.
29 West 35th Street, New York,
New York 10001–2291

Typeset by TecSet Ltd, Wallington, Surrey, UK
Printed in Hong Kong

Library of Congress Cataloging-in-Publication Data
Reviews on immunoassay technology.
Includes bibliographies.
1. Immunoassay—Technique.   2. Immunoenzyme
technique.   I. Pal, S. B., 1928–
QP519.9.I42R48   1988   616.07′56   88–16190
ISBN 0–412–01841–1 (v. 1)
ISBN 0–412–01851–9 (v. 2)

Contents

The Contributors*

R. Anthony (147)
Dept of Pathology
Western Infirmary
Glasgow
Scotland UK

F. B. Bianchi (165)
Istituto di Patologia Medica, Cattedra
   di Clinica Medica II
University of Bologna
Bologna
Italy

R. Braun (177)
Institut für Medizinische Virologie
Ruprecht-Karls-Universität Heidelberg
Im Neuenheimer Feld 324
6900 Heidelberg
FR Germany

J. B. Bury (1)
Dept of Biochemistry
Raadsherenlaan 49
8310 Brugge
Belgium

A. Castro (95 and 111)
University of Miami School of Medicine
South Campus
12500 SW 152nd Street
Building B
Miami
FL 33177
USA

J. Coolen (59)
TNO Institute for Experimental
   Gerontology
PO Box 5815
2280 HV Rijswijk
The Netherlands

C. Crespi (165)
Istituto di Patologia Medica
   Cattedra di Clinica Medica II
University of Bologna
Bologna
Italy

C. Deen (59)
TNO Institute for Experimental
   Gerontology
PO Box 5815
2280 HV Rijswijk
The Netherlands

G. Dunkler (177)
Institut für Medizinische Virologie
Ruprecht-Karls-Universität Heidelberg
Im Neuenheimer Feld 324
6900 Heidelberg 324
FR Germany

G. Fahraeus-Van Ree (195)
Thyroid Research Laboratory
Health Sciences Center
St John's
Newfoundland
Canada A1B 3V6

N. R. Farid (195)
Thyroid Research Laboratory
Health Sciences Center
St John's
Newfoundland
Canada A1B 3V6

S. A. Gaffar (123)
University of California at San Diego
UCSD Cancer Center
T-011, Department of Medicine
La Jolla
CA 92093
USA

---

*Numbers in parentheses adjacent to the contributors' names indicate the first page of their contribution(s)

M. C Glassy (123)
California Biotherapeutics Inc
11025 N. Torrey Pines Road
La Jolla
CA 92037
USA

J. J. Haaijman (59)
TNO Medical Biological Laboratory
PO Box 45
2280 AA Rijswijk
The Netherlands

A. Hamilton (147)
Dept of Pathology
Western Infirmary
Glasgow
Scotland

T. W. Jungi (31)
Institute for Clinical and Experimental
    Cancer Research
University of Berne
Tiefenau Hospital
3004 Berne
Switzerland

T. Kröse (59)
TNO Institute for Experimental
    Gerontology
PO Box 5815
2280 HV Rijswijk
The Netherlands

J. Kühn (177)
Reprecht-Karls-Universität Heidelberg
Im Neuenheimer Feld 324
6900 Heidelberg
FR Germany

N. Monji (95 and 111)
Genetic Systems Corporation
3005 First Avenue
Seattle
WA 98121
USA

L. Morrison (147)
Dept of Pathology
Western Infirmary
Glasgow
Scotland

K. Munk (177)
Repurecht-Karls-Universität Heidelberg
Im Neuenheimer Feld 324
6900 Heidelberg
FR Germany

M. Musiani (165)
Istituto di Microbiologia
University of Bologna
Bologna
Italy

J. Radl (59)
TNO Institute for Experimental
    Gerontology
PO Box 5815
2280 HV Rijswijk
The Netherlands

M. Rosseneu (1)
Dept of Clinical Biochemistry
AZ St-Jan van het OCMW
Ruddershove 10
8000 Brugge
Belgium

P. Tazzari (165)
Istituto di Ematologia 'L. & A.
    Seragnoli'
University of Bologna
Bologna
Italy

K. Whaley (147)
Dept of Pathology
Western Infirmary
Glasgow
Scotland

D. Zauli (165)
Istituto di Patologia Medica Cattedra
    di Clinica Medica II
Policlinico S. Orsola
Via Massarenti 9
40138 Bologna
Italy

J. Zijlstra (59)
TNO Institute for Experimental
    Gerontology
PO Box 5815
2280 HV Rijswijk
The Netherlands

Preface

Immunology is a rapidly developing scientific discipline, as a result of which many new techniques are now available. On this basis it was decided to publish this series of monographs which we have called *Reviews on Immunoassay Technology*, which is targeted mainly at immunologists and other laboratory workers. The first volume contains 10 chapters by 28 authors with wide experience in immunoassay, and it is hoped that readers will find the information presented interesting and thought provoking.

Much credit goes to The Macmillan Press Ltd for making the necessary arrangements for the publication of this series. I should also like to take this opportunity of thanking Dr. D. Donaldson, MRCP, FRCPath, Consultant Chemical Pathologist, East Surrey Hospital, Redhill, Surrey, UK, for his helpful suggestions during the preparation of this volume, and Mrs. M. R. Lingard-Pal for her assistance as an honorary editorial secretary.

Ulm, 1987   S. B. P.

1. Apolipoprotein Quantitation by ELISA: Technical Aspects and Clinical Applications

J. B. BURY AND M. Y. ROSSENEU

INTRODUCTION

The structure of the major apolipoproteins and their specific functions in lipo-protein metabolism have been extensively studied (Jackson *et al.*, 1976; Mahley *et al.*, 1984; Eisenberg, 1984; Scanu *et al.*, 1982). The quantitation of apolipo-proteins by chromatographic means is cumbersome and bioassays hardly exist. Therefore, one has to rely on the differential quantitation of specific apolipo-proteins by immunological techniques (Lippel, 1983). Several immunoassays have already been described (Lippel, 1983; Steinberg *et al.*, 1983; Rosseneu *et al.*, 1983a), among which are radial immunodiffusion (RID), electroimmuno-diffusion (EID), immunonephelometric assay (INA) and radioimmunoassay (RIA).

Applicability of the immunodiffusion technique to apolipoprotein quanti-tation is limited by differences in the diffusion constants between the purified apolipoproteins and the various lipoprotein classes, thereby obscuring the assay standardization. In addition, these assays have a limited sensitivity compared with RIA, require large amounts of antisera and are not easily automated. In contrast, the INA, based on the proportionality between the antigen concentra-tion and intensity of light scattered by the insoluble antigen–antibody complex, is fast, precise, simple and easily automated. However, the apolipoproteins belong to several lipoprotein classes of different size and with different kinetics of antigen–antibody complex formation. Therefore, application of this technique is restricted to endpoint laser nephelometry of apolipoproteins present in normolipidaemic plasma. The accuracy of the INAs decreases with increasing turbidity of hypertriglyceridaemic samples, owing to high blanks. Therefore, these samples have to be pretreated with detergents, lipoprotein lipase or organic solvents (Bury *et al.*, 1985; Rosseneu *et al.*, 1981a).

The most sensitive technique for apolipoprotein measurement is RIA (Blum, 1983). Most assays are, however, time consuming and suffer from the major drawbacks associated with the use of radioisotopes, i.e. the high cost and short shelf-life of reagents, the expensive gamma counters and the biohazards which attend the preparation, use and disposal of isotope-labelled reagents.

Therefore, alternative analytical techniques have been developed, whereby the radioisotope was replaced by an enzyme (Scharpé *et al.*, 1978; Oellerich, 1984), a fluorochrome (Hemmilä, 1985) or another indicator (Schall and Tenoso, 1981). Since the introduction in 1971 of the enzyme immunoassay (EIA) by Avrameas and Guilbert (1971), Engvall and Perlmann (1971) and Van Weemen and Schuurs (1971), multiple variations of this technique have been developed, which can be classified among two main assay types: homogeneous and heterogeneous assays. When the activity of the enzyme is influenced by the formation of an antigen–antibody complex, the EIA is called homogeneous. This technique has been applied mainly to the quantitation of small molecules such as drugs (Scharpé *et al.*, 1978) and does not require separation of free and bound enzyme. In the heterogeneous assays, however, where the enzyme activity is not influenced by the formation of the antigen–antibody complex, bound and unbound enzyme conjugate have to be separated. In the classical EIA (Avrameas and Guilbert, 1971; Engvall and Perlmann, 1971; Van Weemen and Schuurs, 1971), the antigen or the antibody is attached to an insoluble carrier (solid phase), enabling easy separation of free and bound enzyme. This technique is called the enzyme-linked immunosorbent assay (ELISA) technique, and it can be applied as well to competitive as to non-competitive-assays. In view of the limited stability of apolipoproteins in solution, the competitive ELISA techniques, requiring an antigen–enzyme complex or an antigen-coated solid phase, are of limited use for apolipoprotein quantitation.

Therefore, we chose to develop a sandwich ELISA, using immunoglobulins for both the coating of the solid phase and the preparation of the enzyme conjugate. The principle of the assay is presented in figure 1. After coating with monospecific antibodies (I) and washing, the solid phase is incubated with the test samples containing the antigen for assay (II). The solid phase is then washed, incubated with the monospecific enzyme-labelled antibodies (III) and washed again. The amount of bound enzyme, which is proportional to the amount of antigen in the test solution, is assayed colorimetrically (IV).

ISOLATION OF APOLIPOPROTEINS

The four major lipoprotein classes were obtained by sequential ultracentrifugal flotation from hypertriglyceridaemic plasma for chylomicrons and very low density lipoproteins (VLDL) and from normolipaemic plasma for low density lipoproteins (LDL) and high density lipoproteins (HDL) (Mills *et al.*, 1984). All fractions were subsequently delipidated with ether:ethanol (Mills *et al.*, 1984). The apolipoproteins A-I and A-II were isolated from apo HDL by ion exchange chromatography on diethylaminoethyl cellulose (DEAE cellulose) (Blaton *et al.*, 1977). Water-soluble apo B was prepared from LDL (d = 1.030–1.050 g/ml) as

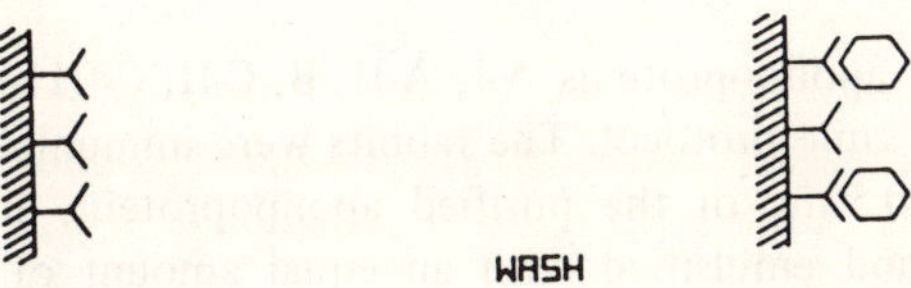

Figure 1   Principle of the sandwich ELISA for apolipoprotein quantitation.

described by Cardin *et al.* (1982). Apo VLDL was fractionated by gel filtration on a Sephacryl S_{200} column (Bury *et al.*, 1985a), yielding three major fractions containing apo B, apo E and apo C. Apo C-III$_0$, apo C-III$_1$ and apo C-III$_2$ were isolated from the apo C-containing fraction by ion exchange chromatography on DEAE cellulose (Bury *et al.*, 1985a), while apo C-II was isolated from the same fraction by chromatofocusing on polybuffer exchanger 94 (Bury *et al.*, 1986a). The apo E-containing fraction of apo VLDL was further purified either by high performance liquid chromatography (HPLC), using size exclusion chromatography on an LKB ultra-pac TSK-G 3000 SW (Vercaemst *et al.*, 1984), or by chromatofocusing on polybuffer exchanger 94 (Bury *et al.*, 1986b).

The purified apolipoproteins were identified by their electrophoretic mobility on polyacrylamide gels containing sodium dodecyl sulphate (Mills *et al.*, 1984), by isoelectric focusing on polyacrylamide gels containing 8 M urea (Mills *et al.*, 1984), by immunodiffusion against specific antisera and on the basis of their specific amino acid composition (Scanu *et al.*, 1982).

PRODUCTION OF ANTISERA

Polyclonal antisera against apolipoproteins A-I, A-II, B, C-II, C-III and E were raised in rabbits using the same protocol. The rabbits were immunized by subcutaneous injection with 0.5 mg of the purified apolipoprotein, dissolved in 0.5 ml 5 mM NH_4HCO_3 and emulsified with an equal amount of complete Freund's adjuvant (Difco Laboratories). Because of the poor solubility of apo B in aqueous buffers, apo B antisera were raised by immunization with LDL, isolated from normolipidaemic plasma at a density range 1.030–1.050 g/ml (Rosseneu *et al.*, 1983a).

Booster injections of 0.2–0.3 mg apolipoprotein, dissolved and emulsified as described above, were given at 3 week intervals until reasonable titres were obtained (usually three boosters). The rabbits were bled 2 weeks after the last injection.

Antiserum titres were determined by immunodiffusion as described by Sewell (1967), while the specificity was checked by double immunodiffusion against purified apolipoproteins A-I, A-II, B, C-II, C-III, E and human serum albumin.

ISOLATION OF SPECIFIC IMMUNOGLOBULINS

The total immunoglobulin fraction was isolated from the antisera by a combination of ammonium sulphate precipitation and anion exchange chromatography on DEAE cellulose (Johnstone and Thorpe, 1982). Affinity-purified antibodies were prepared by immunosorbent chromatography. Affinity chromatography columns were prepared by covalent linkage of 0.5–10 mg of the purified apolipoprotein, dissolved in 5 ml 0.1 M $NaHCO_3$ buffer, pH 8.3, with 0.5 M NaCl, to 3–15 ml CNBr-activated Sepharose 4B (Pharmacia, Uppsala, Sweden) suspended in the same buffer (Pharmacia, 1979). The yield of coupling, determined from the absorbance at 280 nm of the protein solution before and after incubation with the gel, was > 90% for all apolipoproteins. The residual coupling sites of the CNBr-activated Sepharose were blocked by incubation with 0.2 M glycine–HCl buffer, pH 8.0. An apo B–Sepharose matrix was prepared by covalent linkage of LDL (d = 1.030–1.050 g/ml) as a source of apo B (Rosseneu *et al.*, 1983a).

The apolipoprotein-Sepharose gel was incubated for 90 min at room temperature with 3–10 ml of the corresponding antisera and poured into a small column (2 cm × 10 cm). The gel was eluted at a rate of 35 ml/h with a 10 mM sodium phosphate buffer, pH 7.4, containing 0.15 M NaCl, until absorbance of the eluate at 280 nm had reached baseline levels. The immunoglobulins, linked to the Sepharose matrix, were eluted with 20 ml of 0.2 M glycine-HCl buffer, pH 2.6, and collected into 5 ml of 1 M K_2HPO_4. After concentration on a YM 30 Diaflo membrane (Amicon Co., Danvers, MA 01923), the purified immunoglobulins were dialysed against 10 mM sodium carbonate buffer, pH 9.5, and used for the preparation of an antibody-enzyme conjugate (this page). If the immunoglobulins were used for solid phase coating (page 6), the eluate was dialysed against 10 mM sodium phosphate buffer, pH 7.4, containing 0.15 M NaCl and 1 g/l NaN_3, filtered through a 0.45 μm pore-size filter (Millipore Corp., Bedford, MA 01730), and stored at 4°C.

PREPARATION OF THE ENZYME–ANTIBODY CONJUGATE

Several enzymes, including alkaline phosphatase and horse radish peroxidase (HRPO), have been proposed as suitable labels for EIA (Scharpé *et al.*, 1978; Oellerich, 1984). In view of its excellent properties and its easy conjugation with immunoglobulins (Scharpé *et al.*, 1978; Voller *et al.*, 1979), HRPO (E.C. 1.11.1.7) was selected for conjugate preparation. The antibody–enzyme conjugate was prepared by a modification of the periodate coupling procedure described by Nakane and Kawaoi (1974). HRPO is a glycoprotein whose reducing hydroxyl groups can be oxidized by sodium periodate to form the corresponding aldehyde. The free primary alkylamino groups of the immunoglobulins can form a Schiff base with the HRPO aldehyde, thereby covalently linking the two proteins.

Five milligrams HRPO (grade I, RZ > 3.0, Boehringer Mannheim, FRG) was dissolved in 2 ml of 0.3 M $NaHCO_3$ and gently mixed with 100 μl of a 0.1 g/l ethanolic solution of 2,4-dinitro-monofluorobenzene, in order to block the free amino groups of the enzyme. After 2 h incubation at room temperature, 1 ml of 80 mM $NaIO_4$ solution was added. The reaction was stopped after 1 h by the addition of 0.2 ml of glycerol. The incubation mixture was extensively dialysed at 4°C against 10 mM sodium carbonate–bicarbonate buffer, pH 9.5.

One millilitre of a 10 g/l solution of affinity-purified immunoglobulins was dialysed against the same carbonate–bicarbonate buffer and subsequently incubated with the peroxidase aldehyde for 3 h at room temperature. The incubation mixture was dialysed against 0.1 M sodium phosphate buffer, pH 7.4, and stored in 100 μl aliquots without further reduction of the Schiff base or fractionation of free and bound enzyme. After the addition of an equal mount of glycerol, storage was carried out, either at -20°C for conjugates used daily, or at -70°C for longer storage periods. The conjugates, stored at -70°C were stable for at least two years without significant loss of immunologic or enzymatic activity.

Both total immunoglobulins and affinity-purified immunoglobulins are suitable for the preparation of an enzyme–antibody conjugate. However, the low specific activity of the total immunoglobulin fraction requires higher concentrations of conjugated enzyme to obtain a specific response. As a consequence, the non-specific binding is significantly increased. Therefore, the enzyme–antibody conjugates used in the apolipoprotein immunoassays were prepared with affinity-purified immunoglobulins.

COATING, WASH AND ASSAY BUFFERS

Coating of the solid phase is usually performed in alkaline solutions (Voller *et al.*, 1979; Wood and Gadow, 1983). Similar results were, however, obtained with a 10 mM sodium phosphate buffer, pH 7.4, containing 0.15 M NaCl, which was further used throughout the whole assay procedure, for coating, for washing, for antigen or conjugate dilution, and for incubation. In addition, the coating buffer contained 1 g/l NaN_3 as a preservative, whilst the assay buffer contained bovine serum albumin (1 g/l) and the wash buffer contained Tween 20 (0.5 ml/l) to reduce non-specific binding (page 9).

COATING OF THE SOLID PHASE

Although several carriers such as grains of glass, silicone, cellulose or various kinds of plastic materials have been proposed for the solid phase, polystyrene beads and microtitre plates have found a wide application owing to their practical use and reproducible coating properties.

The wells of polystyrene microtitre plates were coated with the specific antibodies by passive adsorption from 110 μl coating buffer containing 1–3 μg immunoglobulins. The plates were sealed with sealing tape (Dynatech, Alexandria, VA 22234) to reduce evaporation and incubated for 3 h at 37°C, followed by overnight incubation at 4°C. In view of possible batch-dependent edge effects (Kricka *et al.*, 1980), the outer rows of the microtitre plates were excluded. The coated plates, stored at 4°C in the presence of the immunoglobulin solution, were stable for three to six months without any significant loss of immuno-reactivity or assay precision.

Before use, the microtitre plates were washed three times with wash buffer and incubated for 1 h at room temperature with 150 μl assay buffer, containing bovine serum albumin to block the residual binding sites. After washing with the wash buffer, the plates were ready for use.

Polystyrene beads with a diameter of 6.5 mm (Seroa, Monaco) were washed with distilled water and coated by immersion in a solution of specific immunoglobulins (10–30 μg/ml coating buffer) and incubated for 3 h at 37°C. As described for the microtitre plates, the residual binding sites were blocked with albumin.

When affinity-purified antibodies were used for coating, the excess immunoglobulins were recycled as they could be used for at least five consecutive coatings.

As the assay precision of the ELISA techniques is mainly determined by reproducibility of the coating (McCullough and Parkinson, 1984b), several polystyrene supports were tested for their use as a solid phase in the apolipoprotein assay: polystyrene beads (Seroa), Greiner and Dynatech microtitre plates, Dynatech MicroELISA plates and Nunc Immunoplates, number I. Although high reproducibility was obtained with polystyrene beads (mean intra-assay coefficient of variation (CV) 4.4%, $n = 10$), the ELISA performed on the microtitre plates, using the same assay conditions (coating concentration, conjugate dilution, incubation time and temperature; pages 8–10), was about 10 times more sensitive (figure 2). In addition, polystyrene beads are not well suited for scaling-up procedures, owing to their lack of practical use and high cost compared with microtitre plates. Among the microtitre plates, the Micro-ELISA plates M 129B (Dynatech) were selected because of their high and reproducible coating.

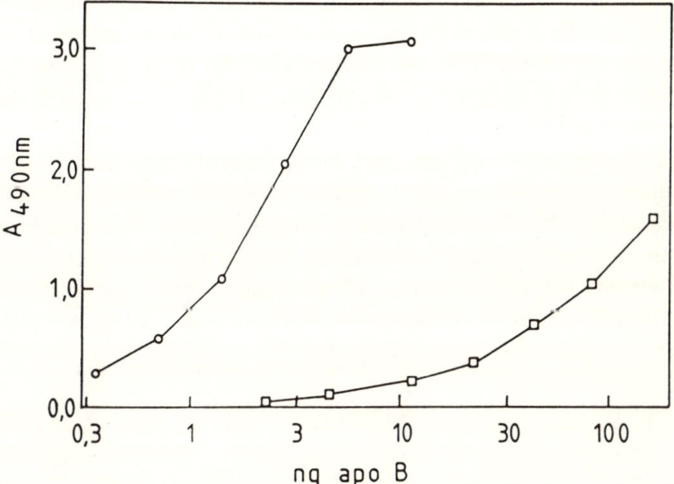

Figure 2 Comparison of the apo B ELISA performed on polystyrene microtitre plates (○) and on polystyrene beads (□) using the same assay conditions.

The selection of either total immunoglobulins or affinity-purified antibodies for solid phase coating was dependent on the apolipoprotein to be assayed. For example, a total immunoglobulin fraction was satisfactory for the apo B ELISA, whereas the use of affinity-purified antibodies was essential in most other apolipoprotein assays in order to minimize non-specific binding. As such factors are probably dependent on the titre and the affinity of the polyclonal antisera raised, and may differ from one batch to another, it is advisable to use either affinity-purified antibodies or well-characterized monoclonal or oligoclonal antibodies for coating and for the preparation of the enzyme–antibody conjugate.

OPTIMIZING ASSAY CONDITIONS

The optimal coating concentration, conjugate dilution and minimal antigen concentration can be determined by a single chequer-board titration (Voller *et al.*, 1979). For this purpose, the horizontal rows of microtitre plates were coated with increasing antibody concentrations, ranging from 0 to 100 μg immunoglobulins/ml coating buffer. The assay was performed with antigen amounts between 0 and 100 ng, using several conjugate dilutions (1000- to 20 000-fold) in the vertical rows of the microtitre plates. The incubations with antigen and conjugate were performed at 37°C for 2 h. If a slow antigen–antibody formation is to be expected, the incubations can be extended overnight.

Some of the results obtained by chequer-board titration for the apo A-I ELISA are summarized in table 1. They indicate that the non-specific response increases with increasing coating and conjugate concentrations. However, the specific response (expressed as the assay response at given antigen concentrations minus the non-specific response of the assay without antigen) plateaus at increasing coating concentrations. The determination of the optimal coating concentration for the apo A-I ELISA is shown in figure 3. Since the specific response tends to decrease at high coating concentrations (> 100 μg/ml, data not shown), the optimal coating concentration for the apo A-I ELISA was found to be 15–20 μg/ml.

As indicated in table 1, the optimal conjugate dilution is dependent on the assay sensitivity required: using a 2500-fold conjugate dilution, the detection range lies between 0.1 and 3 ng apo A-I per assay, whereas, at a 20 000-fold conjugate dilution, the detection range lies between 3 and 50 ng apo A-I. High

Table 1   The optimal assay parameters are determined by chequer-board titration

Conjugate dilution	Coating concentration								
	5 μg/ml			10 μg/ml			20 μg/ml		
	0 ng	1 ng	10 ng	0 ng	1 ng	10 ng	0 ng	1 ng	10 ng
1000	0.81	2.28	>3.2	1.23	2.29	>3.2	1.41	3.81	>3.2
2500	0.29	1.22	>3.2	0.40	1.64	>3.2	0.53	1.82	>3.2
5000	0.16	0.67	2.98	0.16	0.86	3.13	0.22	1.03	3.16
10000	0.02	0.26	1.04	0.05	0.40	2.14	0.08	0.48	2.36
20000	0.02	0.14	0.55	0.02	0.18	0.87	0.03	0.19	0.98

The data represent absorption measurements at 490 nm, compared with a blank containing 100 μl substrate and 100 μl 2.5 M H_2SO_4. The test solutions contained 0, 1 or 10 ng of antigen as indicated.

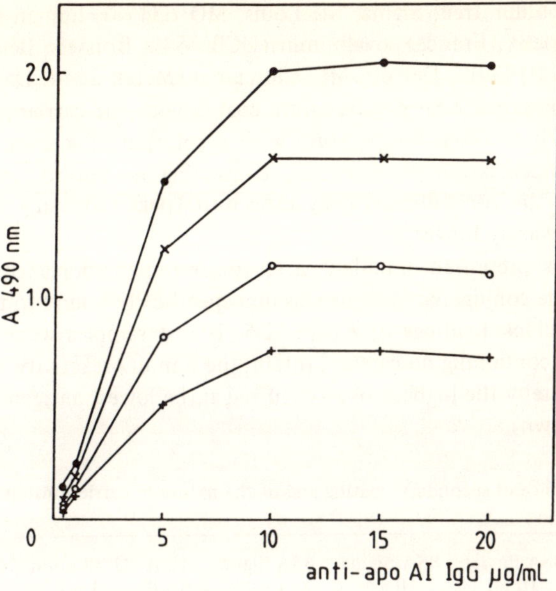

Figure 3   Influence of the coating concentration on the specific response of various amounts of antigen: +, 2.5 ng apo A-I; ○, 5 ng apo A-I; ×, 10 ng apo A-I; ●, 20 ng apo A-I. The assay was performed using the standard assay procedure. (Reproduced with permission from Bury and Rosseneu (1985a).)

conjugate dilutions result, however, in poor slopes of the calibration curves. Therefore, the best combination of a high sensitivity and a low zero-dose response was obtained by using a 7500-fold conjugate dilution, whereby the assay could quantify 0.5–15 ng apo A-I.

INHIBITION OF NON-SPECIFIC BINDING

As a consequence of their hydrophobic character, significant losses of apolipoproteins, as a result of adsorption onto plastic recipients and pipettes, might occur during the manipulation of dilute solutions (Holmquist, 1982a). Such losses should, therefore, be minimized by the presence of a carrier protein in all buffers used for sample dilution and during assay incubations (Livesey and Donald, 1982; Samaké *et al.*, 1983; McCullough and Parkinson, 1984a). In addition, non-specific binding of the antigen and of the enzyme–antibody conjugate to the solid phase should be reduced by blocking any residual binding sites with a non-interfering protein. Widely used albumin preparations might contain some contaminating apolipoproteins (Deckelbaum *et al.*, 1980), requiring the comparison of several carrier proteins such as bovine serum albumin (Poviet grade, Organon Technika, Boxtel, Holland), bovine serum albumin (A-7030 fatty acid and globulin free, Sigma, St. Louis, MO 63178), human serum albumin (Institut Merieux, France), ovalbumin (UCB 4542, Brussels, Belgium), gelatine (Difco-Bacto 0143-02, Detroit, MI) and casein (Merck 2244, Darmstadt, FRG). For this purpose microtitre plates were coated with the carrier protein by incubation for 1 h at room temperature with a solution of a given protein at the specified concentration. Such plates, containing no antibodies, were further processed by the conventional assay procedure (page 13), using the same carrier protein in the assay buffer.

The results, presented in table 2, stress the extreme importance of a secondary coating, as the conjugated enzyme was non-specifically bound to the solid phase, resulting in blank readings of $E_{490} > 2.5$. If test samples were diluted in the assay buffer, containing no carrier protein, the immunoreactivity was reduced by 10–50%, whereby the highest losses occurred at the lowest antigen concentrations (data not shown).

Table 2   Influence of secondary coating and of the nature of carrier protein on non-specific plates binding

Non-coated plates	BSA Poviet 10 g/l	BSA Sigma 10 g/l	BSA Sigma 1 g/l	HSA 1 g/l	Ovalbumin 1 g/l	Casein 1 g/l	Gelatine 1 g/l
2634	423	11	38	658	276	23	687

Tests were performed in microtitre plates, coated with the carrier protein only, using the standard assay procedure for the apo E ELISA, with assay buffers containing the concentrations specified for each protein. Data represent the E_{490} nm readings for tests, performed in the absence of antigen. BSA, bovine serum albumin; HSA, human serum albumin.

As shown in table 2 non-specific binding was inhibited by using casein or a fatty acid- and globulin-free bovine serum albumin preparation (Sigma A-7030). Bovine serum albumin, at a concentration of 1 g/l, was selected as carrier protein in the assay buffers and for the secondary coating of the solid phase, especially in view of its solubility properties.

Non-specific protein–protein interactions were inhibited by washing and soaking the incubated microtitre plates in wash buffer containing Tween 20 (0.5 ml/l). The use of this non-ionic detergent reduced the zero-dose response values by 30–70%, while the intra- and inter-assay coefficients of variation, determined for the apo A-I ELISA, concomitantly decreased from 7.5% to 3.9% and from 12.1% to 7.8% respectively. The combination of a secondary coating with albumin and the use of Tween 20 in the wash buffer decreased the intra-assay coefficient of variation for the apo C-III ELISA from 13.5% to 3.8%.

KINETICS OF THE ANTIGEN–ANTIBODY REACTION

The temperature-dependent kinetics of the antigen–antibody reaction were investigated by performing the assay (page 13), with incubation periods of either 30 min, 1 h, 2 h or 4 h at room temperature, 37°C or 45°C, or of 4 h at

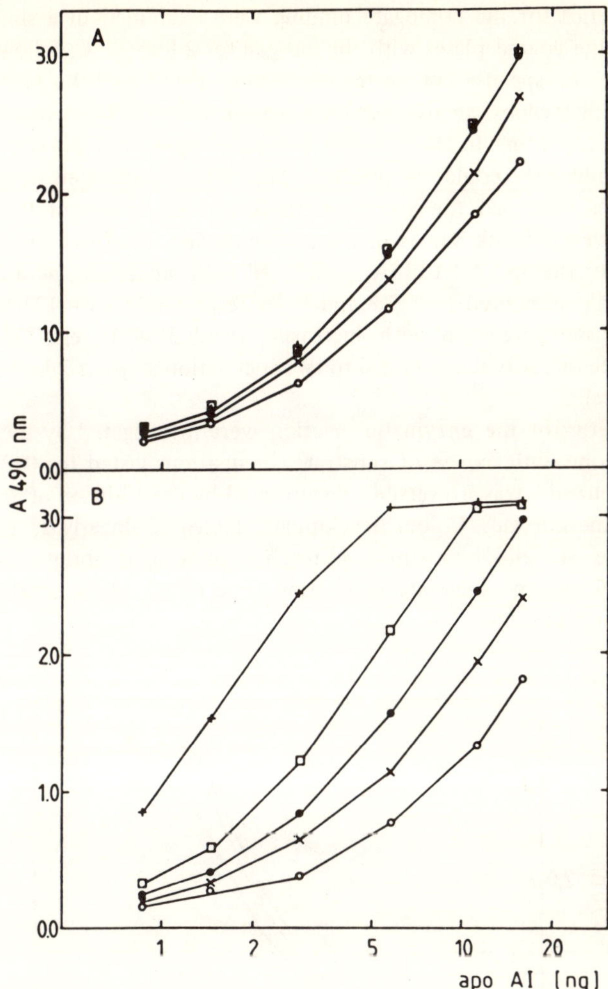

Figure 4 Kinetics of the antigen–antibody reaction for the apo A-I ELISA. Incubation conditions with the antigen (A) and with the antibody–enzyme conjugate (B) were 30 min (○), 1 h (×), 2 h (●) or 4 h (□) at 37°C or 4 h at 37°C followed by 16 h at 4°C (+). The assay was performed according to the standard assay procedure. (Reproduced with permission from Bury and Rosseneu (1985a).)

37°C, followed by an overnight incubation at 4°C. As demonstrated in figure 4A for the apo A-I ELISA, stable values were reached after the antigen was incubated for 2 h at 37°C. The same plateau was reached after 3 h for tests performed at room temperature. Increasing the incubation temperature up to 45°C did not further enhance the reaction kinetics.

The kinetics for the conjugate binding were examined in a similar way by incubating the coated plates with the antigen for 2 h at 37°C, followed by incubation with the specific conjugate for 30 min, 1 h, 2 h or 4 h at 37°C, or 4 h at 37°C, followed by an overnight incubation at 4°C. The assay was further carried out according to the standard procedure (page 13). As shown in figure 4B, no equilibrium could be reached. The use of prolonged conjugate incubation times increased the assay sensitivity and the slopes of the calibration curves. However, blank values increased simultaneously. In addition, the intra-assay CV for the apo A-I ELISA, performed with incubation periods of 2 h or 4 h at 37°C, amounted to 3.9% and 7.3% respectively ($N = 12$), indicating a decreased assay precision with increasing incubation times. Therefore, the ELISA procedure was standardized to two incubation steps of 2 h at 37°C for all apolipoproteins.

The kinetics of the enzymatic reaction were investigated by incubating the bound enzyme with excess of substrate. Incubations lasted for 0–30 min after which the enzyme was irreversibly denaturated by the addition of 2.5 M H_2SO_4 at 2 min time intervals. Colour development increased linearly as a function of time during the initial 6–8 min, to reach a plateau at about 20–25 min. A standardized enzyme–substrate incubation time of 30 min was selected for all apolipoprotein assays.

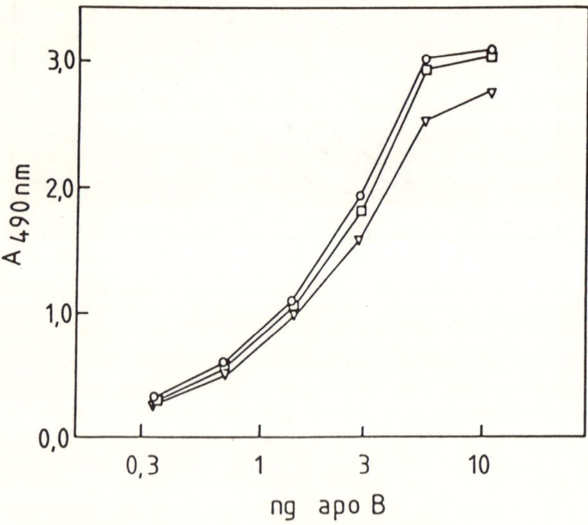

Figure 5 Combinations of several assay parameters yield the same assay sensitivity. The apo B ELISA was performed with two incubation steps of 2 h at 37 °C and a conjugate dilution of 1:10 000 (□), incubation steps of 3 h at 23°C and a conjugate dilution of 1:10 000 (○) or incubation steps of 16 h at 4°C and a conjugate dilution of 1:30 000 (▽).

As indicated in figure 5, an assay with the same detection limits can be obtained by the proper combination of conjugate concentration and incubation time and temperature. The choice of the assay conditions will, therefore, be dependent on the assay requirements, such as high sensitivity or fast acquisition of the results; it might become limited by the availability of some of the reagents, such as coating antibodies and enzyme–antibody conjugates.

GENERAL ASSAY PROCEDURE

The optimization of the assay parameters (pages 6–10) resulted in a common assay procedure, applicable to the quantitation of all apolipoproteins tested: apo A-I, apo B, apo C-II, apo C-III and apo E.

Tests Performed on Microtitre Plates

One hundred microlitres of the appropriate dilutions of a primary or a secondary standard, containing either 0.5–10 ng of purified apolipoprotein or 100 μl of diluted test samples, were pipetted in duplicate into the wells of a precoated and washed microtitre plate. The assay precision was increased by the use of an automatic diluter (Microlab 1000 Hamilton, Bonaduz, Switzerland). The plates were sealed with sealing tape (Dynatech), incubated for 2 h at 37°C and washed five times with wash buffer as described under page 9. The wells of the microtitre plates were shaken dry and filled with 100 μl of affinity-purified antibody-enzyme conjugate, diluted with assay buffer. The optimal conjugate dilution was determined by the chequer-board titration (page 8) and was usually around 5000- to 10 000-fold. After sealing, the plates were incubated for another 2 h at 37°C and washed as described above.

A substrate solution, containing H_2O_2 (0.2 g/l) and o-phenylenediamine dihydrochloride as a proton donor (3 g/l) in 0.1 M sodium phosphate–citrate buffer, pH 5.6, was freshly prepared; 100 μl of substrate was pipetted at timed intervals into the wells of the microtitre plates and incubated at room temperature in the dark. After 30 min the enzyme–substrate reaction was stopped by adding 100 μl 2.5 M H_2SO_4 (analytical grade, Merck, Darmstadt, FRG) to each well. Within 2 h, the absorption of the substrate solutions was read from each well at 490 nm, using a Chromo Scan EIA reader (Bio-Tek instruments, Burlington, VT 05401).

A calibration curve was obtained by plotting the absorbance at 490 nm as a function of the logarithm of the apolipoprotein concentration of the primary or the secondary standard. The results could also be calculated on a desk computer from the best-fitting least-squares parabola.

Tests Performed on Polystyrene Beads

When the ELISA was performed on polystyrene beads, the same assay procedure was essentially used with the following modifications. The incubation volumes were increased up to 300 μl, whereas the detectable antigen concentrations amounted to 5-100 ng of apolipoprotein per assay. The enzyme–substrate reaction was blocked by the addition of 2.0 ml 1 M H_2SO_4 following which the absorbance was read on a Quantum 1 Dual Wavelength Analyser (Abbott Instruments, Irving, TX 75062). The polystyrene beads were washed with a Pentawash II system (Abbott).

ASSAY STANDARDIZATION

The specific association of plasma apolipoproteins with lipids, tending to form stable lipid–protein complexes, complicates the standardization of apolipoprotein immunoassays. As more than 95% of the plasma apolipoproteins are located inside lipoproteins, a number of their antigenic sites might be masked by lipids. As a consequence, their actual plasma concentrations might be underestimated. Moreover, apolipoproteins belong to various lipoproteins of different sizes, compositions and surface pressures. This might influence the availability of some apolipoprotein epitopes and yield results varying with the plasma lipoprotein patterns.

Pretreatment of a sample with the aim of releasing the apolipoproteins from the lipoprotein complexes, by either partial or total delipidation using organic solvents, or with the aim of exposing the buried epitopes by treatment with lipase, detergents or denaturants, seems to be a prerequisite for the proper quantitation of some apolipoproteins (Lippel, 1983; Steinberg *et al.*, 1983; Rosseneu *et al.*, 1983a). As the requirements for sample pretreatment depend both on the nature of the apolipoprotein and on the immunological technique, no consensus has been reached so far. The sample pretreatments have recently been extensively reviewed for the apo A-I (Steinberg *et al.*, 1983) and apo B (Rosseneu *et al.*, 1983a) immunoassays. Therefore, we will focus on some general directions for the quantitation of apolipoproteins C and E.

As these apolipoproteins are present in both triglyceride-rich lipoproteins and in HDL (Jackson *et al.*, 1976; Mahley *et al.*, 1984; Eisenberg, 1984; Scanu *et al.*, 1982), special attention has to be paid to exposure of their antigenic sites. The influence of the plasma lipid concentration on the epitope expression of apolipoproteins C and E was investigated by their quantitation in normolipidaemic, hypercholesterolaemic and hypertriglyceridaemic samples, both before and after delipidation. For apolipoprotein immunoassays, delipidation was mostly performed with either ether–ethanol (Scanu and Edelstein, 1971) or diisopropyl-ether–*n*-butanol (Cham and Knowles, 1976). In contrast to the latter procedure, proposed by Cham and Knowles (1976), the ether–ethanol extraction induces precipitation of the apolipoproteins, which have to be resolubilized. Buffers containing urea or guanidinium chloride (GdmCl) can be used for this purpose, thereby enhancing the exposure of masked apolipoprotein epitopes.

The influence of triglyceride-rich lipoproteins on the immunoreactivity of exchangeable apolipoproteins (apo C and apo E) might also be investigated by the incubation of plasma with chylomicron-like triglyceride microemulsions such as Intralipid (Kabi Vitrum, Uppsala, Sweden).

If such treatments suggest that some of the apolipoprotein epitopes are masked in the lipoprotein complexes, sample pretreatment is required in order to obtain exact apolipoprotein concentrations. As organic solvent extraction of plasma is quite cumbersome, alternative approaches are possible, such as partial delipidation by the addition of tetramethylurea, triglyceride hydrolysis by lipoprotein lipase, addition of denaturants (8 M urea or 6 M GdmCl), or detergents (Tween 20, Triton X-100, Apovax, sodium decyl sulphate, sodium dodecyl sulphate, sodium cholate etc.).

A second major problem in the standardization of immunoassays arises from self-association of apolipoproteins on exposure to aqueous buffers. Such protein-protein associations influence the overall folding of the polypeptide backbone and might therefore affect the immunological properties of the primary apolipoprotein standard (Osborne *et al.*, 1983). As the formation of these apolipoprotein oligomers is reversible and is dependent on the protein concentration, pH, temperature and ionic strength of the buffer, their presence in the primary standards should be avoided by using low protein concentrations of 10 mg/l or less (Osborne *et al.*, 1983). This is most easily achieved for the most sensitive immunoassays, such as RIA or ELISA.

Apolipoprotein aggregates can also be irreversibly formed during the lyophilization or prolonged storage of apolipoproteins in concentrated solutions (Osborne *et al.*, 1983). The primary standards should be freshly prepared in aqueous buffers, containing low concentrations of either denaturants (0.3 M GdmCl) or detergents (0.1 g/l Apovax) in order to reduce protein-protein interaction. Alternatively, lyophilized apolipoproteins, stored under nitrogen at $-20°$C, can be solubilized in a buffer containing 3 M GdmCl or 4 M urea, dialysed against the assay buffer (without carrier protein), and filtered through a micro-pore sized filter ($0.22\ \mu$m). The same apolipoprotein solution should be freshly used both as a primary standard in the immunoassay and for quantitative determination of the primary standard by amino acid analysis. The concentration of the primary standard can further be assayed by the Folin–Lowry procedure (Lowry *et al.*, 1951) and by the absorbance measurement of the purified protein at 280 nm, using the theoretical extinction coefficients based on amino acid composition (Scanu *et al.*, 1982).

The numerous difficulties encountered in apolipoprotein immunoassay standardization with primary standards favour the general and controlled use of a secondary standard, distributed by the Lipid–Apoprotein Subcommittee of the Standardization Committee of the International Union of Immunochemical Societies (Cooper *et al.*, 1985). As such, standards are not yet available for the apolipoproteins C and E; a pool of normolipidaemic plasma, aliquoted

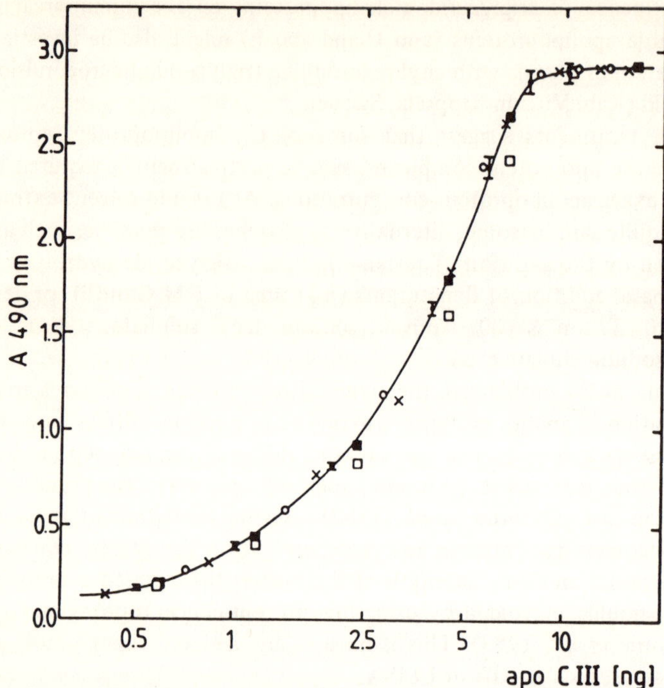

Figure 6   Calibration curves for the apo C-III ELISA: purified apolipoprotein (X), normolipidaemic plasma (⬢) (mean ± S.D.), normolipidaemic delipidated plasma (○) and plasma from a Fredrickson type V patient before (■) and after (□) delipidation. (Reproduced with permission from Bury and Rosseneu (1985b).)

and stored at $-20°C$, was routinely used as a secondary standard and control (Rosseneu *et al.*, 1983a).

The ELISA assays were standardized with freshly purified apolipoproteins, solubilized in a 10 mM sodium phosphate buffer, pH 7.4, containing 0.15 M NaCl and either 0.1 g/l of the non-ionic detergent Apovax or 0.4 M urea (apo E ELISA). For the apo B ELISA, the primary standard consisted of LDL (d = 1.030–1.050 g/ml), freshly isolated from normolipidaemic plasma by sequential ultracentrifugation (Rosseneu *et al.*, 1981b; Rosseneu *et al.*, 1983a).

A prerequisite for a reliable immunoassay is the parallelism of the primary and the secondary standards. As illustrated in figure 6 for the apo C-III ELISA, the calibration curves, constructed with purified apo C-III$_2$ and with plasma obtained from a normolipidaemic subject and from a subject with a severe Fredrickson type V hyperlipoproteinaemia (triglycerides 47.3 g/l and cholesterol 8.9 g/l) were identical. The CV, determined from the apo C-III concentrations of six different dilutions of the same normo- and hyperlipoproteinaemic plasma, spanning the whole assay range, were 3.9% and 4.6% respectively, stressing the good parallelism with the primary calibration curve. Similar results were obtained for the other apolipoprotein immunoassays.

As the apolipoproteins C and E are distributed among various lipoprotein classes, the parallelism between the response of the purified apolipoprotein and that of the lipoproteins has to be investigated. Calibration curves were constructed with increasing amounts of chylomicrons, VLDL, LDL and HDL freshly isolated from plasma by sequential ultracentrifugation. Figure 7 illustrates the analogous behaviour of the four major lipoprotein classes in the apo C-II ELISA. The CV, determined for the different dilutions ($N = 6$) used to construct the lipoprotein standard curves, amounted to 4.0%, 2.4%, 7.1% and 7.1% respectively, indicating good parallelism with the primary apolipoprotein standard. Parallel curves were also obtained for the apo A-I (Bury and Rosseneu, 1985a), apo B, apo C-III (Bury and Rosseneu, 1985b), and the apo E assays (Bury *et al.*, 1986b). On the basis of their total protein content, determined by the Lowry assay (Lowry *et al.*, 1951), the chylomicrons isolated from a Fredrickson type V patient contained 16.2% apo C-II, 38.1% apo C-III and 3.2% apo E, whereas the lipoproteins isolated from a normolipidaemic patient contained 6.8% apo C-II, 36.1% apo C-III and 6.4% apo E for the VLDL ($d < 1.006$ g/ml), 0.26% apo C-II, 0.52% apo C-III and 1.42% apo E for the LDL ($d = 1.030$–1.060 g/ml) and 0.67% apo C-II, 3.4% apo C-III and 1.01% apo E for the HDL (1.07–1.18 g/ml). The agreement of these values with previously published data (Jackson *et al.*, 1976; Mahley *et al.*, 1984; Eisenberg, 1984; Scanu *et al.*, 1982), stresses the validity of the apolipoprotein immunoassays.

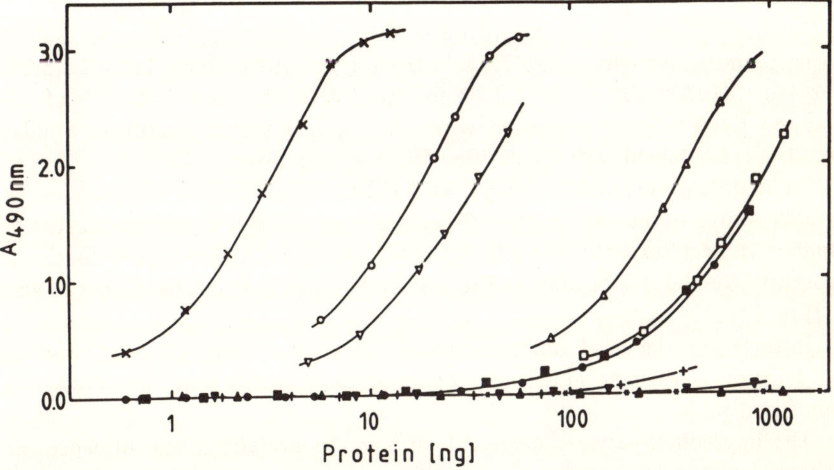

Figure 7   Apo C-II ELISA. Parallelism between the standard curves constructed with purified apolipoprotein (X) and those constructed with chylomicra (O), VLDL (▽), LDL (□) and HDL (△). The cross-reactivity with apolipoproteins A-I (▼), A-II (▲), B (■), C-III (●) and E (+) and human serum albumin (∗) is negligible. (Reproduced with permission from Bury *et al.* (1986a).)

The influence of organic solvent extraction on apolipoprotein immunoreactivity in native plasma and in isolated lipoprotein fractions was further investigated using the extraction procedure proposed by Cham and Knowles (1976). As indicated in figure 6, for the apo C-III ELISA, delipidation did not influence the shape of the calibration curves constructed either with native plasma or with its isolated lipoprotein fractions. Similar results were obtained for the other assays (Bury *et al.*, 1986a; Bury *et al.*, 1986b; Bury and Rosseneu, 1985a). The apolipoprotein recovery from delipidated normolipidaemic and hyperlipoproteinaemic plasma amounted to 97.4% ± 9.1% for apo A-I, 98.8% ± 7.8% for apo C-II, 96.4% ± 4.3% for apo C-III and 101.2% ± 9.8% for apo E. Delipidation of normolipidaemic and hyperlipoproteinaemic plasma with ether:ethanol (Scanu and Edelstein, 1971), and the subsequent resolubilization in assay buffer containing 8 M urea, resulted in a significant loss of 5–15% apo A-I, 5–20% apo C-II and C-III, and 10–25% apo E. Using the alternative lipidation technique, by incubating native plasma 1 h at 37°C with equal amounts of a commercially available triglyceride–phospholipid micro-emulsion (i.e. Intralipid 10%, final triglyceride concentration 50 g/l), did not result in a major decrease in the immunoreactivity of the exchangeable apolipoproteins (apolipoproteins C and E (Eisenberg, 1984)). Their recovery amounted to 102.3% ± 7.5% for apo C-II, 99.4% ± 3.1% for apo C-III and 91.0% ± 5.4% for apo E ($N = 4$). These results indicate that the antigenic sites of all the apolipoproteins measured are fully exposed to the antisera used in the ELISA technique performed as described above (page 13).

In contrast to other immunoassays, the addition of denaturing agents or detergents did not increase the immunoreactivity of plasma apolipoproteins. A 100-fold predilution of plasma with assay buffers, containing 4 M urea, resulted in an immunoreactivity of 96.2% ± 11.0% for apo A-I ($N = 6$), 111.4% ± 5.0% for apo C-II ($N = 10$), 98.6% ± 4.7% for apo C-III ($N = 10$) and 103.9% ± 5.2% for apo E ($N = 6$), as compared with the response before treatment. Similar results were obtained with the purified apolipoprotein standards.

Some detergents (Apovax 0.1 g/l, Tween 20 0.5 ml/l) had no influence on the ELISA assay, except for a 15–19% decrease of the apo E immunoreactivity. Sodium dodecylsulphate (0.1 g/l) decreased the apo C-III and apo E immunoreactivity by about 70% and 50% respectively, whereas it increased that of apo C-II by 11%.

In summary, the apo E immunoreactivity seems to be reduced in the presence of detergents, whereas most other apolipoprotein assays were not influenced significantly.

The interaction between detergents and apolipoproteins might influence the exposure of some epitopes, as suggested by a recent study with monoclonal antibodies against apo C-I, using ELISA (Wong *et al.*, 1985). Differences in polyclonal antisera might, therefore, account for the different response of the antigens to pretreatment. It is, therefore, recommended that the parallelism between primary and secondary standards and the effect of delipidation should be checked whenever a new batch of antisera is used.

The Tween 20 detergent, which is present in the wash buffers used in the ELISA procedure, might influence the exposure of apolipoprotein epitopes in plasma lipoproteins immunochemically linked to the solid phase. Excluding the detergent from the wash buffer significantly reduced the immunoreactivity of plasma apo A-I, apo C-II and apo E, whereas apo C-III was not influenced. This might account for the discrepancy between our sandwich ELISA technique and other immunoassays, which require sample pretreatment (Bury *et al.*, 1986a; Bury *et al.*, 1986b; Bury and Rosseneu, 1985a; Bury and Rosseneu, 1985b).

QUALITY CONTROL

The development and applicability of an immunoassay requires a thorough investigation of its selectivity, precision and accuracy, and lasting quality control.

The selectivity of the ELISA assays was tested by performing the assay in the presence of an excess of potentially interfering substances. As illustrated in figure 7 for the apo C-II assay, the cross-reactivity with other apolipoproteins and other serum proteins such as albumin was always less than 1% (Bury *et al.*, 1986a; Bury *et al.*, 1986b; Bury and Rosseneu, 1985a; Bury and Rosseneu, 1985b). As selectivity of the immunoassays is primarily dependent on specificity of the antisera used, each new batch of antiserum was checked.

The assay precision was determined by the intra- and inter-assay CVs at low, intermediate and high plasma concentrations of the antigen. As indicated by their low intra-assay CVs, presented in table 3, the sandwich ELISA might be considered to be a precise technique for apolipoprotein quantitation. Three plasma pools, with apolipoprotein concentrations evenly distributed over the whole assay range, were used for internal quality control. These control plasma were aliquoted and stored at $-20°C$. Their inter-assay CVs for the indicated number of consecutive runs are summarized in table 3.

Table 3   Precision of the various apolipoprotein ELISA assays, expressed as the coefficient of variation (CV) at low, intermediate and high plasma concentrations

	Apolipoprotein				
	A-I	B	C-II	C-III	E
Intra-assay CV	$N = 12$	$N = 12$	$N = 12$	$N = 12$	$N = 12$
Low concentration	3.5	3.4	3.0	4.2	3.9
Medium concentration	3.9	2.9	2.6	3.8	2.8
High concentration	3.7	3.8	3.4	2.1	5.8
Inter-assay CV	$N = 16$	$N = 15$	$N = 48$	$N = 49$	$N = 36$
Low concentration	9.6	6.3	4.5	9.8	8.6
Medium concentration	7.5	4.9	7.2	5.8	10.8
High concentration	8.9	5.6	8.9	6.3	10.1

If control values deviated more than 2 S.D. from the control mean, results were considered as suspect, and the assays were repeated. If these deviations remained, or increased as a function of time, the assays were recalibrated with a fresh reference pool. Plasma samples with apolipoprotein concentrations outside the calibration curves were reanalysed using the appropriate dilution.

To determine the accuracy of the ELISAs, the apolipoprotein concentrations were assayed both by ELISA and by another immunological technique, such as INA (Rosseneu *et al.*, 1981a; Bury *et al.*, 1985a; Rosseneu *et al.*, 1981b). The correlation coefficients of the least-squares regression lines between both techniques, amounted to $r = 0.97$ ($N = 50$) for apo B, $r = 0.94$ ($N = 100$) for apo A-I (figure 8) and $r = 0.98$ ($N = 79$) for apo C-III. No statistically significant difference could be obtained between the two immunoassay techniques, using a paired t test. Of the added amounts of purified apo A-I and apo C-III to normo-lipidaemic and hypertriglyceridaemic plasma ($N = 8$), 97% ± 6% and 102% ± 5% were respectively recovered.

If INA was not available, the assay accuracy was determined using the admixture technique proposed by Grannis and Miller (1976). For this purpose, plasma samples (pool A), containing low concentrations of the respective antigen, were mixed at various ratios (e.g. 0%, 20%, 40%, 60%, 80%, 100% pool A) with plasma samples containing high apolipoprotein concentrations (pool B). In order to obtain equidisparate specimens (Grannis and Miller, 1976), the plasma mixtures were several-fold diluted, using equidisparate volumes as demonstrated in table 4

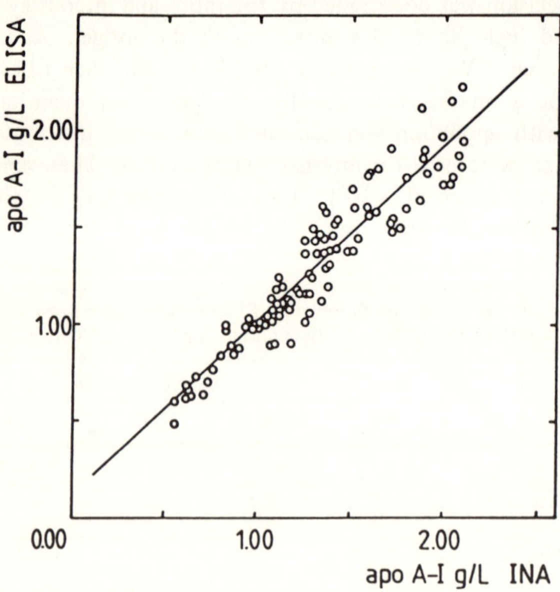

Figure 8   Correlation between the ELISA and an INA for the quantitation of apo A-I in human plasma. $Y = 0.913X + 0.104; r = 0.94; N = 100$.

Table 4 Plasma dilutions used in the accuracy tests performed, according to Grannis and Miller (1976)

	1° dilution			2° dilution		
	Sample		Assay buffer	Sample		Assay buffer
Set I						
A	15.0 μl	+	1000 μl	25.0 μl	+	1000 μl
B	17.5 μl	+	1000 μl	25.0 μl	+	1000 μl
C	20.0 μl	+	1000 μl	25.0 μl	+	1000 μl
D	22.5 μl	+	1000 μl	25.0 μl	+	1000 μl
E	25.0 μl	+	1000 μl	25.0 μl	+	1000 μl
Set II						
F	20.0 μl	+	1000 μl	20.0 μl	+	1000 μl
G	25.0 μl	+	1000 μl	20.0 μl	+	1000 μl
H	30.0 μl	+	1000 μl	20.0 μl	+	1000 μl

'Equidisparate specimen' were obtained from the combination of series A with E, B with D, and F with H. The apo E concentrations were calculated using a dilution factor of 2091 for all samples.

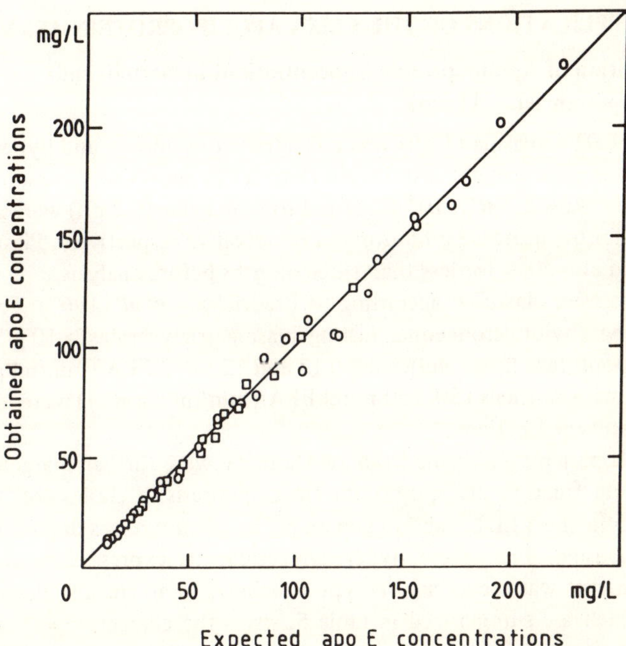

Figure 9 Assay accuracy determined by the admixture technique proposed by Grannis and Miller (1976). Correlation between the expected and obtained (ELISA) apo E concentrations. Values for set I (○) and set II (□) are shown. $Y = 0.997X + 1.008$; $r = 0.997$; $N = 48$.

for the apo E ELISA. The apolipoprotein assay was performed by the conventional assay procedure (cf. page 6), whereas apo E concentrations were calculated using a dilution factor of 2091 for all admixtures. As shown in figure 9 for the apo E assay, the expected apolipoprotein concentrations, calculated from the known concentrations of pool A and B and from the admixture and dispensing ratios, showed a linear correlation with the apolipoprotein concentrations determined by ELISA ($r = 0.94$, $N = 48$). The recovery, expressed as the 'obtained apolipoprotein concentrations multiplied by 100% divided by the calculated concentrations', amounted to $96.9\% \pm 7.5\%$ ($N = 44$) for the apo A-I assay, $100.0\% \pm 4.6\%$ ($N = 44$) for the apo C-II assay and $101.8\% \pm 5.7\%$ ($N = 44$) for the apo E assay. The percentage difference, calculated from the formula of Grannis and Miller (Grannis and Miller, 1976, equation 4) using the equidisparate specimen, amounted to $-3.98\% \pm 2.98\%$ ($N = 18$) for the apo A-I assay, $2.48\% \pm 1.57\%$ for the apo C-II assay ($N = 18$) and $1.78\% \pm 4.61\%$ ($N = 17$) for the apo E assay. Although Grannis and Miller (1976) proposed a $\pm 3\%$ difference limit for chemical assays, the obtained values should be acceptable for an immunological technique.

APPLICATIONS OF THE ELISA APOLIPOPROTEIN ASSAYS

Determination of Apolipoprotein Concentrations in Normo- and Hyperlipoproteinaemic Plasma

Disodium EDTA plasma (1 g/l) was collected from normal and hyperlipidaemic subjects after an overnight fast. DTNB (Sigma Chemical Co., 2 mmol/l), Trasylol (Bayer, Leverkusen, FRG, 10^4 IU/l) and sodium azide (0.2 g/l) were added as an LCAT inhibitor, protease inhibitor and preservative respectively. Plasma samples were stored at $-20°C$ for less than three months before analysis.

Subjects were classified according to Fredrickson *et al.* (1967). Two children with fasting chylomicronaemia, fasting plasma triglycerides > 10 g/l and postheparin lipoprotein lipase deficiency (15 and 12 nmol FFA/(min/ml plasma)) as compared with normals (50–150 nmol FFA/(min/ml plasma)) were identified as Fredrickson type I patients.

Type III patients, suffering from xanthomata, were further characterized by a floating beta fraction on lipoprotein electrophoresis, a cholesterol:triglyceride ratio > 0.5 in the VLDL fraction and an E_2/E_2 phenotype as determined by isoelectric focusing. The severe hypertriglyceridaemia expressed by most of the type V patients was secondary to type I diabetes or to chronic alcoholism. The results, which are summarized in table 5, stress the clinical importance of apolipoprotein quantitation.

The Fredrickson type I patients were characterized by significantly decreased plasma concentrations of apo A-I and apo B, but had normal apo A-I:apo B ratios. The exchangeable apolipoproteins (apo C-II, apo C-III and apo E) were about 3-fold increased as compared with normals.

Table 5 Plasma lipid (g/l) and apolipoprotein (mg/l) concentrations in normolipidaemic (N) and dyslipoproteinaemic subjects (classified according to Fredrickson *et al.*, 1967), as determined by ELISA

Type	Number	TG	TC	A-I	B	C-II	C-III	E	A-I:B
N	30	0.69	1.95	1330	950	33	120	36	1.47
		± 0.21	± 0.30	± 160	± 21	± 7	± 33	± 5	± 0.37
I	2	22.90	2.58	720	480	96	311	96	1.53
II$_A$	22	1.17	3.30	1250	1730	66	193	58	0.71
		± 0.20	± 0.48	± 150	± 280	± 18	± 49	± 15	± 0.11
II$_B$	24	2.38	3.26	1170	1800	76	325	67	0.64
		± 0.86	± 0.29	± 230	± 280	± 22	± 41	± 10	± 0.11
III	3	5.51	4.54	1260	2710	134	401	239	0.52
		± 0.72	± 0.40	± 40	± 970	± 10	± 45	± 53	± 0.24
IV	26	2.63	2.36	1140	1420	76	266	57	0.77
		± 1.23	± 0.28	± 170	± 210	± 23	± 54	± 10	± 0.16
V	7	38.39	6.81	1100	3300	195	997	333	0.34
		± 25.1	± 3.13	± 400	± 1200	± 143	± 584	± 88	± 0.11
Hypo-β	2	0.26	1.21	1220	115	13	33	25	11–12

TG, triglycerides; TC, total cholesterol.

In type II patients, the apo B plasma concentrations were severely increased whereas the apo A-I concentrations tended to be decreased, resulting in highly significantly decreased apo A-I:apo B ratios ($p < 0.001$). Within this group of hypercholesterolaemic patients, a strongly positive correlation existed between plasma triglyceride and plasma apo C-II ($r = 0.50$), apo C-III ($r = 0.66$) and apo E ($r = 0.47$) concentrations, so that a distinction between type II$_A$ and type II$_B$ patients could be made on the basis of the increased plasma concentrations of these apolipoproteins.

In addition to their 2–3-fold increased apo B plasma levels, the Fredrickson type III patients were characterized by their extreme apo E plasma concentrations, about 6-fold the normal values, whereas apo C-II and apo C-III increased about 4-fold above normal values.

In type IV patients, the apo A-I:apo B ratio was significantly reduced ($p < 0.001$), whereas apo C-II, apo C-III and apo E were increased by a factor of about 2–3.

In agreement with the plasma lipids, the most pronounced increase in plasma apolipoproteins was observed in Fredrickson type V patients. Because of their severely increased apo B, and decreased apo A-I plasma concentrations, the apo A-I:apo B ratios were reduced to 0.34 ± 0.11. The apo C-II, apo C-III and apo E concentrations were 5–10-fold increased. As opposed to a positive correlation with apo C-III and apo E, the plasma triglycerides were inversely correlated with apo C-II ($r = -0.22$).

In two well-documented hypo-beta-lipoproteinaemic patients, the apo B plasma concentrations were strongly reduced, whereas the apo A-I concentrations were normal, resulting in apo A-I:apo B ratios of > 10. In addition, the apo C-II and apo E concentrations were reduced by about 50%, whereas the apo C-III plasma concentrations were decreased about 4-fold compared with normals.

In essence, these results demonstrate a reduced apo A-I:apo B ratio in most hyperlipoproteinaemic subjects, whereas apo C and apo E proteins are increased most significantly in the hypertriglyceridaemic state.

The correlation between plasma lipids and apolipoprotein concentrations was investigated in a small group of 32 normo- and Fredrickson type II and IV hyperlipidaemic patients. Plasma lipids were evenly distributed between 0.27 and 4.13 g/l for the triglycerides (mean ± S.D.: 1.94 ± 1.08 g/l) and between 1.25 and 4.02 g/l for total cholesterol (2.56 ± 0.66 g/l). Plasma apo A-I, apo B, apo C-II, apo C-III and apo E were assayed by ELISA, while triglycerides, total and HDL cholesterol were quantitated by enzymatic techniques (Rosseneu *et al.*, 1983a). The LDL cholesterol concentrations were calculated by the Friedewald formula (Friedewald *et al.*, 1972). The linear correlations, expressed as the Pearson correlation coefficient, are presented in table 6.

Plasma triglycerides showed a highly significant, positive correlation with plasma apo C-II, apo C-III and apo E concentrations, and a highly significant, negative correlation with apo A-I and with HDL cholesterol. No correlation was obtained between the apo C-II:apo C-III ratio and the plasma triglyceride concentrations. Total plasma cholesterol was highly correlated with plasma apo B ($r = 0.85$) and with LDL cholesterol calculated by the Friedewald formula ($r = 0.97$). As a consequence, the apo A-I:apo B ratio showed a highly significant, negative correlation with total plasma cholesterol and with LDL cholesterol. HDL cholesterol was highly positively correlated with apo A-I and highly negatively correlated with apo C-II, apo C-III and apo E. HDL cholesterol, expressed as a percentage of total cholesterol, showed the same type of correlation, whereas its negative correlation with apo B was significantly increased. In analogy with HDL cholesterol, apo A-I was negatively correlated with apo C-II, apo C-III and

Table 6   Linear correlation coefficients (*r*) between the plasma concentrations of triglycerides (TG), total cholesterol (TC), percentage and absolute HDL-cholesterol (%HDLC and HDL-C), and LDL-cholesterol (LDL-C), calculated by the Friedewald formula (Friedewald *et al.*, 1972) and the plasma concentrations of apolipoproteins A-I, B, C-II, C-III and E, and the apolipoprotein ratios A-I:B and C-II:C-III (C2:C3)

r	TG	TC	%HDLC	A-I	B	C-II	C-III	E	A-I:B	C2:C3	HDL-C	LDL-C
TG	1.00	0.28	−0.60	−0.42	0.32	0.76	0.72	0.72	−0.31	−0.60	−0.06	0.17
TC	0.28	1.00	−0.60	0.03	0.85	0.24	0.54	0.26	−0.47	−0.57	0.01	0.97
%HDLC	−0.60	−0.60	1.00	0.40	−0.68	−0.64	−0.74	−0.52	0.71	0.28	0.75	−0.66
A-I	−0.42	0.03	0.40	1.00	−0.06	−0.49	−0.23	−0.37	0.16	−0.38	0.61	−0.02
B	0.32	0.85	−0.68	−0.06	1.00	0.36	0.59	0.32	−0.63	−0.48	−0.17	0.85
C-II	0.76	0.24	−0.64	−0.49	0.36	1.00	0.81	0.80	−0.47	0.10	−0.62	0.20
C-III	0.72	0.54	−0.74	−0.23	0.59	0.81	1.00	0.65	−0.51	−0.46	−0.51	0.50
E	0.72	0.26	−0.52	−0.37	0.32	0.80	0.65	1.00	−0.33	0.08	−0.51	0.20
A-I:B	−0.31	−0.47	0.71	0.16	−0.63	−0.47	−0.51	−0.33	1.00	0.29	0.30	−0.49
C2:C3	−0.06	−0.57	0.28	−0.38	−0.48	0.10	−0.46	0.08	0.29	1.00	−0.14	−0.54
HDL-C	−0.60	0.01	0.75	0.61	−0.17	−0.62	−0.51	−0.51	0.30	−0.14	1.00	−0.10
LDL-C	0.17	0.97	−0.66	−0.02	0.85	0.20	0.50	0.20	−0.49	−0.54	−0.10	1.00

For 30 degrees of freedom, the *r* values corresponding to significance limits at 5% and 1% are 0.36 and 0.48 respectively.

apo E whereas apo B was positively correlated with these variables. The plasma concentrations of apo C-II, apo C-III and apo E were highly significantly and positively intercorrelated, whereas a negative correlation existed between these apolipoproteins and the apo A-I:apo B ratio.

These results stress the metabolic relationship existing between plasma lipids and apolipoproteins and, therefore, their significance for clinical chemistry assays. Decreased apo A-I:apo B ratios might be used as a discriminator for coronary artery disease and the development of atherosclerosis (De Backer *et al.*, 1982; Maciejko *et al.*, 1983; Brunzell *et al.*, 1984; Rosseneu and Bury, 1986). Plasma concentrations of apo C and apo E proteins are very useful to classify dyslipoproteinaemias correctly and might yield additional information

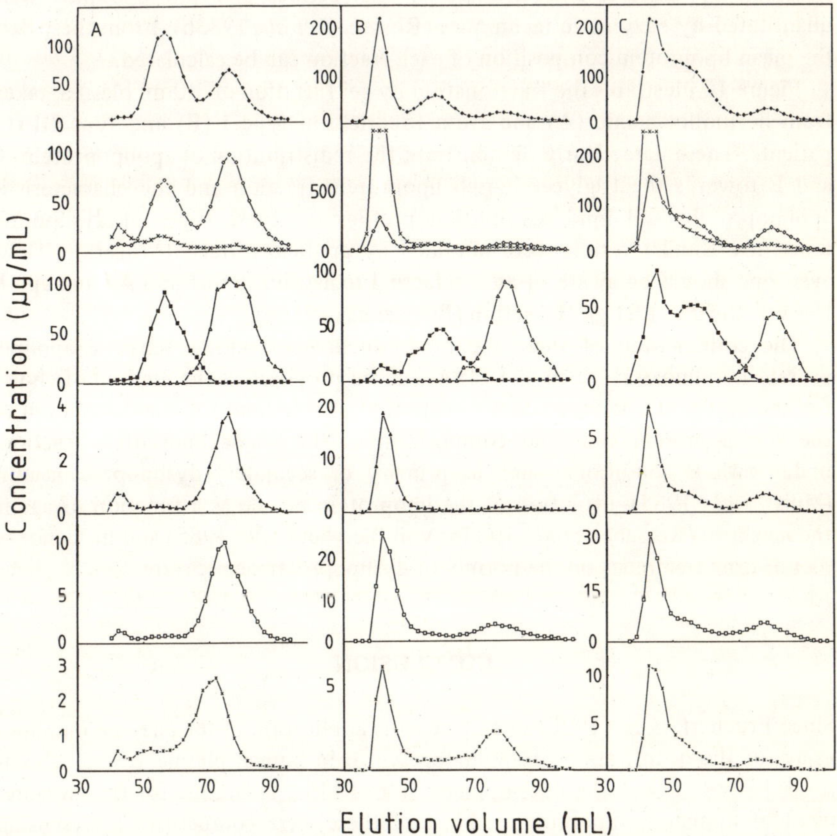

Figure 10 Lipid and apolipoprotein profiles in a normolipidaemic subject (A) and patients with Fredrickson type I (B) and type III (C) hyperlipoproteinaemia. Fresh plasma (1 ml) was separated on a Sepharose 6B column and lipids and apolipoproteins were measured in all fractions. From top to bottom: cholesterol (♦), triglycerides (X) and phospholipids (○), apolipoproteins B (■) and A-I (Δ), apolipoproteins C-II (▲), C-III (□) and E (∗).

about triglyceride metabolism (Bury *et al.*, 1985a; Bury *et al.*, 1986a; Bury *et al.*, 1986b; Bury and Rosseneu, 1985b).

Apolipoprotein Distribution

In the investigation of their metabolism, lipoproteins can be fractionated either by gel filtration or by sequential or gradient ultracentrifugation. Lipoproteins were separated from 1 ml fresh plasma by gel filtration on a Sepharose 6BCL column (Pharmacia) (Bury and Rosseneu, 1985b) or from 0.5 ml plasma by isopycnic centrifugation in a sodium chloride–sucrose gradient (Rosseneu *et al.*, 1983b). Apo A-I, apo B, apo C-II, apo C-III and apo E were quantitated in all fractions by ELISA, and cholesterol, triglycerides and phospholipids were quantitated by enzymatic techniques (Rosseneu *et al.*, 1983b). From these data the mean lipoprotein composition of each fraction can be calculated.

Figure 10 illustrates the fractionation by gel filtration of 1.0 ml plasma, taken from normolipidaemic (A) and from Fredrickson type I (B) and type III (C) patients. These data clearly demonstrate the redistribution of apolipoproteins C and E towards the triglyceride-rich lipoprotein fraction and the characteristic apolipoprotein and lipid distribution profiles for these types of dyslipoproteinaemia. Similar results were obtained by gradient ultracentrifugation. However, one should be aware of an artefactual redistribution of apo A-I and apo E towards the $d > 1.21$ g/ml fraction (Bury *et al.*, 1986b).

The combination of these separation techniques with a sensitive apolipoprotein immunoassay, such as ELISA, can be proposed as the method of choice for the study of apolipoprotein distribution profiles and for the calculation of the apolipoprotein and lipid composition of the major lipoprotein fractions under various conditions, such as primary or secondary dyslipoproteinaemia (Muls *et al.*, 1985), evolution of the lipoprotein profile as a function of age in the newborn (Rosseneu *et al.*, 1983b; Van Biervliet *et al.*, 1985) and influence of diet or drug treatment on the normo- or dyslipoproteinaemic state.

CONCLUSION

Since Fruchart *et al.* (1978) introduced the application of the enzyme immunoassay for the quantitation of apolipoprotein B in human plasma, several laboratories have described the development of an ELISA technique for the measurement of human apolipoproteins. Most of these were competitive assays using solid phases coated with either LDL (Fruchart *et al.*, 1978; Vander Heiden *et al.*, 1983) or purified apolipoproteins (Stein and Pesce, 1983), or using an enzyme, conjugated either with total lipoprotein fractions such as VLDL (Holmquist, 1980) or LDL (Holmquist, 1980) or with purified apolipoproteins (Dufaux *et al.*, 1983). The heterogeneity and instability of these reagents, however, favours the use of immunoglobulins for coating as well as for the preparation of an enzyme conjugate in a sandwich-type ELISA. As described above and in agreement with literature reports (Bury *et al.*, 1986a; Bury *et al.*, 1986b; Bury and Rosseneu 1985a; Bury and Rosseneu, 1985b; Fievet *et al.*, 1984; Fruchart *et al.*, 1984; Koren *et al.*, 1985), the sensitivity, precision and accuracy of this type of assay meet the requirements for a good immunological technique. Results are obtained within one day and the adaptability of the ELISA technique to automation makes it suitable for large scale population studies.

In this report, we have attempted to review the methodological details of the development and quality control of a sandwich ELISA and to document its general applicability to the quantitation of the various apolipoproteins in human plasma and in the lipoprotein fractions.

REFERENCES

Avrameas, S., Guilbert, B. (1971). Dosage enzymo-immunologique de protéines à l'aide d'immunoadsorbants et d'antigènes marqués aux enzymes. *C.R. Acad, Sci. Ser. D*, **273**, 2705–2709

Blaton, V., Vercaemst, R., Rosseneu, M., Mortelmans, J., Jackson, R. L., Gotto, A. M. (1977). Characterization of baboon plasma high-density lipoproteins and of their major apoproteins. *Biochemistry*, **16**, 2157–2163

Blum, C. B. (1983). Radioimmunoassay of apolipoproteins. In Lippel, K. (ed.), *Proceedings of the workshop on apolipoprotein quantification*, NIH publ. 83-1266, Bethesda, 242–250

Brunzell, J. D., Sniderman, A. D., Albers, J. J., Kwiterovich, P. O. Jr. (1984). Apolipoproteins B and A-I and coronary artery disease in humans. *Arteriosclerosis*, **4**, 79–83

Bury, J., De Keersgieter, W., Rosseneu, M., Belpaire, F., Christophe, J. (1985). Immunonephelometric quantitation of the apolipoprotein C-III in human plasma. *Clin. Chim. Acta*, **145**, 249–258

Bury, J., Rosseneu, M. (1985a). Quantitation of human serum apolipoprotein A-I by enzyme immunoassay. *Clin. Chem.*, **31**, 247–251

Bury, J., Rosseneu, M. (1985b). Enzyme linked immunosorbent assay for human apolipoprotein C-III. *J. Clin. Chem. Clin. Biochem.*, **23**, 63–68

Bury, J., Michiels, G., Rosseneu, M. (1986a). Human apolipoprotein C-II quantitation by sandwich enzyme linked immunosorbent assay. *J. Clin. Chem. Clin. Biochem.*, **24**, 457–463

Bury, J., Vercaemst, R., Rosseneu, M., Belpaire, F. (1986b). Quantitation of human apolipoprotein E by enzyme linked immunosorbent assay. *Clin. Chem.*, **32**, 265–270

Cardin, A. D., Witt, K. R., Barnhart, C. L., Jackson, R. L. (1982). Sulfhydryl chemistry and solubility properties of human plasma apolipoprotein B. *Biochemistry*, **21**, 4503–4511

Cham, B. E., Knowles, B. R. (1976). A solvent system for delipidation of plasma or serum without protein precipitation. *J. Lipid Res.*, **17**, 176–181

Cooper, G. R., Smith, S. J., Wiebe, D. A., Kuchmak, M., Hannon, W. H. (1985). International survey of apolipoprotein A1 and B measurement (1983–1984). *Clin. Chem.*, **30**, 223–228

De Backer, G., Rosseneu, M., Deslypere, J. P. (1982). Discriminative value of lipids and apoproteins in coronary heart disease. *Atherosclerosis*, **42**, 197–203

Deckelbaum, R. J., Olivecrona, T., Fainaru, M. (1980). The role of different albumin preparations on production of human plasma lipoprotein-like particles in vitro. *J. Lipid Res.*, **21**, 425–434

Dufaux, B., Ilsemann, K., Assmann, G. (1983). Competitive enzyme immuno-assay for apolipoprotein A-II. *J. Clin. Chem. Clin. Biochem.*, **21**, 39–43

Eisenberg, S. (1984). High density lipoprotein metabolism. *J. Lipid Res.*, **25**, 1017–1058

Engvall, E., Perlmann, P. (1971). Enzyme-linked immunosorbent assay (ELISA). Quantitative assay of immunoglobulin G. *Immunochemistry*, **8**, 871–874

Fievet, C., Koffigan, M., Ouvry, D., Marcovina, S., Moschetto, Y., Fruchart, J. C. (1984). Noncompetitive enzyme-linked immunoassay for apolipoprotein B in serum. *Clin. Chem.*, **30**, 98–100

Fredrickson, D. S., Levy, R. I., Lees, R. S. (1967). Fat transport in lipoproteins: an integrated approach to mechanisms and disorders. *New Engl. J. Med.*, **276**, 32–44, 94–103, 148–156, 215–226, 273–281

Friedewald, W. T., Levy, R. J., Fredrickson, D. S. (1972). Estimation of the concentration of low-density lipoprotein cholesterol in plasma without use of the preparative ultracentrifuge. *Clin. Chem.*, **18**, 488–509

Fruchart, J. C., Desreumaux, C., Dewailly, P., Sezille, G., Jaillard, J., Carlier, Y., Bout, D., Capron, A. (1978). Enzyme immunoassay for human apolipoprotein B the major protein moiety in low density and very low density lipoproteins. *Clin. Chem.*, **24**, 455–459

Fruchart, J. C., Fievet, C., Ouvry, D., Koffigan, M., Beucler, I., Ayrault-Jarrier, M., Du Barry, M., Marcovina, S. (1984). Enzyme-linked immunoassay on microtitre plates for human apolipoprotein B. *La Ricerca Clin. Lab.*, **14**, 569–574

Grannis, F. G., Miller, W. G. (1976). On the design of clinical chemistry quality-control sera. *Clin. Chem.*, **22**, 500–512

Hemmilä, I. (1985). Fluoroimmunoassays and immunofluorometric assays. *Clin. Chem.*, **31**, 359–370

Holmquist, L. (1980). Quantitation of human serum very low density apolipo-proteins C-I C-II C-III and E by enzyme immunoassay. *J. Immunol. Meth.*, **34**, 243–251

Holmquist, L. (1982a). Loss of human serum apolipoproteins C and E during manipulation of diluted solutions. *J. Lipid Res.*, **23**, 357–359

Holmquist, L. (1982b). Quantitation of human serum apolipoprotein B by enzyme immunoassay. *Clin. Chim. Acta*, **121**, 327–336

Jackson, R. L., Morrisett, J. D., Gotto, A. M. (1976). Lipoprotein structure and metabolism. *Physiological Reviews*, **56**, 259–276

Johnstone, A., Thorpe, R. (1982). *Immunochemistry in practice*, Blackwell Scientific Publications, Oxford

Koren, E., Puchois, P., McConathy, W. J., Fesmire, J. D., Alaupovic, P. (1985). Quantitative determination of human plasma apolipoprotein A-I by a non-competitive enzyme-linked immunosorbent assay. *Clin. Chim. Acta*, **147**, 85–95

Kricka, L. J., Carter, T. J. N., Burt, S. M., Kennedy, J. H., Holder, R. L., Halliday, M. I., Telford, M. E., Wisdom, G. B. (1980). Variability in the adsorption properties of microtitre plates used as solid supports in enzyme immunoassay. *Clin. Chem.*, **26**, 741–744

Lippel, K. (1983). *Proceedings of the workshop on apolipoprotein quantification*, NIH Publication 83-1266, Bethesda

Livesey, J. H., Donald, R. A. (1982). Prevention of adsorption losses during radioimmunoassay of polypeptide hormones: effectiveness of albumins gelatin caseins Tween 20 and plasma. *Clin. Chim. Acta*, **123**, 193–198

Lowry, O. H., Rosenbrough, N. J., Farr, L., Randall, R. J. (1951). Protein measurement with the folin phenol reagent. *J. Biol. Chem.*, **193**, 265–275

Maciejko, J. J., Holmes, D. R., Kottke, B. A., Zinsmeister, A. R., Dinh, D. M., Mao, S. J. T. (1983). Apolipoprotein A-I as a marker of angiographically assessed coronary-artery disease. *New. Engl. J. Med.*, **309**, 385–389

Mahley, R. W., Innerarity, T. L., Rall, S. C. Jr., Weisgraber, K. H. (1984). Plasma lipoproteins: apolipoprotein structure and function. *J. Lipid Res.*, **25**, 1277–1294

McCullough, K. C., Parkinson, D. (1984a). The standardization of a 'spot-test' ELISA for the rapid screening of sera and hybridoma cell products I. The determination of the optimum buffering system. *J. Biol. Stand.*, **12**, 67–74

McCullough, K. C., Parkinson, D. (1984b). The standardization of a 'spot-test' ELISA for the rapid screening of sera and hybridoma cell products II. The determination of binding capacity binding ratio and coefficient of variation of different ELISA plates in sandwich and indirect ELISA. *J. Biol. Stand.*, **12**, 75–86

Mills, G. L., Lane, P. A., Weech, P. K. (1984). A guidebook to lipoprotein technique. In Burdon, R. H. and Knippenberg, P. H. (eds.) *Laboratory techniques in biochemistry and molecular biology*, Elsevier, Amsterdam

Muls, E., Rosseneu, M., Bury, J., Lamberigts, G., De Moor P. (1985). Hyperthyroidism influences the distribution and apolipoprotein A composition of the high density lipoproteins in man. *J. Clin. Endocrin. Metab.*, **61**, 882–889

Nakane, P. K., Kawaoi, A. (1974). Peroxidase-labeled antibody. A new method of conjugation. *J. Histochem. Cytochem.*, **22**, 1084–1091

Oellerich, M. (1984). Enzyme-immunoassay: a review. *J. Clin. Chem. Clin. Biochem.*, **22**, 895–904

Osborne, J. C., Brewer, H. B., Bronzert, T. J., Schaefer, E. J., Tate, R. L. (1983). Molecular properties of plasma apolipoproteins. In Lippel K. (ed.) *Proceedings of the workshop on apolipoprotein quantification*, NIH publ. 83-1266, Bethesda, 179–199

Pharmacia (1979). CNBr-activated Sepharose 4B. In *Affinity chromatography: principles and methods*, Pharmacia Fine Chemicals, Uppsala

Rosseneu, M., Vinaimont, N., Vercaemst, R., De Keersgieter, W., Belpaire, F. (1981a). Standardization of immunoassays for the quantitation of plasma apo B protein. *Anal. Bioch.*, **116**, 204–210

Rosseneu, M., Vercaemst, R., Vinaimont, N., Van Tornout, P., Henderson, L. O., Herbert, P. N. (1981b). Quantitative determination of human plasma apolipoprotein A-I by laser immunonephelometry. *Clin. Chem.*, **27**, 856–859

Rosseneu, M., Vercaemst, R., Steinberg, K. K., Cooper, G. R. (1983a). Some considerations of methodology and standardization of apolipoprotein B immunoassays. *Clin. Chem.*, **29**, 427–433

Rosseneu, M., Van Biervliet, J. P., Bury, J., Vinaimont, N. (1983b). Isolation and characterization of lipoprotein profiles by density gradient ultracentrifugation. *Ped. Res.*, **17**, 788–794

Rosseneu, M., Bury, J. (1986). Apolipoprotein assays for the diagnosis of hyperlipidemias. In Naito, H. (ed.) *Recent aspects on diagnosis and treatment of lipid disorders: impact on prevention of atherosclerotic diseases*, A. R. Liss, New York

Samaké, H., Rajkowski, K. M., Cittanova, N. (1983). The choice of buffer protein in steroid (enzyme-) immunoassay. *Clin. Chim. Acta*, **130**, 129–135

Scanu, A. M., Edelstein, C. (1971). Solubility in aqueous solutions of ethanol on the small molecular weight peptides of the serum very low density and high density lipoproteins: relevance to the recovery problem during delipidation of serum lipoproteins. *Anal. Biochem.*, **44**, 576–588

Scanu, A. M., Edelstein, C., Shen, B. W. (1982). Lipid–protein interactions in plasma lipoproteins. Model: high density lipoproteins. *Lipid–Protein Interact.*, **1**, 259–316

Schall, R. S. Jr., Tenoso, H. J. (1981). Alternatives to radioimmunoassay: labels and methods. *Clin. Chem.*, **27**, 1157–1164

Scharpé, S. L., Cooreman, W. M., Blomme, W. J., Laekeman, G. M. (1978). Quantitative enzyme immunoassay: current status. *Clin. Chem.*, **22**, 733–738

Sewell, M. M. H. (1967). A semi-quantitative technique using the LKB immunodiffusion apparatus. *Science Tools*, **14**, 11–12

Stein, E. A., Pesce, A. J. (1983). Enzyme linked immunoassays for apolipoproteins: advantages problems and prototype assay. In Lippel K. (ed), *Proceedings of the workshop on apolipoprotein quantification*, NIH publ. 83-1266, Bethesda, 319–331

Steinberg, K. K., Cooper, G. K., Graiser, S. G., Rosseneu, M. (1983). Some considerations of methodology and standardization of apolipoprotein A-I immunoassays. *Clin. Chem.*, **29**, 415–426

Van Biervliet, J. P., Rosseneu, M., Bury, J., Caster, H., Stul, M., Lamote, R. (1985). Apolipoprotein and lipid composition of plasma lipoproteins in neonates during the first month of life. *Ped. Res.*, **20**, 324–328

Van Weemen, B., Schuurs, A. (1971). Immunoassay using antigen–enzyme conjugates. *FEBS Lett.*, **15**, 232–236

Vander Heidern, G. L., Sasse, G. A., Yorde, D. E., Madiedo, G., Barboriak, J. J. (1983). Examination of a competitive enzyme-linked immunoassay (CELIA) technique and a laser nephelometric immunoassay technique for the measurement of apolipoprotein B. *Clin. Chim. Acta*, **135**, 209–218

Vercaemst, R., Bury, J., Rosseneu, M. (1984). Isolation of human apolipoprotein E by high performance liquid chromatography. *J. Lipid Res.*, **25**, 876

Voller, A., Bidwell, D. E., Bartlett, A. (1979). The enzyme linked immunosorbent assay (ELISA). Dynatech Europe, Guernsey

Wong, L., Anderson, P. D., Gallaher, W. R., Roheim, P. S. (1985). Monoclonal antibodies to rat C apolipoproteins: production and characterization of a unique antibody whose binding to apo C-I is inhibited by nonionic detergents. *J. Lipid Res.*, **26**, 528–539

Wood, W. G., Gadow, A. (1983). Immobilisation of antibodies and antigens on macro solid phases. A comparison between adsorptive and covalent binding. A critical study of macro solid phases for use in immunoassay systems. Part I. *J. Clin. Chem. Clin. Biochem.*, **21**, 789–797

2. Recent Progress in the Quantitation of Phagocytosis

T. W. JUNGI

GENERAL INTRODUCTION

Since the discovery of phagocytosis by Metchnikoff, this process has been recognized as being an important mechanism for the defence and self-preservation of multicellular organisms. In higher vertebrates, specialized cells (the so-called professional phagocytes), namely polymorphonuclear leukocytes (PMNs) and mononuclear phagocytes, fulfil this task. Operationally, phagocytosis can be divided into several phases: (i) recognition and binding of the prey to be ingested, (ii) actual ingestion, and (iii) elimination of the engulfed particle. In order to recognize the material to be internalized, a variety of specific binding sites are expressed on the phagocyte surface which specifically bind to surface determinants of the target, e.g. β-glucan on microorganisms (Czop and Austen, 1985). Some of these determinants are host-derived humoral factors ('opsonins') fixed to the target surface, e.g. antibodies or split products of the complement component C3 (Newman *et al.*, 1980; Wright and Silverstein, 1982). Thus, for optimal performance of phagocytosis, not only cellular but also humoral requirements must be satisfied. Depending on the cellular state, the type of receptors triggered and the intensity of triggering, this binding event is transduced to the motile apparatus in a manner which promotes ingestion and enclosure of the particle within a phagocytic vacuole; alternatively, binding to receptors may not be followed by ingestion (Newman *et al.*, 1980; Wright and Silverstein, 1982; Pommier *et al.*, 1983). Once engulfed, the particle must be killed (if it is a live organism), and finally eliminated by digestion. Again, depending on the cellular state and the type of particle which has been internalized, either killing is performed rapidly or the particle resists or subverts elimination (Wilson *et al.*, 1980). Thus it becomes evident that an experimental system measuring phagocytosis must allow determination of attachment, ingestion, killing and elimination both separately and independently, and must permit assessment of both humoral and cellular aspects of phagocytosis. Since these events occur concomitantly in a multicellular system, it is not always an easy task to satisfy these criteria.

Broadly, two types of approaches have been taken in order to assess phagocytosis. First, in an *in vitro* system in which phagocytes and targets are allowed to interact, either in suspension or by adherence, the number of particles becoming associated with phagocytes is assessed. Particles attached to the surface, but which have not actually been ingested, must be separated from ingested targets, must be eliminated before analysis or must be controlled in some other way. Alternatively, it has to be verified that the number of attached, non-ingested particles is negligible. Phagocyte-associated particles are followed microscopically or, alternatively, targets are labelled in some way, in order to facilitate quantitation. In the case of microorganisms, particles are quantified by colony counting of cultured phagocyte lysates. In the second type of approach, a metabolic event associated with phagocytosis is measured. Although these measurements are often much simpler than the former and lend themselves to clinical application and development of screening assays, it has to be verified to what extent phagocytosis and the metabolic event in question are really related. This applies even more to attempts to relate microbial killing to biochemical parameters. Evolutionary development has provided an antimicrobial defence system comprising multiple backup systems; for a given pathogen, several different systems may contribute, these being poorly represented by measurement of any single biochemical component.

Thus, it may be concluded that there is not a single, ideal phagocytosis system. Depending on the problem under study, advantages and disadvantages will be weighed differently. If one is interested in the study of functional aspects of phagocytes, one may choose a system with model target particles with which one finds it easy to work. If one wishes to elucidate the role of humoral opsonins in general, one has to select a system in which these opsonins have been shown to be of importance. If, however, one needs to elucidate cellular and humoral requirements for the ingestion and killing of a given pathogen, one cannot avoid working with that particular pathogen, however unsuitable it may be for analysis; most probably, several different assay systems will have to be used in order to reach clear conclusions. This approach is crucial, since even closely related organisms may be dealt with in quite different ways by phagocytes (Lehrer, 1975). The problem of studying antimicrobial defence *in vitro* is further complicated by the fact that many contributing factors can be mimicked poorly *in vitro*; thus, bacteria attached to either biological or artificial surfaces are dealt with by phagocytes in a quite different way to bacteria in suspension (Lee *et al.*, 1983; Vaudaux *et al.*, 1985).

In the subsequent two sections of this chapter, there will be a review of the methodology used in attempting either direct assessment of phagocytosis (page 33), or the measurement of phagocytosis-related biochemical events (page 39). Recent non-isotopic methods, lending themselves to clinical application, will be emphasized. The final section describes a sensitive screening assay, developed in our own laboratory, for quantitating ingestion of opsonized erythrocytes by using mononuclear phagocytes.

THE *IN VITRO* SYSTEMS USED FOR DIRECT ASSESSMENT OF PHAGOCYTOSIS

Microscopy

Obviously, microscopic examination is the most straightforward approach for surveying phagocytosis. It is, however, hampered by time-consuming evaluation, particularly if, in addition to rating response of the phagocyte subpopulation, the number of ingested particles per phagocyte is also measured. Although it appears at first glance very easy to discriminate between attachment and ingestion, by microscopic observation, in practice this is often difficult, particularly if the target particles are considerably smaller than the phagocytes. It is not surprising, therefore, that the most widely used phagocytosis system involves erythrocytes as model targets, since attached, non-ingested erythrocytes can be eliminated prior to analysis, either by hypotonic lysis or by treatment with 0.83% ammonium chloride (Czop and Austen, 1985; Newman *et al.*, 1980; Wright and Silverstein, 1982; Pommier *et al.*, 1983). The use of erythrocytes has a number of additional advantages. Without prior opsonization, they fail to bind to phagocytes except under special circumstances (Czop *et al.*, 1978) and therefore lend themselves to studies on the interaction of opsonins with phagocytes. By enzymatic removal of sialic acid from the erythrocyte surface, or by selecting erythrocytes poor in sialic acid, another class of receptors mediating phagocytosis, now called β-glucan receptors (Czop and Austen, 1985), could be demonstrated (Czop *et al.*, 1978). By surface treatment with tannin (Biegel and Rabinovitch, 1983; Herbert, 1978), chromium chloride or other methods (Herbert, 1978), erythrocytes can adsorb other proteins not normally bound by red blood cells, thus allowing study of the interaction of any protein (bound to a particle) with phagocytes (Pommier *et al.*, 1983). As will be shown below, erythrocytes are also appropriate targets for spectrometric and radiometric phagocytosis assays. Once ingested, erythrocytes maintain their integrity for sufficient time to allow particle counting within the phagocytes. A recent improvement of the widely used rosetting and erythrophagocytosis technique (Jungi and Baradun, 1985) utilizes siliconized slides containing 12 reaction fields spared from siliconization for the subsequent application of adherent phagocytes. The advantage of this modification lies in the requirement of very small cell numbers (10^4 phagocytes/test) and in the high reproducibility due to the uniform washing procedure applicable to such slides.

Other particles commonly used in phagocytosis studies are latex spheres of diameter ca. 0.5–2.0 μm. However, in contrast to erythrocytes, latex beads stick to cells, and attached, non-ingested particles are difficult to remove from the cellular surface by simple washing. Nevertheless, the solubility of latex in xylene has been used to develop a procedure for quantitatively removing extracellular latex beads (Van Furth and Diesselhoff-Den Dulk, 1980).

Among the microorganisms most often used in microscopic assays are several *Candida* species, for these are clinically important. *Candida* blastospores are large enough to permit easy counting. Attachment has been differentiated from ingestion by using stains which do not accumulate in phagocytes, such as trypaneosin (Lehrer, 1981) or FITC-labelled Con A (Richardson *et al.*, 1982). The studies on microscopic assessment of phagocytosis of bacteria, mycoplasma and protozoa, however, are too numerous to be mentioned. Often, special staining procedures, including fluorescent staining, have been used to facilitate microscopy.

Electron Microscopy

It is evident that electron microscopy (EM) is not the standard method for studying phagocytosis. It has been used for providing unequivocal proof that the targets under study are not only bound but also actually ingested, for following ingestion of constituents too small for light microscopic observation and for investigating the exact mechanism of ingestion and the exact intracellular localization of endocytosed material (Edelson *et al.*, 1982; Kaplan, 1977). Recently, the uptake of iron particles has been studied by scanning EM, in both the secondary and the back scattered imaging modes (Soligo and de Harven, 1982; Warheit *et al.*, 1983; Kaplan, 1977). These methods allow the distinction between attachment and ingestion to be made.

Spectrometry

Oil droplets containing the dye red O and coated with proteins were used as model particles in a spectrometric assay (Stossel *et al.*, 1973). These droplets do not attach to phagocytes but, on appropriate opsonization, they become readily engulfed by PMNs (Stossel *et al.*, 1973) or mononuclear phagocytes (Weston *et al.*, 1975; Ueda *et al.*, 1981). Photometry of lysed phagocyte monolayers has been used, not only for determining the phagocytic capacity but also for assessing the initial rate of uptake by PMNs (Stossel, 1973).

Erythrophagocytosis has been assessed spectrometrically by reading the lysed phagocyte monolayer at 405 or 412 nm (Cooper *et al.*, 1984; Rummage and Leu, 1985). The low sensitivity of these methods has been overcome by exploiting the pseudoperoxidase activity of haemoglobin (Jungi, 1985). As will be shown later, the sensitivity of the spectrometric assay could be increased by a factor of >30 by allowing phagocyte lysates to react with the appropriate substrates. The possibility of quantitating the uptake of erythrocytes in the range between 10^3 and 10^6 renders the assay more sensitive than isotopic procedures. In another spectrometric system latex beads coated with alkaline phosphatase were used as targets (Osterholz *et al.*, 1984). All these recent methods were adapted to microtitre plates, thus permitting automated reading of the assay plate in an ELISA reader photometer. Despite the advantage of being rapid and relatively simple to perform, these assays have the disadvantage that results reflect the behaviour of the whole cell population, and no information regarding individual cells is provided.

Fluorimetry and Cytofluorography

Using particles tagged with a fluorescent marker, cytofluorography has been used to study phagocytosis of latex beads (Schroeder and Kinden, 1983), glutaraldehyde-fixed sheep erythrocytes (Loike and Silverstein, 1983), *Staphylococcus aureus* (Horn *et al.*, 1985), yeast particles and immunoglobulin aggregates (Sahlin *et al.*, 1983) at the individual cell level. The procedure is rapid if a computer-centred spectrofluorimeter or photometer interphased to a computer is available (Schroeder and Kinden, 1983; Sahlin *et al.*, 1983). Since the intensity of the emitted light depends on the pH of the medium, fluorimetry can provide information regarding the pH values within phagocytic vacuoles (Sahlin *et al.*, 1983; Bassøe *et al.*, 1983). However, it precludes quantitation of ingested targets on the basis of the fluorescence of extracellular particles. Intracellular particles, therefore, must be counted (Horn *et al.*, 1985) or else the extracellular pH has to be adjusted to the value within the phagolysosomes (Sahlin *et al.*, 1983).

Discrimination between attached and internalized particles has been achieved elegantly by the use of quenching dyes. Acid dyes, such as amido black, and direct dyes, e.g. trypan blue, do not enter the phagolysosomes; however, some of these dyes bind with high affinity to extracellular fluorescent particles and cause a significant degree of quenching whereas the internalized particles still emit the unquenched signal (Sahlin *et al.*, 1983). Using this principle, glutaraldehyde-fixed erythrocytes ingested by murine macrophages fluoresced chartreuse, while their extracellular trypan blue-quenched counterparts showed a shift in fluorescence to red (Loike and Silverstein, 1983). Similarly, when PMNs were exposed to *Saccharomyces cerevisiae* or heat-aggregated immunoglobulin, then treated with trypan blue, amido black or another dye and finally inspected cytofluorimetrically at an appropriate pH, a highly quenched signal was obtained from extracellular FITC-labelled yeast particles and immunoglobulin aggregates respectively, compared with the signal emitted by internalized counterparts (Sahlin *et al.*, 1983).

Another method exploited the finding that acridine orange shows green fluorescence when associated with double-stranded DNA and red fluorescence when in contact with denatured or depolymerized DNA or with RNA (Kasten, 1967). This principle was applied to differentiation between dead and viable bacteria ingested by PMNs (Smith and Rommel, 1977; Pantazis and Kniker, 1979). In a recent improvement of this assay (Horn *et al.*, 1985), a combination of Gram staining, acridine orange staining and fluorescence microscopy of the dry-mounted phagocytosis slides permitted one to distinguish between non-fluorescent extracellular *Staphylococcus aureus*, viable ingested particles (green) and killed, intracellular bacteria (red).

Flow Cytometry

The method of choice for a rapid simultaneous analysis at population and at single cell level is flow cytometry. In recent years, several attempts at assessing phagocytosis by this procedure have been published. In the first reports of this kind, latex beads were the target particles (Dunn and Tyrer, 1981; Steinkamp *et al.*, 1982; Fujikawa-Yamamoto and Wada, 1983; Glass *et al.*, 1984). In one study, the resolution was sufficiently high to allow determination of the frequency with which cells ingest a given number of particles (Steinkamp *et al.*, 1982).

In a study involving heat-killed, FITC-labelled *Staphylococcus aureus* and acridine orange-stained peripheral blood mononuclear cells, flow cytometry and narrow angle light scattering measurements provided a number of parameters related to phagocytosis, including assessment of the proportion of non-phagocytic cells and number of particles associated with the phagocytes (Bassøe *et al.*, 1983). The latter, however, was found to be poorly represented by the ratio of acridine orange to green fluorescence; it was found that the green fluorescence intensity of bacteria-associated FITC was considerably more susceptible to low pH than that of latex-associated FITC. It was concluded that the relatively low level of fluorescence emitted by phagocyte-associated bacteria was related to the low pH of phagocytic vacuoles. A decrease in fluorescence could be prevented by pre-storing the PMNs for 24 h prior to phagocytosis.

In a study involving heat-killed *Saccharomyces cerevisiae* and postlabelling of the incubation mixture with acridine orange, the red-to-green fluorescence ratio provided information regarding the degree of association of PMNs with yeast particles (Dérer *et al.*, 1983). The limitation of this procedure lies in its relatively low sensitivity (threshold ≈25% ingesting cells) and in the inability to correct for associated, non-ingested particles.

In a recent study (Bjerknes, 1984) the fluorescence quenching procedure (see page 35) has been combined with the flow cytometric investigation of interaction of viable organisms with phagocytes. Bjerknes (1984) also achieved the simultaneous determination of intracellular killing by using a second dye, ethidium bromide, for selectively labelling killed organisms inside cells. Given the advantages of rapidity for analysis and requirement of low cell numbers, flow cytometry is highly attractive for further phagocytosis studies and lends itself to clinical application.

Bioluminescence

Instead of using an experimental label, recent reports (Barak *et al.*, 1983; Barak *et al.*, 1984) have described the use of a light-emitting bacterial variant (*Vibrio cholerae*, var. *albensis*). Following a phagocytosis phase in suspension, the decrease in bioluminescence with time correlated with the decrease in viable organisms, as assessed by colony counting. The method is appropriate for determination of the killing of bacteria rather than for assessment of their attachment and ingestion; attempts to determine the latter have not been reported for this probe.

Colony Counting Methods

These procedures are based on the lysis of a phagocyte population after ingestion and counting of the organisms giving rise to colonies. Although mainly used for assessment of killing and elimination, information regarding phagocytosis, as such, has been obtained with this method. However, since microbial organisms may multiply during the assay, either intracellularly or extracellularly, and since killing may occur during the ingestion phase, a number of controls must be run in parallel in order to permit quantitation of attachment, ingestion and killing *per se*. Moreover, clumping of bacteria may lead to an underestimation of the number of viable organisms on the basis of the number of colonies.

A number of different approaches have been taken to overcome these difficulties. In some systems, a relatively low target-to-effector cell ratio is used, allowing accurate determination of the decrease in the number of colonies in the supernatants of incubation mixtures of bacteria and phagocytes when compared with the colony number of incubates of bacteria alone (Leijh *et al.*, 1979). In order to warrant a sufficiently high incidence of collisions between bacteria and phagocytes in such suspension assays, phagocyte concentrations must be high, and therefore, even in microassays, 10^6 phagocytes per determination are the lower limit (Maródi *et al.*, 1983). The method is only applicable if the rate of attachment without ingestion is low.

In other systems, the number of phagocyte-associated organisms is assessed, and attached but non-ingested organisms are removed. This is achieved by treatment with lysostaphin in the case of *Staphylococcus aureus* (Tan *et al.*, 1971), for it has been reported that this murolytic enzyme does not penetrate the phagocytic cell membrane. However, later investigators came to different conclusions (Pruzanski *et al.*, 1983). In the case of *Escherichia coli*, polymyxin B has been used, and evidence has been provided that intracellular organisms are not affected (Roberts and Ford, 1982). Again, others have disagreed on this (Brown and Percival, 1978). A more elegant procedure seems to be the application of bacteriophages of appropriate specificity for killing extracellular bacteria, as has been done with phage T6 using *Yersinia pestis* and *Shigella flexneri* as target particles (Shaw *et al.*, 1983).

A variant of the colony counting method is the counting of free particles following an interaction phase between opsonized *Saccharomyces cerevisiae* and PMNs (Levinsky *et al.*, 1978). The decrease in the number of free yeast particles, as assessed by a Coulter counter, was interpreted as being due to attachment to phagocytes with subsequent internalization.

Radiometry

A review of the techniques of assessment of phagocytosis, even in a series devoted to non-isotopic methods, would be incomplete without making reference to radiometric methods, since numerous phagocytosis assays have made use of isotopically labelled targets. The first study of this kind involved the uptake of radiolabelled albumin–anti-albumin complexes (Sorkin and Boyden, 1959). The accumulation of non-TCA-precipitable labelled albumin in the supernatant was taken as a measure for internalization and digestion. The method has been rediscovered (Ward and Zvaifler, 1973) and used by many others for answering clinical and experimental questions (Leslie, 1985; Finbloom, 1985).

Erythrophagocytosis has been widely studied using red blood cells labelled with [51]Cr (Newman *et al.*, 1980; Biegel and Rabinovitch, 1983; Jungi and Baradun, 1985; Cooper *et al.*, 1984) or with [111]In (Friedrich and Gliniorz, 1981). These assays have no advantage over the spectrometric test (Jungi, 1985, part 4). Likewise, platelets labelled with ^{51}Cr have been used as phagocyte targets (McMillan *et al.*, 1974; Handin and Stossel, 1974). However, since platelets may bind to phagocytes under physiological (Jungi *et al.*, 1986) and pathological (Yoo *et al.*, 1982) circumstances in the absence of a phagocytic event, differentiation between attachment and ingestion becomes important in this kind of study; this differentiation is not possible with radiometric procedures.

Numerous systems working with viable organisms have used radioactive prelabelling of the targets by adding isotopically labelled nucleotides, amino acids or sugars to the culture medium (Verhoef *et al.*, 1977; Boghossian *et al.*, 1983). The advantages over the colony counting method are obvious: intracellular killing does not lead to an underestimation of ingestion, since the label either remains intracellularly or enters the non-TCA-precipitable fraction of the medium. Extracellular multiplication has little influence on ingestion (because of the dilution of the label in the target population, which is in part compensated for by the increase in target density). The problem of discriminating between attachment and ingestion, when it has arisen, has been solved in the same manner as has been described for the colony counting methods, i.e. by the use of lytic enzymes (Verhoef *et al.*, 1977) or antibiotics (Roberts and Ford, 1982). One group has employed a double labelling procedure for simultaneous, but separate, assessment of the ingestion and killing of *Escherichia coli* (Roberts and Ford, 1982). Here, bacteria internally labelled with ^{14}C-phenylalanine were allowed to interact with adherent PMNs. Following washing and treatment with polymyxin B, phagocytes were lysed, and the lysate was pulse labelled with ^{3}H-thymidine. The latter was incorporated into viable free bacteria, thus allowing calculation of the number of viable (multiplying) bacteria when compared with the ^{3}H-thymidine incorporation into a calibration culture run in parallel. The total number of ingested organisms was deduced from the ^{14}C counts of the phagocyte lysates.

Several radiometric systems have been devised for measuring uptake and/or intracellular killing of *Candida albicans*. Using organisms prelabelled with ^{51}Cr, the ^{51}Cr release was shown to represent a simple measure of uptake and killing (Yamamura *et al.*, 1976; Bistoni *et al.*, 1982). Postlabelling with ^{3}H uridine, harvesting of labelled particles and comparison of ^{3}H incorporation with a calibration curve provided information as to the number of extracellular organisms present at the end of ingestion, thereby allowing calculation of the ingested blastospore number (Yamamura *et al.*, 1977). Release of intracellular organisms with detergents prior to prelabelling served for determining the number of intracellular, viable organisms (Bridges *et al.*, 1980), but it was later found that detergent lysis could lead to alteration of ^{3}H uridine incorporation into blastospores (Husseini *et al.*, 1985).

Electron Spin Resonance Spectroscopy

Besides spectrometric, fluorescent and isotopic labels, spin labels have recently been used to tag phagocytic target particles (Tsuge *et al.*, 1982). These labels were incorporated into liposomes which were offered to phagocyte monolayers for ingestion, and the electron spin resonance signal resulting from phagocyte extracts was determined. Using a murine macrophage cell line, a variety of tempole derivatives were tested but only tempocholine was found to be suitable. By using appropriate inhibitors, a non-phagocytic cell line and microscopy, evidence for liposome internalization was provided. Owing to the suboptimal interaction of the low-density liposomes with the glass-adherent phagocytes and the lack of opsonins in the system, the degree of internalization was low. Despite the relatively high cell numbers required (1.5×10^{6} cells for an optimal response) the system has the potential to be further optimized by appropriate opsonization procedures, by the choice of other effector cells and more intimate interaction of phagocytes with targets.

THE MONITORING OF METABOLIC EVENTS RELATED TO INGESTION

Metabolic Responses of Phagocytes Exposed to Ingestible Stimuli

During the course of ingestion, a number of biochemical events are triggered, either as a result of receptor specific interaction with the target or as a result of ingestion as such. It has long been known that phagocytosis is associated with an alteration of the way hexose is catabolized (hexose monophosphate shunt (HMP)) and there is also a burst in oxygen consumption (respiratory burst). Biochemical studies and investigations of inherited enzyme deficiencies provided evidence that the respiratory burst leads to the generation of microbicidal oxygen radicals, including $\cdot O_2^-$, H_2O_2, OH^-, $OH\cdot$ (reviewed in Babior, 1984, and Badway and Karnowsky, 1980). In the presence of H_2O_2, myeloperoxidase catalyses other microbicidal processes, such as halidination (Klebanoff, 1971) and formation of aldehydes (Strauss *et al.*, 1970). Although a respiratory burst is observed within minutes after contact of phagocytes with appropriate ingestible targets, ingestion may, under special conditions, occur in the absence of a respiratory burst (Schnyder and Baggiolini, 1978). In contrast, appropriate membrane perturbance, receptor triggering (Briheim *et al.*, 1984; Kiyotaki *et al.*, 1978), protein kinase stimulation and Ca^{2+} flux (reviewed in Johnston and Kitagawa, 1985) may all trigger a respiratory burst in the absence of such particle ingestion.

Another series of events related to phagocytic ingestion is the generation of arachidonic acid and the formation of bioactive metabolites of the lipoxygenase and cyclooxygenase pathways (Scott *et al.*, 1980). It is not yet clear how the metabolic events following oxygen consumption and those associated with arachidonic acid metabolism are interdependent.

A further cellular response following the interaction of phagocytes with target particles is the release of lysosomal enzymes (Henson, 1971; Weissman *et al.*, 1972). Again, phagocytosis is but one possible trigger; others are receptor-specific interactions of soluble or surface-bound components. All these events, respiratory oxidative burst, triggering of arachidonic acid metabolism and enzyme release, occur rapidly and, therefore, lend themselves to the development of indirect phagocytosis assays and/or microbial killing assays. I shall review assays related to the metabolic burst triggered by ingestible particles, thus allowing rapid and reproducible measurement of samples containing low numbers of phagocytes.

Measurement of Oxygen Consumption

Oxygen consumption can be readily measured polarographically, using a Clarc-type oxygen electrode (DeChatelet and Parce, 1981). A Japanese group (Nakamura *et al.*, 1978) has developed a micromethod for detecting inherited oxidase defects, using as little as 1 ml blood pretreated with CO for generating CO haemoglobin prior to stimulation with zymosan. In studies with isolated PMNs, kinetic determinations of O_2 consumption, following triggering with latex beads, were performed (Segal and Coade, 1978). In a spectrometric procedure, haemoglobin was used as oxygen donator, and the decreased absorbance at 438.5 nm was taken as a measure of O_2 consumption by PMNs ingesting zymosan (Markert and Frei, 1979). Although both methods possess sufficient sensitivity, only one sample can be analysed at a time.

Nitroblue–Tetrazolium Reduction and Cytochrome C Reduction

Phagocytes displaying a respiratory burst reduce the dye nitroblue–tetrazolium (NBT) to formazan. Although the exact mechanism is still unclear, evidence has been provided that NBT reduction is an indicator for superoxide generation (Baehner *et al.*, 1976). The NBT test has been used to diagnose chronic granulomatous disease (Baehner and Nathan, 1968) and to indicate the presence of a bacterial infection (Park *et al.*, 1968). The diagnostic value of the latter test has been widely criticized, since much simpler haematological evaluations have proved to be more sensitive than the NBT test (Steigbigel *et al.*, 1974) and a variety of artifacts have been identified; the latter include use of an inappropriate anticoagulant, inadvertent reactivity of damaged cells or endotoxin contamination of samples (Rothwell and Doumas, 1975; Humbert *et al.*, 1973). Despite these shortcomings, the test is widely used in the clinic, and several improvements of the original method have been reported (Rothwell and Doumas, 1975; Humbert *et al.*, 1973; Schopf *et al.*, 1984). There is a qualitative histochemical variant (Park *et al.*, 1968; Steigbigel *et al.*, 1974; Rothwell and Doumas, 1975; Humbert *et al.*, 1973) and a quantitative spectrometric variant of the test (Stossel, 1973; Baehner *et al.*, 1976; Baehner and Nathan, 1968; Rothwell and Doumas, 1975; Humbert *et al.*, 1973; Schopf *et al.*, 1984). In the latter, cells exposed to ingestible particles in suspension in the presence of NBT are then separated from the substrate, and the formazan accumulated within phagocytes is extracted and measured photometrically at 580 nm. Like other assays performed in suspension, relatively high phagocyte numbers and target numbers are required.

The alternative procedure for assessment of superoxide radicals generated during the respiratory burst is the SOD-inhibitable reduction of cytochrome C, a test comparable in sensitivity with the quantitative NBT test (Johnston, 1981; Babior *et al.*, 1973). In both tests the ratio between measured response, in both the presence and the absence of a phagocytic stimulator, is often lower than that obtained with the assays described below.

H_2O_2 Generation

The most commonly used assay of H_2O_2 production by phagocytes is measurement of the loss in fluorescence of scopoletin when exposed to H_2O_2 in the presence of horse radish peroxidase (HRPO) (Root *et al.*, 1975; Nathan, 1981). A more recent fluorimetric assay is based on the H_2O_2-dependent, HRPO-catalysed oxidation of homovanillic acid to a fluorescent dimer (Rossi *et al.*, 1980; Ruch *et al.*, 1983). Although the sensitivity of both assays is high, the latter procedure avoids some of the disadvantages of the scopoletin method (measurement of disappearance of an unstable substrate rather than generation of a relatively stable product) and may be adapted to the automated reading of microtitre plates. In a spectrometric procedure, the shift in absorption undergone by yeast cytochrome C peroxidase when forming a complex with H_2O_2 is determined (Boveris *et al.*, 1972). Despite the high sensitivity, the assay is seldom used, since it requires double-beam spectrometry and an enzyme not commercially available. In a more recent spectrometric assay, adapted to automated reading of microtitre plates, accumulation of the oxidation product of phenol red is measured at 610 nm (Pick and Mizel, 1981). This method, however, is less sensitive than the former procedures.

Chemiluminescence

The radical species generated during the respiratory burst emit light which can be measured in a luminometer or in a scintillation counter in the single-photo-multiplier or in the out-of-coincidence mode (Allen *et al.*, 1972). The response is recorded over a certain period of time, thus allowing determination of the time-dependent changes in the rate of luminescing radical generation. The recorded signal is relatively weak, and high cell numbers are required. The signal, however, can be amplified by using luminescent substrates. This permits reduction in the number of cells per assay by a factor of 10 to 100, thereby making possible the analysis of paediatric samples (Mills *et al.*, 1979) and blood from neutropenic individuals (Stevens *et al.*, 1978).

Depending on the luminescent substrate used, different radicals can be preferentially monitored. Luminol, the most widely used amplifier in phagocytosis systems, appears to be largely myeloperoxidase dependent (DeChatelet *et al.*, 1982; Faden and Maciejewski, 1981; Seim, 1983), as evidenced by an exquisite azide susceptibility of the reaction and by the failure of cells from myeloperoxidase-deficient patients to respond. However, participation of the lipoxigenase products has recently been suggested (Cheung *et al.*, 1983; Rush and Keown, 1984) on the basis of susceptibility of the reaction to inhibitors of arachidonic acid metabolism. This hypothesis still awaits definitive proof. Lucigenin, in contrast, seems to reflect generation of superoxide anion production (Allen, 1981) and thus resembles the NBT reduction assay.

Chemiluminescence measurements have been performed with whole blood (DeChatelet and Shirley, 1981; Selvaraj *et al.*, 1982; Tono-Oka *et al.*, 1983) and – preferably (Faden and Maciejewski, 1981; Bruchelt and Schmidt, 1984) – with isolated PMNs (Allen *et al.*, 1972; Mills *et al.*, 1979; Stevens *et al.*, 1978; DeChatelet *et al.*, 1982; Cheung *et al.*, 1983; Rush and Keown, 1984) or mononuclear phagocytes (Seim, 1983; Williams and Cole, 1981; Kanegasaki *et al.*, 1981; Braun *et al.*, 1981). In clinical research, two particular aspects must be considered. Firstly, it was hoped that alterations in phagocyte function, either inherited (DeChatelet and Shirley, 1981) or acquired (Selvaraj *et al.*, 1982; Williams and Cole, 1981; Kanegasaki *et al.*, 1981; Braun *et al.*, 1981; Barbour *et al.*, 1980), would be detected by this measurement. Secondly, by using opsonized particles as stimulatory targets, defects in the opsonic capacity (Vernon *et al.*, 1984) or pathologically elevated degrees of opsonization (Deschamps-Latscha *et al.*, 1984) should be sought. By using patient–control combinations, both aspects can be studied simultaneously (Mills *et al.*, 1979; Stevens *et al.*, 1978; Wilson *et al.*, 1978). A further control for phagocyte responsiveness is the triggering of cells with soluble stimuli of the protein C kinase, such as phorbol myristate acetate (DeChatelet and Shirley, 1981) or calcium ionophores which trigger the oxidative burst in the absence of a phagocytic event (Johnston and Kitagawa, 1985). Opsonized particles used as chemiluminescing triggers include pneumococci (Allen and Liebermann, 1984), streptococci (Hemming *et al.*, 1976), *Escherichia coli* (Stevens and Young, 1977; Allen, 1977), yeast particles (Vernon *et al.*, 1984), platelet-carrying autoantibodies (Deschamps-Latscha *et al.*, 1984), virus-infected antiviral-antibody-coated target cells (Weber and Peterhans, 1983), IgG aggregates (Rush and Keown, 1984), antibody-coated erythrocytes (Mossman *et al.*, 1981), latex beads coated with luminol (Uchida *et al.*, 1985) and others. The stimulatory targets most often used are opsonized zymosan particles, which are among the strongest stimuli available. The selection of this target, however, may be inappropriate for detecting subtle functional defects of phagocytes. Opsonized zymosan interacts with a number of cellular receptor systems, including Fc receptors, C3b receptors and β-glucan receptors, which may all mediate generation of luminescing radicals. A defect in the recognition by one type of receptor may be compensated for by intact or increased function of another. Furthermore, as the response may be expected to depend on the number of receptors involved, more information may be gained from experiments with suboptimally sensitized particles. In a recent study involving *Pneumococcus aeruginosa* and human PMNs, the quantitative relationship of antibody-dependent triggering of Fc receptor-mediated chemiluminescence has been carefully analysed by studying the kinetics of the response (Allen and Liebermann, 1984), an approach recommendable for future studies.

It has to be realized that phagocytosis is not assayed directly, and a number of factors involved in transduction of the recognition signal into generation of light have to be controlled for. For example, target particles may themselves participate in the generation of light, be it by amplifying the response caused by phagocyte-derived radicals or by acting as scavengers of these radicals. An artifact to be considered when working with cell line cells as stimulators is the capacity of mycoplasma to induce chemiluminescence by an as-yet unknown mechanism, thereby falsely suggesting that the cell line itself has triggered radical generation, whereas it could merely be due to contamination with mycoplasma (Peterhans *et al.*, 1984). However, by appropriate selection of the analytical conditions, chemiluminescence proves to be a powerful tool for evaluating the interaction of opsonized targets and phagocytes.

SPECTROMETRIC SCREENING ASSAY OF ERYTHROPHAGOCYTOSIS

Reagents

Medium 'MHA'

Dulbeccos's MEM without sodium bicarbonate, 10x (Seromed, Fakola, Basle, No. 0423), diluted with 9 parts H_2O bidest., supplemented with 4-(2-hydroxyethyl)-piperazine-1-ethane sulphonic acid (HEPES) (1 M, pH 8), final concentration 40 mM, and BSA solution (Boseral S, 30%; Organon Technika, Turnhout, Belgium), final concentration 0.5%. This medium (MHA) is prepared fresh each day.

Washing Buffer

Physiological saline containing 0.01 M Na_2HPO_4–NaH_2PO_4, pH 7.4 (PBS) and supplemented with 1.05 mM Mg^{2+}, 0.9 mM Ca^{2+}, 3 mM NaN_3.

Lysis Buffer

2 parts washing buffer and 7 parts H_2O dest.

Acetate Buffer, pH 5.5

9 parts acetic acid, 1 M, and 10 parts NaOH, 1 M.

Substrate Solutions

3,3′,5,5′-tetramethylbenzidine (TMB; Sigma, St. Louis, MO, No. T-2885) is dissolved in absolute ethanol to yield a stock solution of 2 mg/ml. Each day, 1 part of stock solution, kept in the dark, is mixed with 19 parts of sodium phosphate buffer (PB) 0.1 M, pH 5.5, and 4 μl H_2O_2 (30%) per ml are added. *o*-tolidine (Fluka, Buchs, Switzerland) is dissolved in acetic acid, 1 M, and brought to pH 5.5 by adding 10 parts NaOH, 1 M, per 9 parts *o*-tolidine. From this stock solution, which is stored in the dark, a working solution of 0.08 mg/ml is made using acetate buffer, pH 5.5; to this solution 4 μl H_2O_2 (30%) are added per ml *o*-tolidine. Diaminobenzidine (DAB) is made freshly by dissolving 0.4 mg/ml DAB (Sigma, No. D-5637) in PBS (0.01 M, pH 7.4) and adding 4 μl H_2O_2 per ml DAB.

Sodium Dodecylsulphate Solutions

A stock solution of sodium dodecylsulphate (SDS) is made in PBS when working with DAB, or in PB 0.1 M, pH 5.5, when working with TMB or *o*-tolidine. The stock solution is diluted with the corresponding solvent either to 0.3% (macrophage assays) or to 0.1% (monocyte assays).

Cetavlon–Amido Black Solution

0.1 M citric acid containing 0.05% amido black and 1% cetavlon (*N*-acetyl-*N,N,N*-trimethylammonium bromide; Merck, Darmstadt, FRG, No. 2342) (Nakagawara and Nathan, 1983).

Procedure

Opsonization of Erythrocytes

In all our studies, opsonization with IgG or with IgM and complement has been performed according to conventional methods (Czop and Austen, 1985; Newman *et al.*, 1980; Wright and Silverstein, 1982; Pommier *et al.*, 1983; Jungi and Baradun, 1985), using either sheep erythrocytes (E^s) or human red blood cells (E^h). Using affinity-purified, ^{125}I-labelled anti-E^s antibodies, sigmoid curves were obtained when phagocytic indices were plotted as a function of the logarithm of the number of antibodies per E^s (Jungi, 1985). Alternatively, tannin-treated erythrocytes (E-T) may be used (Biegel and Rabinovitch, 1983). On preincubation of E-T with IgG, efficient opsonization is obtained; furthermore, phagocytosis is inhibitable by high amounts of IgG, suggesting that an Fc receptor-mediated mechanism is operative.

Preparation of Phagocytes

In our laboratory, freshly isolated monocytes, monocytes matured to macrophages *in vitro* or macrophages obtained from bronchoalveolar lavages are routinely used. The method is nevertheless applicable to other phagocytic cells. For assays with fresh monocytes, mononuclear cell suspensions are prepared according to standard methods (Jungi and Baradun, 1985; Bøyum, 1968). Macrophages cultured *in vitro* are prepared as described elsewhere (Jungi, 1985; Andreesen *et al.*, 1983).

Phagocytosis Test

The above-mentioned phagocytes are resuspended in medium MHA after washing (2.5×10^6 mononuclear cells/ml, 0.3×10^6 cultured macrophages/ml or 0.5×10^6 alveolar macrophages/ml respectively), and 100 μl of the suspension are placed into each well of microtitre plates (Nunc, Roskilde, Denmark, No. 001-67008A). Following an adherence phase of 1 h (monocytes) or 2 h (macrophages), cells are washed with washing buffer, using a Nunc Immunowash 12 washing comb connected interchangeably with washing buffer or with lysis buffer by a Y valve. Washing buffer is then replaced by 50 μl MHA. Next, 50 μl of a 1% suspension of appropriately opsonized erythrocytes are added, control wells receiving either 50 μl MHA or unsensitized erythrocytes. Plates are incubated for 1 h at 37°C in humidified air. Thereafter, microtitre plates are washed, using the Immunowash again. Then, washing buffer is replaced by lysis buffer which is substituted by washing buffer once more 30 s later. After 5 min, a further washing step is performed. Next, monolayers are sucked dry and 100 μl SDS solution is added. After 30 min, 150 μl of substrate are added, the content of the wells then being mixed, and the plate finally read in an ELISA reader 5 to 30 min later, depending on the actual substrate used and the ambient temperature.

One set of wells is reserved for the calibration curve which allows conversion of the recorded optical density (OD) into the number of ingested erythrocytes per well. Here, no erythrocytes are present during the ingestion phase, but a known number of erythrocytes, in 50 μl saline, are added prior to lysing the monolayers with 50 μl double-strength SDS solution. Erythrocyte numbers may be determined spectrometrically or microscopically.

A further set of control monolayers receiving no erythrocytes is used for determining the number of phagocytes per well. Here, instead of SDS solution, 100 μl of cetavlon–amido black (Nakagawara and Nathan, 1983) are added to the wells, their content then being vigorously mixed, and the released nuclei are finally counted in a haematocytometer. Phagocyte nuclei are readily distinguishable from the nuclei of lymphocytes which may contaminate the monolayer.

Critical Comments

Choice of the Medium

The proportion of mononuclear phagocytes adhering to the surface of microtitre wells and the phagocytic capacity depend on the choice of medium. MEM provides better adherence than RPMI 1640. The presence of protein is essential for optimal performance of phagocytosis. While the highest proportion of adherent cells is obtained by supplementing the medium with 2% of heated (30 min 56°C) homologous serum, the addition of serum containing IgG during adherence phase should be avoided if Fc receptor-mediated phagocytosis is to be studied. The IgG moiety adhering to the microtitre well surface effectively mimics the presence of immobilized immune complexes (Michl *et al.*, 1979) and leads to Fc receptor modulation, thereby inducing phagocytosis blockade within 1 h. This blockade lasts for several days (Kurlander, 1980; Jungi and von Below, in preparation). Therefore, IgG-free serum albumin or foetal bovine serum (FBS) are recommendable. Using 0.5% bovine serum albumin, 65–75% of added monocytes can be recovered at the end of the assay, 20% being non-adherent already at the beginning. When FBS is used, the proportion of adherent cells is somewhat lower. The use of media buffered with HEPES, without sodium bicarbonate, is recommended.

Choice of Cell Numbers

The number of cells applied to the microtitre wells should not be less than 5×10^4 monocytes/well, or 3×10^4 macrophages/well. With lower cell numbers, loss of cells during the assay is overproportionally high.

The Kinetics of the Phagocytic Response

In its simplest form, the assay is carried out as an endpoint assay. Although the endpoint of ingestion is usually reached less than 30 min after addition of the erythrocytes, 60 min is routinely employed. For longer incubation times, a decrease in the number of ingested particles is observed, particularly with macrophages. This may be due to intracellular inactivation of the pseudoperoxidase of haemoglobin. Phagocytosis rate determinations would require additional manipulations, since exact temperature control within microtitre wells and an accelerated sedimentation of erythrocytes onto the monolayer would be a prerequisite.

Choice of Target Particles and Density

Routinely, either E^s and E^h are used, but the method can be adapted to any other kind of erythrocytes. The offered number of target particles is a large excess ($\approx$ 200-fold in the case of E^s).

Choice of Detergent for Lysing Phagocyte Monolayers

By trying a wide variety of detergents, only SDS met the two requirements of lysing the monolayer completely and being compatible with the substrate buffer systems used.

Choice of Substrate

Among various peroxidase substrates tested, three were found to be useful for the erythrophagocytosis test (table 1). Although it is essential to work at defined ionic strength and at precisely defined pH, buffers other than those recommended in table 1 might also be found suitable. The possibility of reading absorbance at 405 nm or 412 nm (Cooper *et al.*, 1984; Rummage and Leu, 1985) prior to the addition of substrate, together with the use of substrates of differing sensitivities, permits a wide range of ingested erythrocytes to be tested, between 10^3 E^s and $> 10^6$ E^s per well.

Time between Substrate Addition and Reading

There is no need to stop the reaction if the time differences between addition of substrate and the reading of individual wells are kept identical. Depending on the strength of reaction, reading is performed between 5 and 30 min after substrate addition. Using DAB and reading at 360 nm, the linear relationship between OD and number of E^s per well is limited to an early phase of the reaction. Furthermore, endogenic peroxidase does not contribute to substrate conversion during the first 30 min, but may lead to an elevated background later on.

Table 1   Choice of conditions for performing spectrophotometric erythrophagocytosis test

Number of E^S per well expected[a] $((E^S) \times 10^{-3})$	Detergent for lysing monolayer[b] $(100\ \mu l)$	Substrate $(150\ \mu l)$	Photometry wavelengths $\lambda_{Test}, \lambda_{Ref}$ (nm)	Range of linearity[c] $((E^S) \times 10^{-3})$
> 100	SDS in PBS		405	Whole range
20–800	SDS in PBS	0.4 mg DAB–ml PBS	450–490	_[d]
10–400	SDS in PBS	0.4 mg DAB–ml PBS	360	0–300
1–200	SDS in PB, 0.1 M, pH 5.5	0.1 mg TMB–ml PB, 0.1 M, pH 5.5	405, 550 or 650, 550	0–100
2–200	SDS in PB, 0.1 M, pH 5.5	0.08 mg *o*-tolidine– ml acetate buffer, pH 5.5	405, 550	0–80

[a] Depending on haemoglobin concentration per cell, these numbers vary for erythrocytes of other species.
[b] Final concentration of SDS: 0.3% (macrophage assays) or 0.1% (monocyte assays).
[c] Defined as linear regression with $r^2 \geq 0.99$.
[d] $OD = a \times (E^S)^2 + b \times (E^S)$ in the range 0–400 where (E^S) is the number of E^S per well and a and b are constants of the reaction.

Accuracy and Reproducibility

The spectrometrically determined phagocytic indices were found to correlate well with those measured in parallel in a ^{51}Cr release assay (Jungi, 1985) as long as the ingestion phase did not exceed 30–60 min. The reproducibility was found to be very good when either human monocytes or macrophages were used in combination with IgG-sensitized sheep or human erythrocytes.

Conclusions

The described method offers an objective non-isotopic alternative to the widely used microscopic and radiometric erythrophagocytosis tests. It exceeds the sensitivity of the ^{51}Cr assay when TMB or *o*-tolidine is used as substrate, and it allows the use of erythrocytes as targets (e.g. from clinical isolates) without involvement of further manipulations. Adaption to microtitre plates permits rapid reading of the assay in an ELISA reader and automated processing of the data, thus making the test well suited for screening programs.

REFERENCES

Allen, R. C. (1977). Evaluation of serum opsonic capacity by quantitating the initial chemiluminescence response from phagocytizing polymorphonuclear leukocytes. *Infect. Immunity*, **15**, 828–833

Allen, R. C. (1981). In DeLuca, M. and McElroy, W. (eds.), *Bioluminescence and Chemiluminescence*, Academic Press, New York, 63–73

Allen, R. C. and Liebermann, M. M. (1984). Kinetic analysis of microbe opsonification based on stimulated polymorphonuclear leukocyte oxygenation activity. *Infect. Immunity*, **45**, 475–482

Allen, R. C., Stjernholm, R. L. and Steele, R. H. (1972). Evidence for the generation of an electronic excitation state(s) in human polymorphonuclear leukocytes and its participation in bactericidal activity. *Biochem. Biophys. Res. Comm.*, **47**, 679–684

Andreesen, R., Picht, R. and Löhr, G. W. (1983). Primary cultures of human blood-borne macrophages grown on hydrophobic teflon membranes. *J. Immunol. Methods*, **56**, 295–304

Babior, B. M. (1984). The respiratory burst of phagocytes. *J. Clin. Invest.*, **73**, 599–601

Babior, B., Kipnes, R. S. and Curnutte, J. T. (1973). Biological defense mechanisms. The production by leukocytes of superoxide, a potential bactericidal agent. *J. Clin. Invest.*, **52**, 741–744

Badway, J. A. and Karnowsky, M. L. (1980). Active oxygen species and the function of phagocytic leukocytes. *Annu. Rev. Biochem.*, **49**, 695–726

Baehner, R. L., Boxer, L. A. and Davis, J. (1976). The biochemical basis of nitroblue tetrazolium reduction in normal human and chronic granulomatous disease polymorphonuclear leukocytes. *Blood*, **48**, 309–313

Baehner, R. L. and Nathan, D. G. (1968). Quantitative nitroblue tetrazolium test in chronic granulomatous disease. *N. Engl. J. Med.*, **278**, 971–976

Barak, M., Ulitzur, S. and Merzbach, D. (1983). The use of luminous bacteria for determination of phagocytosis. *J. Immunol. Methods*, **64**, 353–363

Barak, M., Ulitzur, S. and Merzbach, D. (1984). Elucidation of the phagocytosis mechanism with the aid of luminous bacteria. *J. Med. Microbiol.*, **18**, 65–72

Barbour, A. G., Allred, C. D., Solberg, C. O. and Hill, H. R. (1980). Chemiluminescence by polymorphonuclear leukocytes from patients with active bacterial infection. *J. Infect. Dis.*, **141**, 14–26

Bassøe, C.-F., Laerum, O. D., Glette, J., Hopen, G., Haneberg, B. and Solberg, C. O. (1983). Simultaneous measurement of phagocytosis and phagosomal pH by flow cytometry: role of polymorphonuclear neutrophilic leukocyte granules in phagosome acidification. *Cytometry*, **4**, 254–262

Biegel, D. and Rabinovitch, M. (1983). Measurement of phagocytosis utilizing ^{51}Cr-labeled tannic acid treated erythrocytes. *J. Immunol. Methods*, **58**, 19–23

Bistoni, F., Baccarini, M., Blasi, E., Puccetti, P. and Marconi, P. (1982). A radiolabel release microassay for phagocytic killing of *Candida albicans. J. Immunol. Methods*, **52**, 369–377

Bjerknes, R. (1984). Flow cytometric assay for combined measurement of phagocytosis and intracellular killing of *Candida albicans. J. Immunol. Methods*, **72**, 229–241

Boghossian, S. H., Wright, G. and Segal, A. W. (1983). The kinetic measurement of phagocyte function in whole blood. *J. Immunol. Methods*, **60**, 125–140

Boveris, A., Oshino, N. and Chance, B. (1972). The cellular production of hydrogen peroxide. *Biochem. J.*, **128**, 617–630

Bøyum, A. (1968). Isolation of mononuclear cells and granulocytes from human blood. *Scand. J. Clin. Lab. Invest.*, **21**, Suppl. 97, 77–89

Braun, D. P., Harris, J. E., Maximovich, S., Marder, R. and Lint, T. F. (1981). Chemiluminescence in peripheral blood mononuclear cells of solid tumor cancer patients. *Cancer Immunol. Immunother.*, **12**, 31–37

Bridges, C. G., DaSilva, G. L., Yamamura, M. and Valdimarsson, H. (1980). A radiometric assay for the combined measurement of phagocytosis and intracellular killing of *Candida albicans. Clin. Exp. Immunol.*, **42**, 226–233

Briheim, G., Stendhal, O. and Dahlgren, C. (1984). Intra- and extracellular events in luminol-dependent chemiluminescence of polymorphonuclear leukocytes. *Infect. Immunity*, **45**, 1–5

Brown, K. N. and Percival, A. (1978). Penetration of antimicrobials into tissue culture cells and leucocytes. *Scand. J. Inf. Dis. Suppl.*, **14**, 251–260

Bruchelt, G. and Schmidt, K. H. (1984). Comparative studies on the oxidative processes during phagocytosis measured by luminol-dependent chemiluminescence. *J. Clin. Chem. Clin. Biochem.*, **22**, 1–13

Cheung, K., Archibald, A. C. and Robinson, M. F. (1983). The origin of chemiluminescence produced by neurophils stimulated by opzonized zymosan. *J. Immunol.*, **130**, 2324–2329

Cooper, P. H., Mayer, P. and Baggiolini, M. (1984). Stimulation of phagocytosis in bone marrow-derived mouse macrophages by bacterial lipopolysaccharide: correlation with biochemical and functional parameters. *J. Immunol.*, **133**, 913–922

Czop, J. K. and Austen, K. F. (1985). Properties of glycans that activate the human alternative complement pathway and interact with the human monocyte β-glucan receptor. *J. Immunol.*, **135**, 3388–3393

Czop, J. K., Fearon, D. T. and Austen, K. F. (1978). Membrane sialic acid on target particles modulates their phagocytosis by a trypsin-sensitive mechanism on human monocytes. *Proc. Natl. Acad. Sci. USA*, **75**, 3831–3835

DeChatelet, L. R., Long, G. D., Shirley, P. S., Bass, D. A., Thomas, M. J., Henderson, F. W. and Cohen, M. S. (1982). Mechanism of the luminol-dependent chemiluminescence of human neutrophils. *J. Immunol.*, **129**, 1589–1593

DeChatelet, L. R. and Parce, J. W. (1981). In Edelson, P. J. and Koren, H. (eds.), *Methods for Studying Mononuclear Phagocytes*, Academic Press, New York, 477–488

DeChatelet, L. R. and Shirley, P. S. (1981). Evaluation of chronic granulomatous disease by chemiluminescence assay of microliter quantities of whole blood. *Clin. Chem.*, **27**, 1739–1741

Dérer, M., Walker, C., Kristensen, F. and Reinhardt, M. C. (1983). A simple and rapid flow cytometric method for routine assessment of baker's yeast uptake by human polymorphonuclear leukocytes. *J. Immunol. Methods*, **61**, 359–365

Deschamps-Latscha, B., Feuillet-Fieux, M.-N., Baruchel, A., Patereau, C. and Nguyen, A.-T. (1984). Activation du métabolisme oxydatif des granulocytes et des monocytes par des plaquettes recouvertes d'IgG provenant de patients porteurs de thrombopénies, *C.R. Acad. Sc. Paris*, **298/III**, 419–422

Dunn, P. A. and Tyrer, H. W. (1981). Quantitation of neutrophil phagocytosis, using fluorescent latex beads. Correlation of microscopy and flow cytometry. *J. Lab. Clin. Med.*, **98**, 374–381

Edelson, P. J., Zwiebel, R. and Cohn, Z. A. (1982). The pinocytosis rate of activated macrophages. *J. Exp. Med.*, **142**, 1150–1164

Faden, H. and Maciejewski, N. (1981). Whole blood luminol-dependent chemiluminescence. *J. Reticuloendothel. Soc.*, **30**, 219–226

Finbloom, D. S. (1985). Binding, endocytosis and degradation of model immune complexes by murine macrophages at various levels of activation. *Clin. Immunol. Immunopathol.*, **36**, 275–288

Friedrich, E. A. and Gliniorz, R. (1981). A rapid new method of measuring phagocytosis and cytotoxicity in macrophage tissue cultures. *J. Immunol. Methods*, **47**, 259–262

Fujikawa-Yamamoto, K. and Wada, M. (1983). Flow cytometry of the phagocytosis of fluorescent microspheres in V79 cells. *Cell Struct. Funct.*, **8**, 373–377

Glass, W., Jenssen, H. L., Mix, E. and Friedrich, A. (1984). Flow cytometric measurements of phagocytosis. I. A methodical and comparative study. *Biochem. Biophys. Acta*, **43**, 187–196

Handin, R. I. and Stossel, T. P. (1974). Phagocytosis of antibody-coated platelets by human granulocytes. *New Engl. J. Med.*, **290**, 989–993

Hemming, V. G., Hall, R. T., Rhodes, P. G., Shigeoka, G. O. and Hill, H. R. (1976). Assessment of group B streptococcal opsonins in human and rabbit serum by neurophil chemiluminescence. *J. Clin. Invest.*, **58**, 1379–1387

Henson, P. M. (1971). The immunologic release of constituents from neutrophil leukocytes. I. The role of antibody and complement on nonphagocytosable surfaces or phagocytosable particles. *J. Immunol.*, **107**, 1535–1546

Herbert, W. J. (1978). In Weir, D. M. (ed.), *Handbook of Experimental Immunology*, Vol. 1, Blackwell, Oxford, 20.1–20.20

Horn, W., Hansmann, C. and Federlin, K. (1985). An improved fluorochrome microassay for the detection of living and nonliving intracellular bacteria in human neurophils. *J. Immunol. Methods*, **83**, 233–240

Humbert, J. R., Gross, G. P., Vatter, A. E. and Hathaway, W. E. (1973). Nitro-blue–tetrazolium reduction by neutrophils: biochemical and ultrastructural effects of methylene blue. *J. Lab. Clin. Med.*, **82**, 20–30

Husseini, R. H., Hoadley, M. E., Hutchinson, J. J. P., Penn, C. W. and Smith, H.

(1985). Intracellular killing of *Candida albicans* by human polymorphonuclear leucocytes: comparison of three methods of assessment. *J. Immunol. Methods*, **81**, 215–221

Johnston, R. B., Jr. (1981). In Adams, D. O., Edelson, P. J. and Koren, H. (eds.), *Methods for Studying Mononuclear Phagocytes*, Academic Press, New York, 489–497

Johnston, R. B., Jr. and Kitagawa, S. (1985). Molecular basis for the enhanced respiratory burst of activated macrophages. *Fed. Proc.*, **44**, 2927–2932

Jungi, T. W. (1985). A rapid and sensitive method allowing photometric determination of erythrophagocytosis by mononuclear phagocytes. *J. Immunol. Methods*, **82**, 141–153

Jungi, T. W. and Barandun, S. (1985). Estimation of the degree of opsonization of homologous erythrocytes by IgG for intravenous and intramuscular use. *Vox Sang.*, **49**, 9–19

Jungi, T. W., Spycher, M. O., Nydegger, U. E. and Barandun, S. (1986). Platelet leukocyte interaction. I. Selective binding of thrombin-stimulated platelets to human monocytes, polymorphonuclear leukocytes and related cell lines. *Blood*, **67**, 629–636

Kanegasaki, S., Homma, J. Y., Homma, H. and Washizaki, M. (1981). Enhanced chemiluminescence response of phagocyting monocytes from sarcoidosis patients. *Int. Archs. Allergy Appl. Immun.*, **64**, 72–79

Kaplan, G. (1977). Differences in the mode of phagocytosis with Fc-receptors and C3 receptors in macrophages. *Scand. J. Immunol.*, **6**, 797–807

Kasten, F. H. (1967). Cytochemical studies with acridine orange and the influence of dye contaminants in the staining of nucleic acids. *Int. Rev. Cytol.*, **21**, 141–202

Kiyotaki, C., Shimizu, A., Watanabe, S. and Yamamura, Y. (1978). Superoxide production from human polymorphonuclear leucocytes stimulated with immunoglobulins of different classes and fragments of IgG bound to polystyrene dishes. *Immunology*, **35**, 613–618

Klebanoff, S. J. (1971). Iodination of bacteria: a bactericidal mechanism. *J. Exp. Med.*, **126**, 1063–1078

Kurlander, R. J. (1980). Reversible and irreversible loss of Fc receptor function of human monocytes as a consequence of interaction with immunoglobin G. *J. Clin. Invest.*, **66**, 773–781

Lee, D. A., Hoidal, J. R., Clawson, C. C., Quie, P. G. and Peterson, P. K. (1983). Phagocytosis by polymorphonuclear leukocytes of *Staphylococcus aureus* and *Pseudomonas aeruginosa* adherent to plastic, agar, or glass. *J. Immunol. Methods*, **63**, 103–114

Lehrer, R. I. (1975). Fungicidal mechanisms of human monocytes. I. Evidence for myeloperoxidase-linked and myeloperoxidase-independent mechanisms. *J. Clin. Invest.*, **55**, 338–346

Lehrer, R. I. (1981). In Adams, D. O., Edelson, P. J. and Koren, H. (eds.), *Methods for Studying Mononuclear Phagocytes*, Academic Press, New York, 693–708

Leijh, P. C. J., van den Barselaar, M. T., van Zwet, T. L., Dubbeldeman-Rempt, I. and van Furth, R. (1979). Kinetics of phagocytosis of *Staphylococcus aureus* and *Escherichia coli* by human granulocytes. *Immunology*, **37**, 453–465

Leslie, R. G. Q. (1985). Macrophage handling of soluble immune complexes: evaluation of mechanisms involved in the selective clearance of complexes from the circulation. *Mol. Immunol.*, **22**, 513–519

Levinsky, R. J., Harvey, H. A. M. and Paleja, S. (1978). A rapid objective method for measuring yeast opsonisation activity in serum. *J. Immunol. Methods*, **24**, 251–256

Loike, J. D. and Silverstein, S. C. (1983). A fluorescent quenching technique using trypan blue to differentiate between attached and ingested glutaraldehyde-fixed red blood cells in phagocytosing murine macrophages. *J. Immunol. Methods*, **57**, 373–379

Markert, M. and Frei, J. (1979). The energy metabolism of the leucocyte. X. Kinetics of oxygen consumption during phagocytosis by polymorphonuclear leucocytes. A photometric method. *Enzyme*, **24**, 327–336

Maródi, L., Leijh, P. C. J. and van Furth, R. (1983). A micromethod for the separate evaluation of phagocytosis and intracellular killing of *Staphylococcus aureus* by human monocytes and granulocytes. *J. Immunol. Methods*, **57**, 353–361

McMillan, R., Longmire, R. L., Tavassoli, M., Armstrong, S. and Yelenosky, R. (1974). In vitro platelet phagocytosis by splenic leukocytes in idiopathic thrombocytopenic purpura. *New Engl. J. Med.*, **290**, 249–251

Michl, J., Pieczonka, M., Unkeless, J. C. and Silverstein, S. C. (1979). Effects of immobilized immune complexes on Fc and complement-receptor function in resident and thioglycollate-elicited mouse peritoneal macrophages. *J. Exp. Med.*, **150**, 607–621

Mills, E. L., Thompson, T., Björkstén, B., Filopovich, D. and Quie, P. G. (1979). The chemiluminescence response and bactericidal activity of polymorphonuclear neutrophils from newborns and their mothers. *Pediatrics*, **63**, 429–434

Mossmann, H., Schmitz, B., Possart, P. and Hammer, D. K. (1981). Antibody-dependent cell-mediated cytotoxicity in cattle: transfer of IgG subclasses in relation to the protection of the newborn calf. *Adv. Exp. Med. Biol.*, **137**, 279–281

Nakagawara, A. and Nathan, C. F. (1983). A simple method for counting adherent cells: application to cultured human monocytes, macrophages and multinucleated giant cells. *J. Immunol. Methods*, **56**, 261–268

Nakamura, M., Nakamura, M. A., Okamura, J. and Kobayashi, J. (1978). A rapid and quantitative assay of phagocytosis-connected oxygen-consumption by leukocytes in whole blood. *J. Lab. Clin. Med.*, **91**, 568–575

Nathan, C. F. (1981). In Adams, D. O., Edelson, P. J. and Koren, H. (eds.), *Methods for Studying Mononuclear Phagocytes*, Academic Press, New York, 499–510

Newman, S. L., Musson, R. A. and Henson, P. M. (1980). Development of functional complement receptors during *in vitro* maturation of human monocytes into macrophages. *J. Immunol.*, **125**, 2236–2244

Osterholz, J., Luckenbach, A., Bross, K. J., Munder, P. G., Löhr, G. W. and Andreesen, R. (1984). A new quantitative assay for the determination of the phagocytic activity of cells from the human monocyte–macrophage lineage. *Blut*, **49**, 226 (abstract)

Pantazis, C. G. and Kniker, W. T. (1979). Assessment of blood leukocyte microbial killing by using a new fluorochrome microassay. *J. Reticuloendothel. Soc.*, **26**, 155–170

Park, B. N., Fikrig, S. M. and Smithwick, E. M. (1968). Infection and nitroblue-tetrazolium reduction by neutrophils. *Lancet*, **II**, 532–534

Peterhans, E., Bertoni, G., Köppel, P., Wyler, R. and Keller, R. (1984). Antibody-free target cells stimulate chemiluminescence in polymorphonuclear leukocytes: an artifact due to mycoplasma contamination. *Eur. J. Immunol.*, **14**, 201–203

Pick, E. and Mizel, D. (1981). Rapid microassay for the measurement of superoxide and hydrogen peroxide production by macrophages in culture using an automatic enzyme immunoassay reader. *J. Immunol. Methods*, **46**, 211–226

Pommier, C. G., Inada, S., Fries, L. F., Takahashi, T., Frank, M. M. and Brown,

E. J. (1983). Plasma fibronectin enhances phagocytosis of opsonized particles by human peripheral blood monocytes. *J. Exp. Med.*, **157**, 1844–1854

Pruzanski, W., Saitos, S. and Nitzan, D. W. (1983). The influence of lysostaphin on phagocytosis, intracellular bactericidal activity and chemotaxis of human polymorphonuclear cells. *J. Lab. Clin. Med.*, **102**, 198–305

Richardson, M. D., Kearns, M. J. and Smith, H. (1982). Differentiation of extracellular from ingested *Candida albicans* blastospores in phagocytosis tests by staining with fluorescein-labelled concanavalin A. *J. Immunol. Methods*, **52**, 241–244

Roberts, P. J. and Ford, J. M. (1982). A new combined assay of phagocytosis and intracellular killing of *Escherichia coli* by polymorphonuclear leukocytes. *J. Immunol. Methods*, **49**, 193–207

Root, R. K., Metcalf, J., Oshino, N. and Chance, B. (1975). H_2O_2 release from human granulocytes during phagocytosis. I. Documentation, quantitation, and some regulating factors. *J. Clin. Invest.*, **55**, 945–955

Rossi, F., Bellavite, B., Dobrina, A., Dri, T. and Zabucchi, G. (1980). In van Furth, R. (ed.), *Mononuclear Phagocytes: Functional Aspects*, Martinus Nijhoff, The Hague, 1187–1213

Rothwell, D. D. and Doumas, B. T. (1975). The effect of heparin and EDTA on the NBT test. *J. Lab. Clin. Med.*, **85**, 950–956

Ruch, W., Cooper, P. H. and Baggiolini, M. (1983). Assay of H_2O_2 production by macrophages and neutrophils with homovanillic acid and horseradish peroxidase. *J. Immunol. Methods*, **63**, 347–357

Rummage, J. A. and Leu, R. W. (1985). Photometric microassay for quantitation of macrophages Fc and C3b receptor function. *J. Immunol. Methods*, **77**, 155–163

Rush, D. N. and Keown, P. A. (1984). Human monocyte chemiluminescence triggered by IgG aggregates. Requirement of phospholipase activation and modulation by Fc receptor ligands. *Cell. Immunol.*, **87**, 252–258

Sahlin, S., Hed, J. and Rundquist, I. (1983). Differentiation between attached and ingested immune complexes by a fluorescence quenching cytofluorometric assay. *J. Immunol. Methods*, **60**, 115–124

Schnyder, J. and Baggiolini, M. (1978). Role of phagocytosis in the activation of macrophages. *J. Exp. Med.*, **148**, 1449–1457

Schopf, R. E., Mattar, J., Meyenburg, W., Scheiner, O., Hammann, K. P. and Lemmel, E.-M. (1984). Measurement of the respiratory burst in human monocytes and polymorphonuclear leukocytes by nitroblue–tetrazolium reduction and chemiluminescence. *J. Immunol. Methods*, **67**, 109–117

Schroeder, F. and Kinden, D. A. (1983). Measurement of phagocytosis using fluorescent latex beads. *J. Biochem. Biophys. Methods*, **8**, 15–27

Scott, W. A., Zrike, J. M., Hamill, A. L., Kempe, J. and Cohn, Z. A. (1980). Regulation of arachidonic acid metabolites in macrophages. *J. Exp. Med.*, **152**, 324–335

Segal, A. W. and Coade, S. B. (1978). Kinetics of oxygen consumption by phagocytosing human neurophils. *Biochem. Biophys. Res. Comm.*, **84**, 611–617

Seim, S. (1983). Role of myeloperoxidase in the luminol-dependent chemiluminescence response of phagocytosing human monocytes. *Acta Path. Microbiol. Immunol. Scand. Sect. C*, **91**, 123–128

Selvaraj, R. J., Sbarra, A. J., Thomas, G. B., Cetrulo, C. L. and Mitchell, G. W., Jr. (1982). A microtechnique for studying chemiluminescence response of phagocytes using whole blood and its application to the evaluation of phagocytes in pregnancy. *J. Reticuloendothel. Soc.*, **31**, 3–16

Shaw, D. R., Maurelli, A. T., Goguen, J. D., Straley, S. C. and Curtis, R., III (1983). Use of UV-inactivated bacteriophage T6 to kill extracellular bacteria in tissue culture infectivity assay. *J. Immunol. Methods*, **56**, 75–83

Smith, D. L. and Rommel, F. (1977). A rapid micro method for the simultaneous determination of phagocytic–microbicidal activity of human peripheral blood leukocytes in vitro. *J. Immunol. Methods*, **17**, 241–247

Soligo, D. and de Harven, E. (1982). Iron carbonyl, a tracer for phagocytosis in scanning electron microscopy. *J. Reticuloendothel. Soc.*, **32**, 201–207

Sorkin, E. and Boyden, S. V. (1959). Studies on the fate of antigens in vitro. I. The effect of specific antibody on the fate of I^{131} trace labeled human serum albumin in vitro in the presence of guinea pig monocytes. *Immunol.*, **82**, 332–339

Steigbigel, R. T., Johnson, P. K. and Remington, J. S. (1974). The nitroblue-tetrazolium reduction test versus conventional hematology in the diagnosis of bacterial infection. *New Engl. J. Med.*, **290**, 235–238

Steinkamp, J. A., Wilson, J. S., Saunders, G. C. and Stewart, C. C. (1982). Phagocytosis: flow cytometric quantitation with fluorescent microspheres. *Science*, **215**, 64–66

Stevens, P., Winston, D. J. and van Dyke, K. (1978). In vitro evaluation of opsonic and cellular granulocyte function by luminol-dependent chemiluminescence: utility in patients with severe neutropenia and cellular deficiency states. *Infect. Immunity*, **22**, 41–51

Stevens, P. and Young, L. S. (1977). Quantitative granulocyte chemiluminescence in the rapid detection of impaired opsonization of *Escherichia coli*. *Infect. Immunity*, **16**, 796–804

Stossel, T. P. (1973). Evaluation of opsonic and leukocyte function with a spectrophotometric test in patients with infection and with phagocytic disorders. *Blood*, **42**, 121–130

Stossel, T. P., Alper, C. A. and Rosen, F. S. (1973). Serum-dependent phagocytosis of paraffin oil emulsified with bacterial lipopolysaccharide. *J. Exp. Med.*, **137**, 690–705

Strauss, R. R., Paul, B. B., Jacobs, A. A. and Sbarra, A. J. (1970). Role of the phagocyte in host-parasite interactions. XXII. H_2O_2-dependent decarboxylation and deamination by myeloperoxidase and its relationship to antimicrobial activity. *J. Reticuloendothel. Soc.*, **7**, 754–761

Tan, J. S., Watanakunakorn, C. and Phair, J. P. (1971). A modified assay of neutrophil function; use of lysostaphin to differentiate defective phagocytosis from impaired intracellular killing. *J. Lab. Clin. Med.*, **78**, 316–322

Tono-Oka, T., Ueno, N., Matsumoto, T., Ohkawa, M. and Matsumoto, S. (1983). Chemiluminescence of whole blood. 1. A simple and rapid method for the estimation of phagocytic function of granulocytes and opsonic activity in whole blood. *Clin. Immunol. Immunopathol.*, **26**, 66–75

Tsuge, I., Kiyotaki, C., Yamamura, Y., Ito, M., Tokuma, Y. and Shimizu, A. (1982). A quantitative assay of phagocytosis using liposomes with trapped spin labels. *J. Reticuloendothel. Soc.*, **31**, 405–413

Uchida, T., Kanno, T. and Hosaka, S. (1985). Direct measurement of phagosomal reactive oxygen by luminol-binding microspheres. *J. Immunol. Methods*, **77**, 55–61

Ueda, M. J., Ito, T., Ohnishi, S. and Okada, T. S. (1981). Phagocytosis by macrophages. I. Kinetics of adhesion between particles and phagocytes. *J. Cell. Sci.*, **51**, 173–188

Van Furth, R. and Diesselhoff-Den Dulk, M. M. C. (1980). Method to prove ingestion of particles by macrophages with light microscopy. *Scand. J.*

Immunol., **12**, 265–269

Vaudaux, P. E., Zulian, G., Huggler, E. and Waldvogel, F. A. (1985). Attachment of *Staphylococcus aureus* to polymethylmethacrylate increases its resistance to phagocytosis in foreign body infection. *Infect. Immunity*, **50**, 472–477

Verhoef, J., Peterson, P. K. and Quie, P. G. (1977). Kinetics of staphylococcal opsonisation, attachment, ingestion and killing by human polymorphonuclear leukocytes: a quantitative assay using [³H] thymidine labeled bacteria. *J. Immunol. Methods*, **14**, 303–311

Vernon, J., Kemp, A. S., van Asperen, P. P., Worsdall, P. and Roy, L. P. (1984). Yeast opsonization and phagocytosis studied by a visual assay and measurement of neutrophil chemiluminescence. *J. Clin. Lab. Immunol.*, **14**, 93–97

Ward, P. A. and Zvaifler, N. J. (1973). Quantitative phagocytosis by neutrophils. I. A new method with immune complexes. *J. Immunol.*, **111**, 1771–1776

Warheit, D. B., Hill, L. H. and Brody, A. R. (1983). Pulmonary macrophage phagocytosis: quantification by secondary and backscattered electron imaging. *Scan. Electron. Microsc.*, **1**, 431–437

Weber, L. and Peterhans, E. (1983). Stimulation of chemiluminescence in bovine polymorphonuclear leucocytes by virus–antibody complexes and by antibody-coated infected cells. *Immunobiol.*, **164**, 333–342

Weissman, G., Zurier, R. and Hoffstein, S. (1972). Leukocytic proteases and the immunologic release of lysosomal enzymes. *Amer. J. Pathol.*, **68**, 539–559

Weston, W. L., Dustin, R. A. and Hecht, S. K. (1975). Quantitative assays of human monocyte-macrophage function. *J. Immunol. Methods*, **8**, 213–222

Williams, A. J. and Cole, P. J. (1981). Human bronchoalveolar lavage cells and luminol-dependent chemiluminescence. *J. Clin. Pathol.*, **34**, 167–171

Wilson, C. B., Tsai, V. and Remington, J. S. (1980). Failure to trigger the oxidative metabolic burst by normal macrophages. Possible mechanism for survival of intracellular pathogens. *J. Exp. Med.*, **151**, 328–346

Wilson, M. E., Trush, M. A., van Dyke, K., Kyle, J. M., Mullett, M. D. and Neal, W. A. (1978). Luminol-dependent chemiluminescence analysis of opsono-phagocytic dysfunctions. *J. Immunol. Methods*, **23**, 315–326

Wright, S. D. and Silverstein, S. C. (1982). Tumor-promoting phorbol esters stimulate C3b and C3b′ receptor-mediated phagocytosis in cultured human monocytes. *J. Exp. Med.*, **156**, 1149–1164

Yamamura, M., Boler, J. and Valdimarsson, H. (1976). A ⁵¹chromium release assay for phagocytic killing of *Candida albicans*. *J. Immunol. Methods*, **13**, 227–233

Yamamura, M., Boler, J. and Valdimarsson, H. (1977). Phagocytosis measured as inhibition of uridine uptake by *Candida albicans*. *J. Immunol. Methods*, **14**, 19–24

Yoo, D., Weems, H. and Lessin, L. S. (1982). Platelet to leukocyte adherence phenomena (platelet satellitism) and phagocytosis by neutrophils associated with in vitro platelet dysfunction. *Acta Haemat.*, **68**, 141–148

ACKNOWLEDGEMENTS

This work was supported by the Central Laboratory, Swiss Red Cross Blood Transfusion Service, Berne, Switzerland, and the Swiss National Science Fund, Grant Number 3.858–85.

3. Monoclonal Antibodies Directed Against Human Immunoglobulins: Preparation and Evaluation Procedures

J. J. HAAIJMAN, J. COOLEN, C. DEEN, C. J .M. KRÖSE,

J. J. ZIJLSTRA AND J. RADL

INTRODUCTION

Monoclonal antibodies (Mabs) are prepared by immunizing an animal (generally a mouse or rat) and fusing the spleen cells, after a given period of time, with a plasmacytoma cell line (Köhler and Milstein, 1975). The fusion mixture is plated out into such numbers of microcultures that the likelihood of obtaining cultures with single fusion events is reasonable (De Blas *et al.*, 1981). Supernatants from individual cultures are tested with a suitable immunoassay for the presence of antibodies with the desired specificity.

Several factors tend to limit efficacy of the Mab technique.

(a) If a native antigen with a number of epitopes is considered, it is accepted that most immunization protocols are likely to change at least some of them. This may be caused by adsorption phenomena, by the addition of non-polar mineral oils or by the presence of other types of adjuvants.

(b) An individual animal will respond only to a selected number of the presented epitopes; the actual selection is based not only on the properties of the antigen molecules, but also the genetic background of the animal, its sex and the age. Which B cell clones are activated during immunization depends not only on the available B cell repertoire, but also on the antigen-presenting cell and T cell compartments.

(c) Any immunoassay sets particular requirements in order for the Mabs to be scored positive. Epitope representation during the test combines with characteristics of individual Mabs.

The three factors mentioned above indicate that, if there is a considerable incongruence between epitope presentation during immunization and during eventual testing, unsatisfactorily low numbers of desired Mabs may be obtained.

The epitope specificity of Mabs can be used to evaluate epitope presentation in different immunoassays. In this approach, Mabs are initially screened, e.g. with ELISA, and subsequently tested in other immunoassays (Haaijman *et al.*, 1984a). It appears that a positive reaction in one immunoassay does not guarantee a positive reaction in another. The conclusion is that all Mabs must be screened for performance in different assays, as was the case for polyclonal reagents (Pabs). One significant difference between Mab and Pab testing is that Pabs are generally screened for the presence of unwanted antibody specificities, whereas the reactivity of Mabs is based on the presence or absence of epitope.

The test for performance inherently requires an 'expected' reactivity pattern (Swaab *et al.*, 1977). The expected pattern can only be communicated if a stringent set of criteria is formulated. In this paper a number of immunoassays are discussed from this point of view.

The examples quoted here are derived from a study of the epitope structure of human immunoglobulins (Igs) with Mabs. The human Ig system consists of five classes: IgM, IgD, IgG, IgA, and IgE. The IgG and IgA classes may be further subdivided into four and two serologically distinct subclasses respectively. Each heavy chain can occur in combination with kappa or lambda light chains. A great variation is encountered in the Ig system with regard to isotypic, allotypic and idiotypic determinants. Moreover, a number of Igs may occur in different forms possessing a greater or lesser degree of polymerization; consequently, on the one hand new epitopes are being introduced, but on the other hand some epitopes that can be recognized in monomeric form may be masked.

The large heterogeneity of the Ig molecules necessitates careful screening of the performance of anti-Ig reagents, especially if these are to be used by more than one investigator and in more than one type of immunoassay.

MATERIALS AND METHODS

Animals

BALB/c mice were bred at the Radiobiological Institute TNO, Rijswijk, The Netherlands. The mice were reared under SPF conditions up to the age of 4 weeks. After that they were housed under normal sanitary conditions. They received food and water *ad libitum*. 8- to 12-week-old animals were used for primary immunizations.

Antigens

Paraproteins were purified from the sera of patients suffering from multiple myelomatosis or Waldenström's disease. Standard gel permeation, ion exchange and affinity chromatography methods were used (Bloemen *et al.*, 1976; Skvaril and Schilt, 1984). The test panel eventually contained representatives of all Ig classes and subclasses. Within each (sub)class, both the lambda and kappa proteins were present. Where appropriate, different molecular forms (e.g. monomers, dimers and polymers) of the Igs were included in the panel. The purified IgG subclass proteins (Skvaril and Schilt, 1984) and the purified J-chain protein (Mestecky *et al.*, 1972) were generously supplied by Dr. F. Skvaril (Bern,

Switzerland) and Dr. J. Mestecky (Birmingham, AL, USA) respectively. Monomer IgM was prepared and purified (Jol-van der Zijde *et al.*, 1983) by Mrs. E. Jol-van der Zijde (Leiden, The Netherlands).

Monoclonal Antibodies

Mice were primed intraperitoneally (i.p.) with two injections of alum-precipitated antigen over the course of 14 days. The first injection contained 100 μg and the second 50 μg of protein. The mice were then rested for at least 30 days and then boosted with 100 μg antigen (alum precipitated) i.p. 3 days before fusion. The SP2/0 cell line (Shulman *et al.*, 1978) served as the fusion partner. Standard methods (Oi and Herzenberg, 1981) were used: the cells were washed once with serum-free MEMS medium (minimal essential medium for spinner cultures. Flow Laboratories, Irvine, Scotland) and cocentrifuged with spleen cells. Polyethylene glycol (PEG, MW 4000, Merck, Darmstadt, FRG; Fazekas de St. Groth and Scheidegger, 1980) was added slowly and incubated with the cells for 1 min. PEG was removed by slow addition of serum-free MEMs medium, centrifuged and taken up in serum-containing selection medium. Finally, the cells were plated at a density of 10^5 nucleated spleen cells/well in 96-well microtitration

Table 1 Monoclonal antibodies discussed in this paper

Clone number	Antigens used for immunization	Mouse Ig isotype	ELISA specificity
89–1.1.11	IgM–K, 19S	G1–K	IgM
152–7.4	IgM–K, 19S	G2a–K	IgM
179–1.1	IgM–L, 7S	G1–K	IgM
158–9R19	IgD–L	G1–K	IgD
116–1.4	IgG4–K	G2b–K	IgG
268–14.1	IgG2–L	G1–K	IgG
268–24.1	IgG2–L	G1–K	IgG
268–27.1	IgG2–L	G1–K	IgG
315–2.2	IgG4–K	G1–K	IgG
86–2.4	IgG3–K	G1–K	IgG3m(U)
69–6.3.2	IgA1–L	G1–K	IgA
69–10.2	IgA1–L	G1–K	IgA
184–6.1	IgA2–L	G1–K	IgA
194–2.1	s–IgA	G1–K	IgA
194–5.1	s–IgA	G1–K	IgA
194–7.1	s–IgA	G1–K	IgA
69–7.1	IgA1–L	G1–K	IgA1
69–11.4	IgA1–L	G1–K	IgA1
16–512–H5	IgA2–L	G1–K	IgA2
194–3.1	s–IgA	G1–K	IgA2m(2)
214–2.1	IgG Fab	G1–K	Kappa
250–9.1	IgE–K	G1–K	Kappa
285–3.1	IgG4–K	G1–K	Kappa
18–412–1.1	IgA2–L	G1–K	Lambda
64–1.4	J-chain	G1–K	J-chain

plates. The selection medium consisted of DMEM (Dulbecco's modification of MEM, Flow) supplemented with 10% foetal calf serum (FCS), 5% horse serum, 1 mM sodium pyruvate, 2 mM sodium glutamate, 1 μg/ml azaserine (Sigma Chemical Co., MO, USA) and 0.1 mM hypoxanthine. Cells were kept at 37°C during the whole hybridization procedure. Proliferation of hybridoma cells was checked by microscopy, and supernatants were tested for antibody activity if the wells were 1/4 to 1/2 confluent. Positive cultures were expanded and submitted to a limiting dilution procedure. For further propagation, clones of undoubted monoclonality were taken. Cells were eventually injected i.p. into BALB/c mice, for the purpose of ascitic fluid production. Table 1 lists the Mabs discussed in this paper, together with their specificities, as revealed by ELISA.

Preparation of Mab Conjugates

The presence of Mab in ascitic fluid was ascertained by agar electrophoresis according to Wieme and immunoelectrophoresis using a panel of polyclonal, monospecific, goat antisera directed against mouse Ig class and subclass determinants (Skvaril and Schilt, 1984). Antibody-rich ascitic fluid samples were pooled, and the Mab was purified by protein-A chromatography according to Ey *et al.* (1978). The purification process was monitored both by immunoelectrophoresis and by the testing of activity (antigen-binding activity) by radioimmunoassay (RIA) or enzyme-linked immunoassay (ELISA). Purified Mabs were conjugated with fluorescein isothiocyanate (FITC), with tetramethyl rhodamine isothiocyanate (TRITC) (FITC and TRITC were obtained from Nordic Immunological Laboratories, Tilburg, The Netherlands) and with biotinyl hydroxysuccinimide (BHS, Sigma). The compounds were dissolved in a small volume of dimethyl sulphoxide (DMSO) (Bergquist and Nilsson, 1974) and added in a ratio of 10 μg hapten/mg protein to a Mab solution of 10 mg/ml (adjusted to pH 9.0 with 1% $NaHCO_3$) (Hijmans *et al.*, 1969). The mixture was stirred for 3 h at room temperature (RT) and overnight at 4°C. Free FITC, TRITC or BHS was removed with a PD-10 column (Pharmacia Fine Chemicals, Uppsala, Sweden).

Anti-mouse Immunoglobulin Reagents and Avidin

Fluorescein- and peroxidase-conjugated goat antiserum directed against mouse Igs was obtained from Nordic Immunological Laboratories; peroxidase-labelled rabbit anti-mouse Ig was from Dakopats, Copenhagen, Denmark. The reagents were performance tested for cross-reactivity with human Igs in ELISA and immunohistology; they were purified over a normal human serum immunoadsorbent when appropriate. The reactivity of the antisera with all mouse Ig (sub)classes was confirmed by ELISA, using an array of purified mouse Ig preparations.

In RIA three antisera were used: a rabbit anti-mouse IgM + IgG, a composite reagent only reactive with the Fc domains of IgM and IgG; monoclonal rat anti-mouse IgG1 (clone 73.E3b); monoclonal rat anti-mouse IgM (clone 151-119.14) (Haaijman, 1982). Peroxidase-conjugated avidin was obtained from Sigma.

Radioimmunoassay

A solid-phase RIA was employed, using established procedures (Tsu and Herzenberg, 1980). Proteins were iodinated (Markwell, 1982) with the help of a solid-phase oxidizer (iodobeads, Pearse Chemical Co., Rockford, IL, USA). Typically, to 20 μg of protein in 100 μl phosphate buffered saline (PBS) was added 0.05 mCi of carrier-free ^{125}I (Amersham, UK) and one iodobead (beads were stored in small aliquots in the dark at 4°C). The mixture was agitated for 10 min at room temperature and free iodine was removed with a PD-10 column.

In the RIA, wells of 96-well flexible polyvinyl plates (Falcon, 3911, Becton Dickinson Labware, CA, USA) were coated with 25 μl of a 100 μg/ml antigen solution for 30 min. Plates were then incubated for 15 min with PBS containing 1% bovine serum albumin (BSA) and 0.02% NaN_3 to block unoccupied adsorption sites. The wells were then washed with PBS and incubated with 20 μl of supernatant or diluted serum–ascites samples. Again, the wells were washed with PBS and the radioactive second step was added (20 x 10^3 counts/min in 20 μl). After 60 min of incubation, the wells were washed and cut loose with a hot wire. The radioactivity bound to the individual wells was quantitated with a gamma counter.

Other incubation schemes than the one described above are referred to in the text.

ELISA

Several protocol designs were employed in ELISA. Details are given in the section entitled 'Results'. Essentially, the following steps were performed.

(1) Individual wells in the flexible polyvinyl 96-well microtitration plates (Falcon, 3911) were coated with 25 μl of suitable antigen solution. Most proteins were coated for 60 min at RT with PBS as diluent. Optimal concentration of the coating antigen solution was checked for in each case: it varied between 2 and 10 μg/ml.

(2) Wash three times with PBS.

(3) Saturation of unoccupied adsorption sites with 1% BSA in PBS for 15 min at RT.

(4) Wash three times with PBS.

(5) Wash once with PBS + 0.2% (w/v) Tween-20.

(6) Incubate for 60 min at RT with 20 μl antibody solution (diluent: PBS + 0.2% (w/v) BSA + 0.2% Tween-20 + 2 μg/ml phenol red).

(7) Wash three times with PBS and once with PBS-Tween.

(8) Incubate for 60 min at RT with 20 μl of optimally diluted peroxidase-labelled rabbit or goat anti-mouse Ig (RAM/PO and GAM/PO from Dakopats and Nordic Immunological Laboratories respectively). The anti-mouse Ig reagents were selected for the absence of cross-reactivity with human Igs. Their reactivity was checked with different purified mouse Ig classes and subclasses. The peroxidase conjugates were diluted in PBS–BSA–Tween–phenol red.

(9) Wash four times with PBS, once with PBS–Tween and once with PBS.

(10) Incubate for 15 min at RT in the dark with 50 μl OPD solution (2 mg/ml orthophenylene diamine-di-hydrochloride, Eastman Kodak Co., NY, USA, in 0.1 M phosphate buffer, pH 6.0, with 50 mM H_2O_2).

(11) Read with Titertek Multiscan MC (Flow Laboratories) at 492 or 450 nm.

Competitition ELISA

Antigen-coated wells were incubated for 45 min with 20 μl samples of diluted ascitic fluid. Subsequently, 20 μl of biotin-labelled Mab was directly added without washing the wells. The optimal dilution of the biotin reagent was established in preliminary experiments. After 45 min, the wells were washed, incubated for 60 min with 20 μl avidin–peroxidase solution (concentration: 2 μg/ml) and developed with OPD.

Cytoplasmic Immunofluorescence Test

The method of Hijmans *et al.* (1969) was used to visualize intracellular Ig in bone marrow plasma cells. In brief, cytocentrifuge slides were prepared from washed bone marrow cells, fixed for 15 min in acid ethanol (95% ethanol, 5% acetic acid) at −20°C and washed three times in PBS at 4°C. The slides were then incubated with appropriately diluted reagents for 30 min in a moist chamber. In the case of the indirect procedure, the sequence of washing and incubation was repeated with an FITC-labelled goat anti-mouse Ig reagent (GAM/Ig/FITC, Nordic Immunological Laboratories). The slides were embedded in buffered glycerol and the coverslips were sealed with paraffin. A Zeiss microscope equipped for selective visualization of fluorescein and rhodamine was used to read the slides. A 40×/1.30 oil immersion objective was combined with 6.3× eyepieces (Haaijman and Slingerland-Teunissen, 1978; Haaijman, 1977).

Membrane Immunofluorescence Assay

Mononuclear cells (MNCs) were collected from normal blood by the Ficoll-Hypaque method (Schuit *et al.*, 1980). The washed cells (10^6 cells in 50 μl) were then incubated with Mab-containing supernatant, diluted ascitic fluid or directly fluoresceinated or rhodaminated Mab. In the case of the indirect technique, the bound Mab was detected by a fluorescein-conjugated goat antiserum against mouse Igs, specifically tailored for this type of application (GAM/mIg/FITC,

Nordic Immunological Laboratories). Cells were eventually washed and viewed with an epi-illumination fluorescence microscope equipped with phase contrast optics. The lymphocytes were located with transmitted light and then screened for positive membrane fluorescence with a 63×/1.30 Ph3 oil immersion objective and 6.3× eyepieces (Schuit *et al.*, 1980).

Cytoplasmic Immunoperoxidase Staining

Small pieces (3 mm × 3 mm × 10 mm) of autopsy and biopsy material were fixed in formalin–acetic acid–mercury chloride (FAM) fixative (Bosman *et al.*, 1977) for 4 h. After a quick rinse in tap water, the blocks were transferred to 70% ethanol. 3 μm thick sections were cut after dehydration and embedding in Paraplast.

Single immunostaining proceeded as follows.

(1) Deparaffination (routine histology).

(2) Blocking of endogenous peroxidase activity by 30 min incubation with methanol-H_2O_2 (9 volumes of methanol + 1 volume of 3% H_2O_2).

(3) 1 min 70% ethanol.

(4) Three 5 min washes in PBS.

(5) Wiping away of excess fluid, and incubation overnight at 4°C in a moist chamber with diluted ascitic fluid containing Mab. About 100 μl of Mab dilution was needed per slide. Mab dilutions were made in PBS with 1% normal rabbit serum.

(6) Three min washes in PBS.

(7) 30 min incubation at room temperature with appropriately diluted peroxidase-conjugated rabbit anti-mouse Ig (Dakopats).

(8) Three 5 min washes in PBS.

(9) 5 min incubation with diaminobenzidine (DAB) (Graham and Karnovsky, 1966) substrate solution: 5 mg DAB in 10 ml TRIS buffer, pH 7.8, with 5 μl 3% H_2O_2. The substrate solution was prepared just prior to use.

(10) Three 2 min washes in PBS.

(11) Counterstaining with haematoxylin for 15 s.

(12) 5 min rinse in tap water.

(13) Dehydration.

(14) Clearing in xylene and mounting in Malinol.

The differences in the double-staining procedure were as follows (steps (1)–(8) as for single staining).

(9) Substrate solution: 5 mg DAB in 10 ml TRIS + 50 μl 3% H_2O_2 + 2 mg $CoCl_2$ (Hsu and Soban, 1982). Incubation for 5 min at RT.

(10) Three 5 min washes in PBS.

(11) Repeat steps (5)–(8) with second Mab containing ascitic fluid.

(12) Incubation with aminoethyl carbazole (AEC) (Graham *et al.*, 1965) substrate solution: 10 mg 3-amino-9-ethyl carbazole in 2.5 ml DMSO; make up with 0.1 M acetate buffer, pH 5.0, to 50 ml (can be stored at 4°C, filter before use).

(13) Three 5 min washes in aqua dest.
(14) Mounting in Aquamount.

Notes on Technique

(A) The AEC reaction product is soluble in polar embedding media.
(B) The brownish-black precipitate from the DAB–CoCl$_2$ reaction is temperature sensitive. Slides were kept at 4°C until they were scored.

Haemagglutination Assays

Passive haemagglutination and haemagglutination inhibition were performed in collaboration with Dr. G. de Lange. Details of the method have been described previously (Giessen *et al.*, 1974). In brief, erythrocytes were sensitized with CrCl$_3$ and coupled with highly purified Ig preparations. The coated erythrocytes were reacted with serially diluted Mab ascitic fluids in the absence (passive haemagglutination) or presence (inhibition) of competing proteins.

Precipitation Assay

Double radial immunodiffusion was performed according to Ouchterlony. Precipitation was enhanced by polyethylene glycol (PEG, MW 6000, final concentration 3%, w/v). The diffusion plates were photographed, washed, dried and stained with amido black (Skvaril and Schilt, 1984). The antigen test panel contained several representatives of the various Ig classes and subclasses. Where appropriate, different molecular forms of Igs were used: monomeric, dimeric and secretory forms of IgA1 and IgA2; monomeric and pentameric forms of IgM.

RESULTS

The Preparation of Mabs Against Human Immunoglobulins

Some notes will be given here on the preparation of the present set of Mabs. A survey of all possible alternatives will not be attempted.

Immunization of a spleen cell donor only serves to push into cycle as many antigen-specific B cells as possible. Normally, two priming injections (two weeks apart) and one booster injection were sufficient to obtain antigen-reactive hybridomas. All injections were given i.p. and the antigens were precipitated on alum. No consistent differences were observed with experiments in which a booster dose of native antigen was given intravenously. The period between priming and boosting appeared to be important; best results were obtained if the mice were rested for more than four weeks.

The fusion between the spleen cells of an immunized donor and the Sp2/0 plasmacytoma line was carried out according to established procedures. The fusion mixture was then plated out into 96-well flat-bottom plates. The seeding density was quite critical: 10^5 nucleated spleen cells/well. Both higher and lower seeding densities gave a lower frequency of growing hybrid cells. For the selection medium azaserine was used rather than aminopterin. Azaserine selectively blocks the guanidine pathway, whereas aminopterin interferes with both guanidine and thymidine biosynthesis. Azaserine dissolves more easily than aminopterin. Moreover, the hybrid cells from Sp2/0 appear to suffer less from azaserine than from aminopterin, although the differences were small. A possible drawback of the use of azaserine is that infection with mycoplasma goes undetected. One of the most sensitive signs of such an infection is the toxicity of the HAT medium (hypoxanthine–aminopterin–thymidine) to hybrid cells, which results from thymidine consumption by the mycoplasma. The plasmacytoma fusion line and established hybridoma lines should therefore be checked regularly for the presence of mycoplasma if azaserine is used routinely (for method see Sinigaglia *et al.*, 1985).

As well as azaserine and hypoxanthine, the selection medium contained 10% selected FCS and 5% horse serum. Different FCS batches were tesed for their ability to sustain hybridoma cell growth under limiting dilution conditions. In our hands, addition of the horse serum increased the yield of hybrid cells significantly. Feeder cells such as peritoneal macrophages (Fazekas de St. Groth and Scheidegger, 1980), thymocytes or unfused spleen cells were not added because in our experience either they did not increase the hybridoma frequency or they even had a negative effect.

RIA and ELISA Techniques

Solid-phase adsorbed antigens were used in RIA and ELISA techniques. Polyvinyl proved superior to polystyrene in binding a range of human Igs. Notably, Igs bound less to polystyrene, although the effect was significant only for a number of individual IgG preparations. Optimal antigen concentrations for the coating of the plates were in the order of 100 μg/ml in RIA and 2–5 μg/ml for ELISA. The antigen requirements, the inherent hazards of working with ^{125}I and the relatively short shelf-life of the radioactively labelled reagents were the three arguments leading us to favour ELISA techniques in most of our experiments.

The choice of antigens in the screening of supernatants depends, of course, on the desired antibody specificity. The primary aim of the first tests is to reduce the number of cultures that have to be carried. If antibodies directed against isotypic determinants of a given Ig heavy chain are desired, the screen should discriminate between this specificity and, for example, anti-light chain, anti-idiotypic, anti-allotypic and anti-subgroup antibodies. Of course, the reactivity should also be excluded with other isotypes than the desired one. Using one purified paraprotein as the antigen, it was found practical to screen the primary tissue culture supernatants first on a heterogeneous Ig preparation. For instance, if a particular IgA1 paraprotein was chosen for immunization, the first screen consisted of purified heterogeneous IgA from colostrum. Anti-idiotypic antibodies remain undetected in this way, providing generally a sufficient reduction in the number of positive supernatants. More discriminatory tests were then performed on supernatants from expanded clones. Final proof of Mab specificity in ELISA, however, can only be ascertained if a sufficient range of antibody concentrations is tested on an elaborate panel of purified paraproteins. The panel should include specimens of each isotype. The isotypes should be represented by at least one kappa and one lambda protein. Proteins of different allotypes are necessary in order to exclude anti-allotypic reactions. It proved impossible, however, to obtain proteins of all known allotypes. Some of our Mabs which reacted anti-isotypically in our test panel turned out to be anti-allotypic in other tests (haemagglutination inhibition).

This was notably so for the 194–3.1 (a-A2m) antibody. This antibody was obtained after immunization with purified heterogeneous secretory IgA. It reacted only with one IgA2 protein from our test panel which belonged to the IgA2m(2) allotype (van Loghem and Biewenga, 1983). More IgA2m(2) proteins were needed to prove the allotypic specificity of 194–3.1 (a-A2m). Because the gene frequency of IgA2m(2) is so low in Caucasians (in contrast to the African and Japanese populations), this was possible only in collaboration with other laboratories. Another example is 86–2.4 (a-G3m), originally believed to be specific for IgG3. Later it was shown that the antibody does not react with the 'St' allotype of IgG3. The 'St' marker is antithetical with the 'U' marker. The 86–2.4 (a-G3m) antibody has to be designated as anti-IgG3m(U). The 'U' marker is highly prevalent in the Caucasian population which explains why all of our IgG3 proteins were of the 'U' allotype.

The specificity of a Mab in an immunological assay such as ELISA depends strongly on the concentration of the antibody. Titration of the antibody was shown to be indispensable in order to obtain a good impression of the antibody specificity (Swaab *et al.*, 1977; Haaijman, 1977). Some antibodies showed strong non-specific binding to irrelevant proteins, whereas others were devoid of such reaction. A typical titration curve of a monoclonal antibody is shown in figure 1. The titration was carried out with three kinds of target antigens. The example concerns Mab 69–7.1 (a-A1) directed against IgA1. IgG3 served as the 'irrelevant' protein to determine the non-specific binding characteristics of 69–7.1 (a-A1). The steepness of the titration curve in the antibody-dependent range appeared generally to be related to the affinity of the Mab.

It should always be kept in mind that adsorption of a protein to a solid surface may cause the appearance or disappearance of certain epitopes. It is not unusual for a Mab to react specifically only with, for example, plastic-adsorbed antigens. Independent tests of antibody specificity are, therefore, obligatory.

Mab 214–2.1 (a-K) was obtained after immunization with Fab fragments of heterogeneous IgG. It reacted strongly with a number of kappa-bearing proteins (figure 2) but also very strongly with a particular IgG1 lambda protein. The correct typing of this latter protein was proven with several anti-lambda Mabs. Mab 214–2.1 (a-K) was purified from ascitic fluid, bound to an ELISA plate and reacted with biotin-labelled Bence-Jones kappa chains in the presence of different IgG paraproteins. Binding of the biotinylated kappa probe was determined with peroxidase-labelled avidin. All kappa-bearing proteins gave competition in this design, whereas none of the lambda proteins did. Also, the IgG1 lambda protein which was positive in the direct binding test was negative in the competition assay. Two-colour immunofluorescence studies on human bone marrow cells confirmed that Mab 214–2.1 (a-K) reacts only with kappa chains. It was tentatively concluded that binding of the IgG1 lambda protein to plastic induces an epitope which mimmics the kappa epitope recognized by the 214–2.1 (a-K).

To circumvent the adsorption-induced epitopes, a 'catching antibody' is sometimes used (Moudallal *et al.*, 1984; Schönherr and Roelofs, 1982). Binding the target antigen(s) via a catching antibody necessarily shields epitopes to be reached by Mabs. It is not clear at this stage what the overall performance

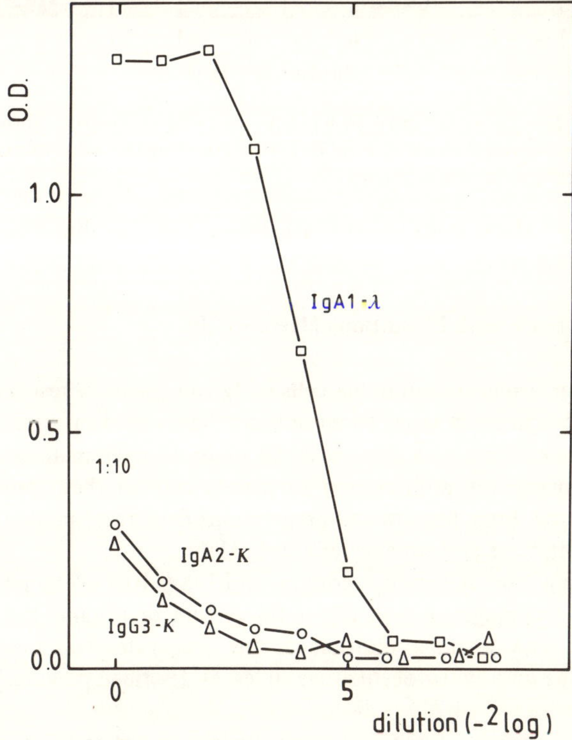

Figure 1 Mab evaluation with ELISA. Purified human immunoglobulins (IgA1-L, IgA2-K and IgG3-K) were coated onto ELISA plates and reacted with different dilutions of Mab 69-7.1 ascitic fluid. Bound antibodies were detected with peroxidase-labelled rabbit anti-mouse Ig.

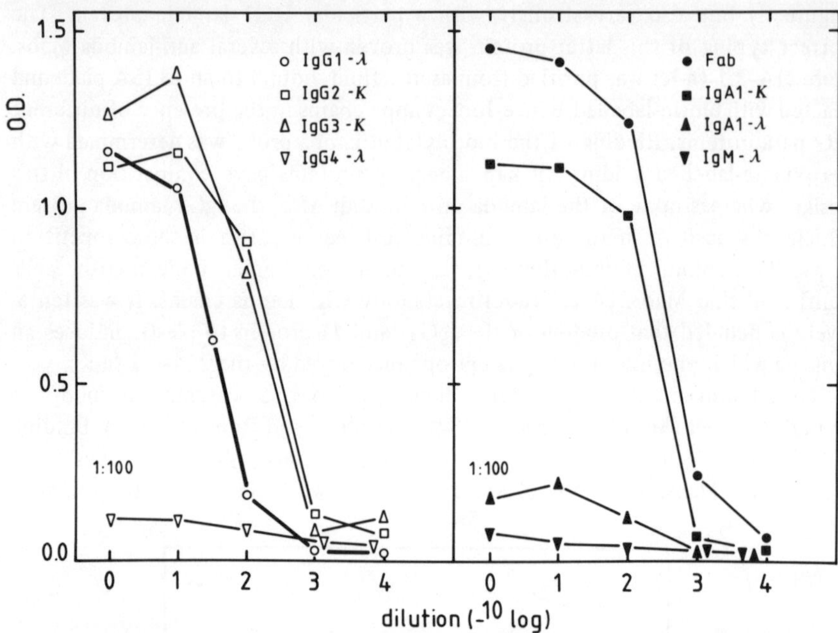

Figure 2   Mab 214-2.1 specificity in ELISA: a strong reaction is observed with a number of kappa proteins and one IgG1-L protein. For the sake of clarity only a selection of titration curves is shown.

characteristics of Mabs, positive with a catching antibody but negative in the direct binding test, are.

Immunofluorescence with Fixed Bone Marrow Cells

In general, cytoplasmic Ig-containing cells (C-Ig cells) show a restriction to one isotype and one light chain type. These cells are then a good substrate for further evaluating the specificity of a given Mab. In multiple myelomatosis and Morbus Waldenström, malignant proliferation of plasma cells or their immediate precursors is observed. Bone marrow cell preparations from these patients were used additionally to test the performance of anti-Ig Mabs.

Mabs meeting our specificity criteria in ELISA–RIA were purified from ascitic fluid and conjugated with either fluorescein or tetramethyl rhodamine isothiocyanate. The working dilution of the conjugates was determined by titration on bone marrow cytocentrifuge slides, as described previously (Hijmans *et al.*, 1971).

Attention was given to the following aspects of the staining pattern: (1) brightness of the positive cells; (2) variation in staining intensity among the positive cells; (3) number of positive cells; (4) distribution of fluorescence over the cell body; (5) non-specific staining, including (a) other plasma cells as revealed by double staining, (b) cells from the myeloid series and (c) small (lymphoid) cells.

The vast majority of Mabs, strongly positive in ELISA, proved to be positive in the cytoplasmic immunofluorescence test (c-IF). Evidently, the acid–ethanol fixative used in c-IF preserves the epitopes on Igs quite well. The concentration or number of these epitopes may, however, vary considerably among cells. This became evident in the large variation in staining intensity using some Mabs of positive cells within one slide. In figure 3 two Mabs directed against IgA are shown, one of which produced little cell to cell variation in staining intensity (Mab 69–6.3.2, a-A) and the other much more (Mab 285–3.1, a-K).

Uneven distribution of the fluorescence was observed in two forms: staining of only the outer rim of the cytoplasm of plasma cells and staining of the total cytoplasm, with the exception of a small perinuclear area. These phenomena are not restricted to Mabs and were originally noted with polyclonal reagents (Schuit, personal communication). The first non-homogeneity appears to be related to conjugate concentration: the phenomenon disappeared on reduction of the working dilution. The second non-homogeneity is probably caused by the Golgi apparatus. Some Mabs stain Igs within the Golgi apparatus brightly whereas others do not. It is worth mentioning here that in some cells that

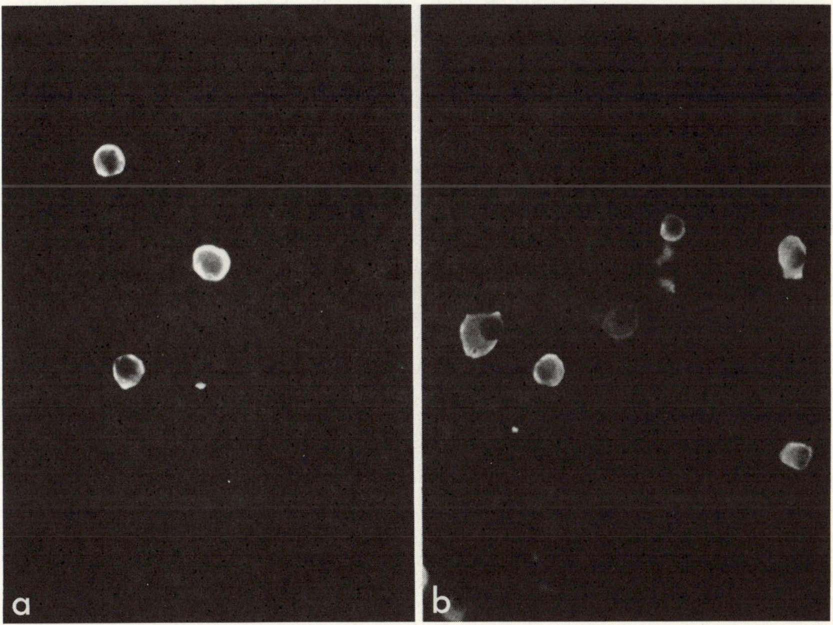

Figure 3   Immunofluorescence micrographs of human bone marrow cells (cyto-centrifuge preparations) treated with Mab 69-6.3.2–FITC (a) and Mab 285-3.1–FITC (b). Note the difference in cell-to-cell variation in the staining.

produce Ig at a high rate (e.g. hybridoma cells) the Golgi apparatus was the only part of the cytoplasm in which Ig could be detected.

Significant differences were observed between the non-specific staining qualities of various Mabs. Staining of plasma cells other than those containing the 'specific' antigen was encountered only occasionally. In those cases, the non-specific reaction was a magnitude less in intensity than the specific reaction. The view that a given reaction was non-specific was only held after excluding a (non-desired) specific reaction by several tests.

The granules of specially eosinophilic granulocytes appear to have a high affinity for a variety of compounds, including at least some conjugated Mabs. The granular staining could normally be distinguished clearly from the evenly distributed fluorescence of plasma cells. The phase contrast image of the cells provides additional information. The phenomenon clearly varies from Mab to Mab. Figure 4 provides examples of the staining of two slides of the same bone marrow with two Mabs: Mab 18–412-1.1 (a-L) directed against lambda light chains in C-IgM and C-IgG cells stains the eosinophilic granules extremely brightly, whereas Mab 69–6.3.2 (a-A) is much less active in this respect.

Distinct ring-like staining of small (lymphoid) cells was observed with some Mabs. It is likely that this is caused by binding of the Mabs to Fc receptors. The staining normally disappeared with dilution of the conjugates to the extent that the specific staining was not affected. Evidently, the non-specific interaction was of low avidity. The common immunochemical denominator was not further investigated for the Mabs producing this phenomenon. In some cases the ring-like staining was of considerable intensity and could not be diminished selectively by dilution (as compared with clear cytoplasmic staining). Membrane-bound Ig was probably the source of this staining (Schuit *et al.*, 1984).

General non-specific staining or stickiness of a conjugate was evident when all nucleated cells were fluorescent. Some of the stickiness may be caused by over-conjugated molecules, and the non-specific staining would disappear on dilution of the conjugate. A new conjugate was prepared if the specific staining was found not to be strong enough after dilution.

The results obtained with the c-IF technique did not always match those obtained in the first ELISA screening. Two examples will be used to illustrate this point. Mab 184–6.1 (a-A) directed against IgA gave brilliant c-IF staining when used in an indirect design with fluorescent goat antiserum to mouse Igs (GAM/Ig/FITC). Directly conjugated, however, the performance of Mab 184–6.1 (a-A) on bone marrow cells was mediocre. As the isothiocyanate group of the fluorochromes reacts almost exclusively with the ϵ aminogroup of lysine, the phenomenon is likely to be caused by the presence of a lysine residue in the antigen binding site of the antibody. Alternatively, the result can be explained by insufficient avidity of 184–6.1 (a-A) and stabilization (cross-linking) by the anti-mouse Ig antibodies. Control experiments with ELISA, however, made this explanation very unlikely. Mab 184–6.1 (a-A) functions very well as a catching antibody for IgA, which is then detected with a non-competing anti-IgA. This

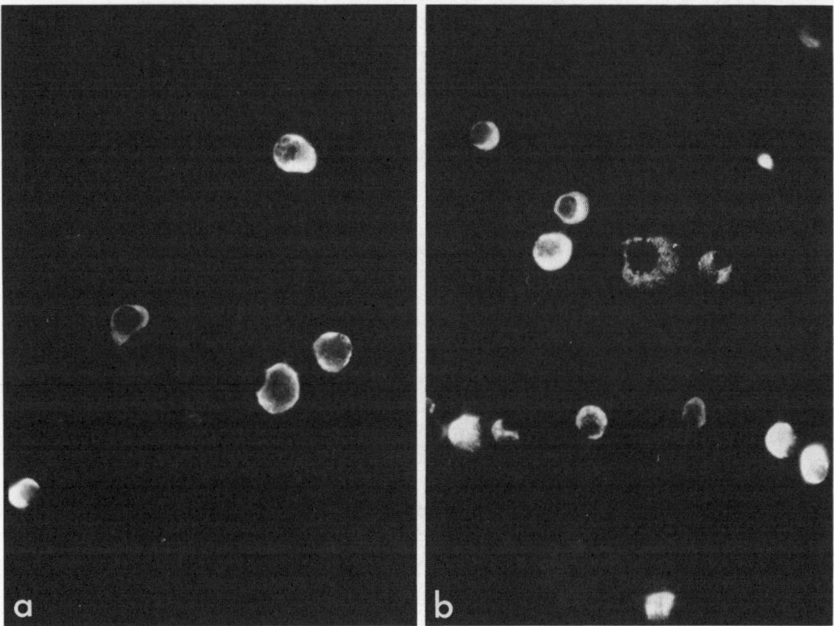

Figure 4   Immunofluorescence micrographs of human bone marrow cells treated with Mab 69-6.3.2–FITC (a) and Mab 18-412-1.1–FITC (b). The 18-412-1.1 conjugate is much more strongly taken up by eosinophilic granulocytes than the 69-6.3.2 conjugate.

assay requires good avidity of the catching antibody. Formal avidity measurements were not performed.

The second example concerns Mab 64–1.4 (a-J) made against purified J-chain. J-chain is a relatively small polypeptide (MW 16 000) present in dimeric IgA and pentameric IgM (Halpern and Koshland, 1970; Mestecky *et al.*, 1971). Free J-chain is also present in immature C-IgG cells and most IgG myeloma cells. Mab 64–1.4 (a-J) was strongly reactive in RIA with the J-chain preparation used for immunization.

Fifteen multiple myelomatosis bone marrow specimens, previously found positive with polyclonal anti-j-chain (Nordic Immunological Laboratories), were tested with Mab 64–1.4 (a-J). Only 2 out of the 15 bone marrows gave a brightly positive staining. The Mab 64–1.4 (a-J) probably recognizes a special form of J-chain or, perhaps, a determinant on the partially degraded J-chain, which might be expressed only in a special form of tumour cells (Haaijman *et al.*, 1984b). The Mab 64–1.4 (a-J) was consequently not accepted as a general purpose reagent.

Immunoperoxidase Staining of FAM-fixed Tissue

An important application of anti-Ig isotype Mabs is the staining of plasma cells *in situ*, i.e. in a histological slide. The topographic localization of positive cells not only gives information to the immunologist, but also is indispensable for the immunopathologist. In the c-IF technique described above, topographical information was lost because cell suspensions were used to prepare cytocentrifuge slides.

Even the rapid and relatively mild fixation with FAM could not prevent the loss of quite a large number of isotypic determinants on Igs. Figure 5 shows the ELISA results of four Mabs directed against IgA, together with the staining pattern for the human duodenum of three of the four Mabs. Many positive plasma cells were revealed by Mab 184-6.1 (a-A) and Mab 194-2.1 (a-A), whereas only few plasma cells were seen with Mab 194-7.1 (a-A).

Two questions should be answered in evaluating the specificity of Mabs in the c-PO technique: (1) does the Mab stain more than the appropriate number of cells containing a given isotype? and (2) does the Mab stain all the cells of a given isotype? Both questions can only be answered conclusively if a reference antiserum is available. For many isotypic determinants on Ig subclasses such reference reagents do not exist. In that case, judicious choice of the target tissues may help to arrive at a preliminary conclusion on specificity. Polyclonal reference antisera were used to establish that Mab 184-6.1 (a-A) and 194-2.1

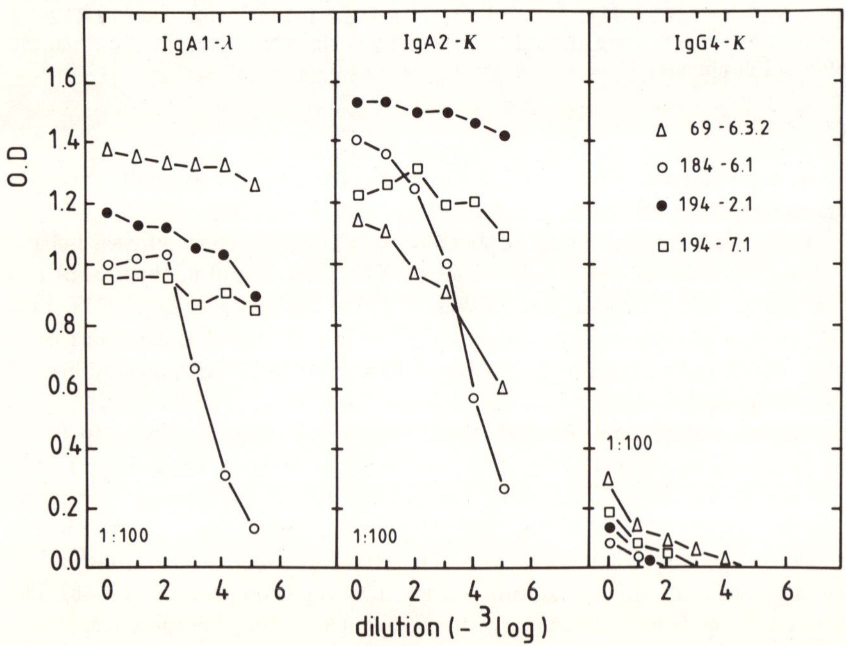

Figure 5 (Part 1)

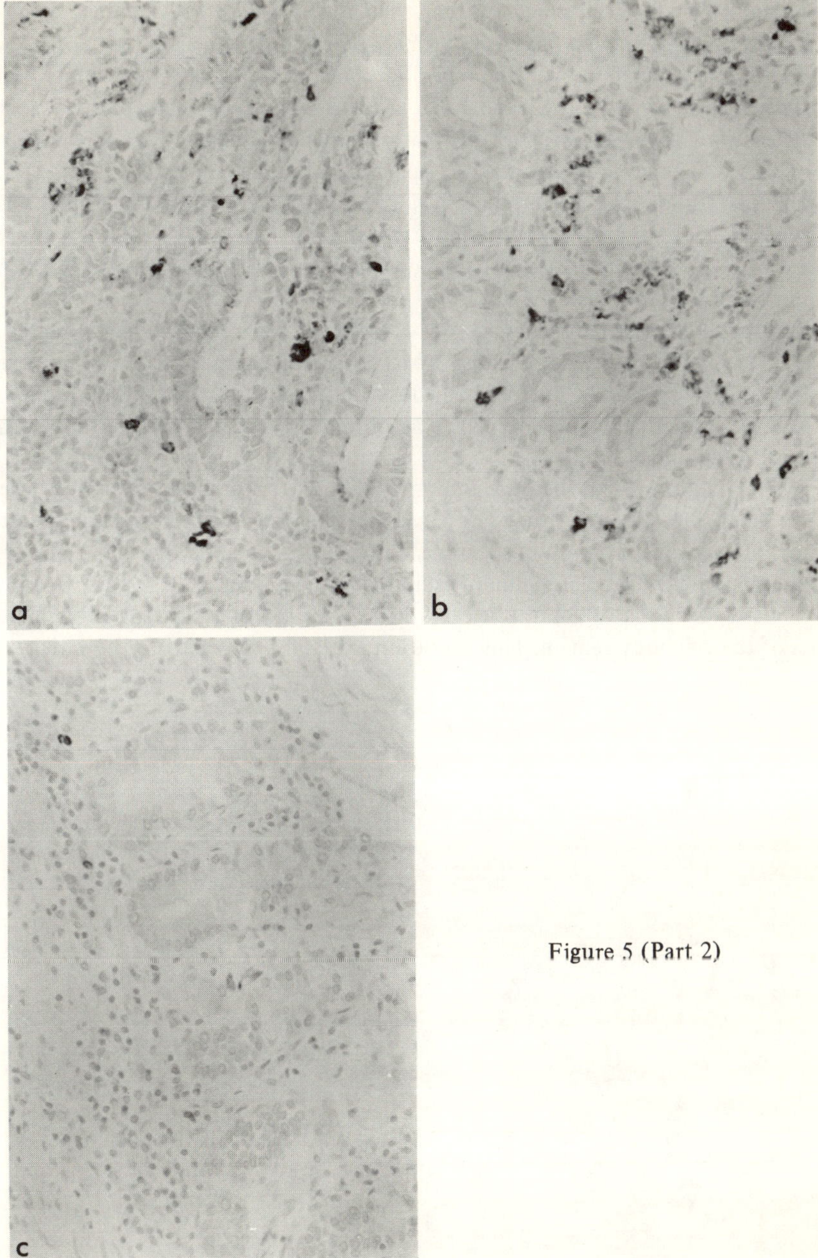

Figure 5 (Part 2)

Figure 5   The performance of Mabs directed against IgA in ELISA and immuno-histology. In the first part of the figure, four anti-IgAs were tested for binding in ELISA to IgA1-L, IgA2-K and IgG4-K. All four Mabs recognize a common IgA epitope. In the second part, three of the four anti-IgAs were tested on FAM-fixed human duodenum. Mabs 184-6.1 (a) and 194-2.1 (b) show many positive C-IgA cells whereas Mab 194-7.1 (c) stains only a small subpopulation of C-Iga cells.

(a-A) stain all c-IgA cells and no other cells. Mab 194–7.1 (a-A) stained a subpopulation of c-IgA cells which were primarily large plasma cells.

Fixation artifacts can be very specific: Mab 69–6.3.2 (a-A) recognizes an epitope present on both IgA1 and IgA2 in ELISA and c-IF. The epitope is lost or at least not accessible after FAM fixation in C-IgA2 cells only, and the Mab 69–6.3.2 (a-A) behaved as an anti-IgA1 specific Mab under those conditions.

The loss of epitopes after the FAM fixation used in these experiments is evident for all isotypes of Ig but most prominently for C-IgG cells: not more than 5–10% of all Mabs ($N = 300$) generated against serum IgGs gave positive immunostaining on slides.

Epitopes preferentially present on FAM-fixed Ig were also encountered. Mab 152–7.4 (a-M) directed against IgM forms an example. It gave mediocre ELISA and c-IF readings but performed extremely well in the c-PO technique. Very strong staining of plasma cells was obtained with Mab concentrations as low as 100 ng/ml.

Several factors other than the intensity of the desired specific staining have to be taken into account for a proper judgement of c-PO performance. These factors include: (a) variation in specific staining, (b) general background staining, (c) staining of extracellular Ig and (d) staining of macrophages.

In tissue sections of 3 μm thickness, plasma cells will be sliced and variable parts of the cell body remain. This condition explained only part of the variation

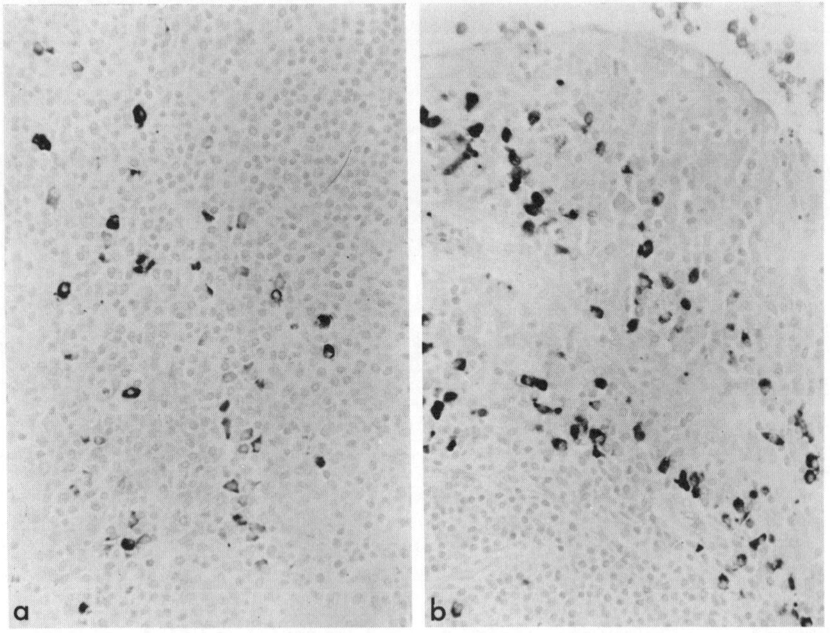

Figure 6   Immunostaining of FAM-fixed human tonsil with Mab 16-512-H5 (a) and Mab 250-9.1 (b). Note the difference in cell-to-cell variation of the staining.

in staining intensity observed with some Mabs. Figure 6 contrasts the staining pattern of Mab 16–512–H5 (a-A2) with that of 250–9.1 (a-K) on human tonsil: the C-K cells all had more or less the same staining intensity, whereas the staining of the C-IgA2 cells varied considerably. To what extent variations in staining intensity were caused by variations in antigen density or by fixation artifacts remained unexplored.

General background staining is a property inherent to a given Mab. Some Mabs do not show any background staining even if they are applied in concentrations of 10 times their working dilution. An example of such an antibody is Mab 158–9R19 (a-D) directed to IgD (figure 7a). The working dilution of this Mab is 2 μg/ml. No significant change in the staining was observed with Mab concentration as high as 200 μg/ml. Other antibodies at such high concentrations interacted vividly with connective tissue and/or with cellular debris (figure 7b). This property became more evident when autopsy material was examined that had been collected more than a few hours post mortem. Appropriate dilution of the ascitic fluid generally reduced the background staining to acceptable levels. With some of our Mabs, however, the specific staining titrated in parallel with the non-specific staining. Such antibodies were classified as unacceptable. Non-specific background staining should not be confused with the signal arriving from extracellular Ig. Extracellular staining was most noted for IgM in the

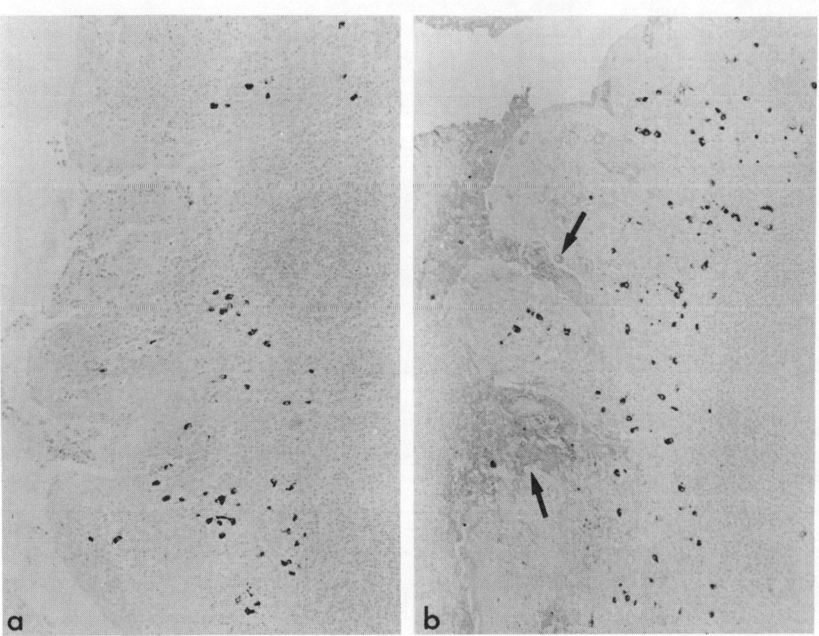

Figure 7 Immunostaining of FAM-fixed human tonsil with Mab 158-9R19 (a) and Mab 69-11.4 (b). Note the difference in non-specific staining (arrows). Both of the Mabs were titrated to give the maximum image contrast.

follicular areas of lymph nodes and tonsils, for IgG in the sub-epithelial area of the tonsil, and for IgA in fresh biopsy material of the colon.

Follicular macrophages are stained by some anti-IgG Mabs. Figure 8 compares two Mabs (268-27.1 (a-G), and 268-14.1 (a-G)) both directed against IgG, one of which gave positive staining with macrophages and the other of which did not. Ingestion of IgG by macrophages is a normal phenomenon and we consider the staining to represent true IgG.

Double enzymatic staining experiments were used to further evaluate a selected number of Mabs. The broad absorption spectra of the commonly employed reaction products in peroxidase cytochemistry do not allow unambiguous distinction of the singly and doubly stained cells. Double staining was, therefore, indicated only if a proof had to be obtained that some Mabs did not react with the same cells.

The Staining of Membrane-bound Ig with Mabs

The membrane form of Igs (m-Igs) differs from the cytoplasmic form in molecular weights (McCune *et al.*, 1980; Singer and Williamson, 1980) and by the addition of a hydrophobic peptide (Oi *et al.*, 1980; Vassalli *et al.*, 1979). Moreover, the Igs anchored in the membrane of the B cell are of monomeric nature;

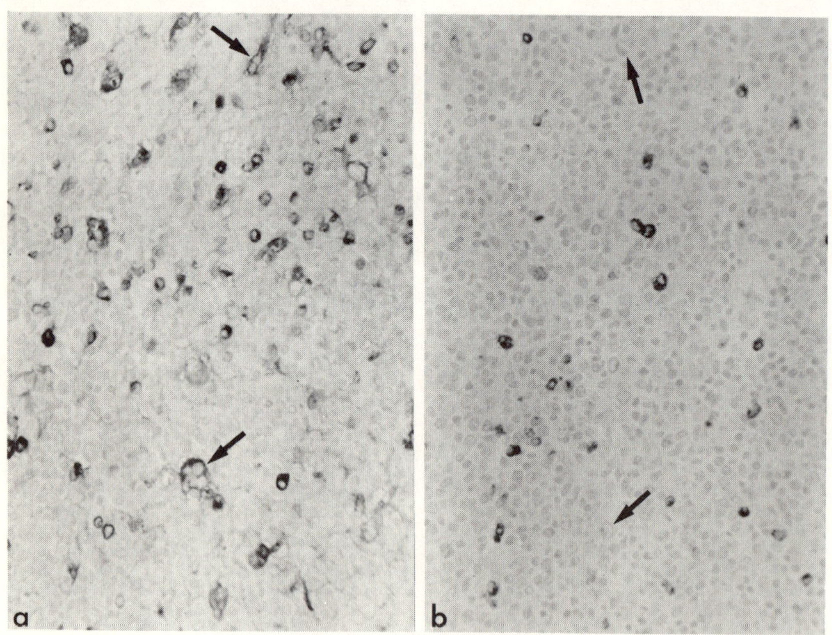

Figure 8   Immunostaining of FAM-fixed human tonsil with Mab 268-27.1 (a) and Mab 268-24.1 (b). Note the difference in 'background' staining of the follicular macrophages (or dendritic cells, arrows).

this is in contrast to the pentameric form of serum IgM and the (predominantly) dimeric form of IgA in secretions. One might theoretically assume that the aligning of m-Ig molecules with their carboxy terminal end fixed in the membrane and the charged groups pointing outwards would lead to reduced accessibility of epitopes near to the CH3 or CH4 domains.

This prediction was not borne out by our series of Mabs, as illustrated by the following two examples.

(1) The m-IgM staining was compared with two Mabs, 89–1.1.11 (a-M) and 179–1.1 (a-M). The former reacted with only a few m-IgM bearing cells, whereas the latter stained the same number of peripheral blood lymphocytes as did a polyclonal reference conjugate (Nordic Immunological Laboratories). A haemagglutination inhibition assay was performed with highly purified fragments of IgM (Bruin *et al.*, 1983). The epitope recognized by Mab 89–1.1.11 (a-M) could be assigned to CH2 and that of Mab 179–1.1 (a-M) to CH3 or CH4 (only a fragment comprising both the third and the fourth domains was available for testing).

(2) Mab 69–11.4 (a-A1) is specific for IgA1 and Mabs 69–6.3.2 (a-A) and 184–6.1 (a-A) for a common IgA epitope. The epitopes recognized by the three Mabs were shown to be highly spatially related in that the epitopes are not independently accessible by Mabs in a competition design (see ahead). Mabs 69–6.3.2 (a-A) and 184–6.1 (a-A) stained m-IgA brightly, whereas Mab 69–11.4 (a-A1) was completely negative.

We concluded that m-Ig reactivity of a Mab is not to be predicted from the position of the epitope it recognizes. All Mabs prepared against secreted forms of Ig (serum or external secretions) should, therefore, be tested for performance in the m-Ig assay (Partridge *et al.*, 1982). For this assay the membrane immunofluorescence test according to Schuit *et al.* (1980) was chosen. This assay involves very mild fixation of peripheral blood lymphocytes with highly diluted formaldehyde. This reduces the unwanted interactions with Fc receptors and appears not to influence the structure of the m-Ig determinants.

The Behaviour of Mabs in Precipitation Assays

Mabs were routinely tested in double radial immunodiffusion (Ouchterlony assays) and immunoelectrophoresis.

The lattice formation necessary to obtain a visible precipitation with Mabs requires the presence of at least two identical epitopes per antigen molecule. This is a necessary, but not sufficient, condition as the following examples show.

(1) Mabs 69–11.4 (a-A1) and 16–512–H5 (a-A2) both precipitate only dimeric and secretory forms of IgA1 and IgA2, respectively. The Mabs were purified from ascitic fluid and applied in a radioimmunoassay in which the purified Mabs were adsorbed to the plate, reacted with monomeric and dimeric IgA preparations, and then followed by addition of radioactive Mab. In the case of Mab 69–11.4 (a-A1), radioactivity was only found if the dimeric form of IgA1 was used in between. Evidently, a single 69–11.4 (a-A1) epitope is present on IgA1

monomer or, alternatively, two epitopes are present but are not accessible for two Mab molecules at the same time. The 16–512–H5 (a-A2) epitope, in contrast, occurs at least twice on IgA2 molecules: both monomer IgA2 and dimer IgA2 produced a good signal in the two-sided assay. Precipitation in agar with the two Mabs was, nevertheless, only observed with dimer and not with monomer IgA1 and IgA2 respectively.

(2) Mab 152–7.4 (a-M) recognizes a determinant present on monomer (7S) IgM, as tested in ELISA. No precipitation was observed, however, with pentameric IgM.

(3) From the spatial structure of Igs, one would assume that epitopes on the constant part of light chains would be spaced sufficiently far apart to allow interaction with two separate Mab molecules. However, in a limited series of

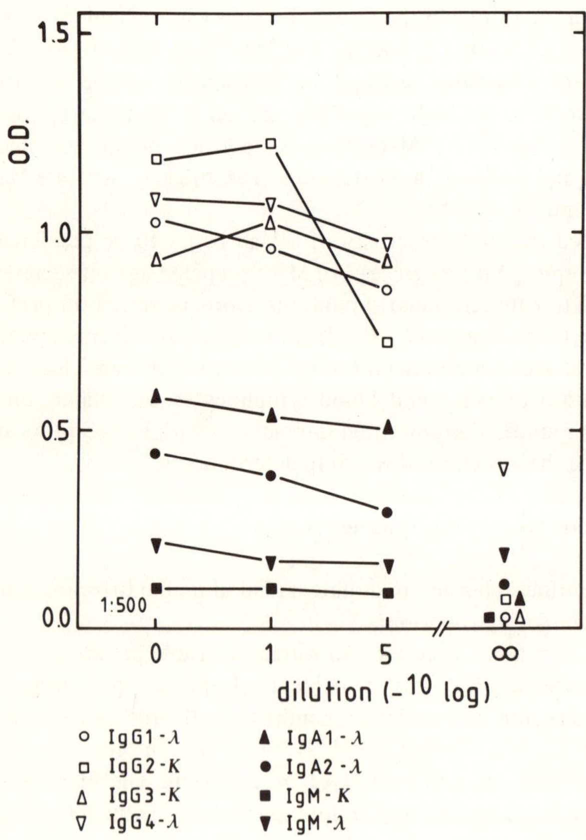

Figure 9   Specificity profile of Mab 268-24.1 in ELISA. A slight but significant binding of Mab 268-24.1 to IgA1-L and IgA2-L is observed.

six anti-light chain antibodies (data not shown), four gave clear precipitation lines in agar. The precipitates dissolved after washing the plates in PBS.

Another example, in which the behaviour in precipitation did not match that in a regular binding assay, was presented by Mab 268–24.1 (a-G). This Mab was raised against IgG1 and recognizes an epitope shared between IgG and IgA. In ELISA (figure 9), binding of Mab 268–24.1 (a-G) to IgG and IgA was observed and the reactions were confirmed by immunostaining on slides containing sections of tonsil and duodenum. Mab 268–24.1 (a-G) reacted only with IgG, however, in precipitation.

Those Mabs that gave a positive precipitation reaction with human Igs were additionally tested for reaction with a selected panel of non-primate mammalian sera. Some Mabs show unexpected cross-reactivity with sera, notably from Artiodactyla and/or Perissodactyla. For example, Mab 116–1.4 (a-G) precipitated not only human IgG but also horse, cow, sheep and goat IgG; Mab 315–2.2 (a-G) precipitates goat IgG; Mab 179–1.1 (a-M) precipitates horse and donkey IgG. Information on this kind of Mab peculiarity (Jefferis *et al.*, 1982) is important if the Mabs are to be used in indirect techniques.

The Recognition of Different Epitopes on One Antigen

As was shown in the preceding sections, Mabs may perform differently in different assay systems. The use of mixtures of two or more Mabs may, therefore, be considered in order to obtain general-purpose reagents. Increased sensitivity due to additive and sometimes superadditive (Ehrlich and Moyle, 1983) signals from the constituent antibodies could be another advantage. This will only be true if the binding of the antibodies to the antigen are independent of each other; in other words, whether the epitopes on the antigen can be reached by two (or more) antibody molecules at the same time.

The accessibility of epitopes was studied in ELISA using purified, biotin-labelled antibodies as probes. The binding of the probe and its possible interference by unlabelled antibodies was quantitated with avidin–peroxidase. The number of probes that have to be made depends on the complexity of the epitope structure. For example, the binding pattern of anti-IgAs (ours and those generously supplied by Dr. R. Jefferis and Dr. D. Delacroix) could be adequately explained by three epitope clusters: Mabs belonging to one cluster inhibit the binding of other cluster members but do not inhibit the binding of Mabs in one of the other clusters (table 2).

Competition depends on antibody avidity and on antibody concentration. In theory, one should choose the Mabs with lowest avidity as labelled probes in order to obtain the most discriminating assay. In many cases, however, data on avidity were not available at the moment of testing. Low-avidity Mabs may give false-negative results if a probe of too high avidity is used and if the concentration of the unlabelled antibody cannot be sufficiently increased. Unequivocal

Table 2   Three independent epitope clusters on human IgA1

194-2.1[a]	184-6.1[a] ———————————— 69-6.3.2[a]		69-10.2[a]
194-2.1	71/2D1 7[b]		69-10.2
194-5.1	N1 F2 J[b]		194-7.1
194-6		69-7.1	B3501 A7[c]
	184-6.1		
	69-6.3.2		
	69-11.4		
	M4 D8 J[b]		
	B3506 B7[c]		

In the competition ELISA, purified IgA1 was adsorbed to the ELISA plate and reacted with different concentrations of the indicated Mabs in the presence of a fixed, limiting, concentration of biotin-labelled Mabs 194-2.1, 69-10.2, 184-6.1 and 69-6.3.2. Binding of the biotin-labelled probe was quantified with peroxidase-labelled avidin. Mabs 184-6.1 and 69-6.3.2 compete with each other, but they recognize spatially distinct epitopes, as some other Mabs do compete with one of the two, but not with the other (e.g. 69-7.1 competes with 69-6.3.2 but not with 184-6.1). The 184-6.1–69-6.3.2 complex is therefore drawn out to accommodate Mabs at the borders and at the centre of the complex.
[a] Labelled antibody probes.
[b] Mabs generously supplied by Dr. R. Jefferis, Medical School, University of Birmingham, UK.
[c] Mabs generously supplied by Dr. D. Delacroix, Université Catholique de Louvain, Brussels, Belgium.

results in our hands were only to be obtained with Mabs in the form of ascitic fluids which were applied in different dilutions.

The design used here provides information on the accessibility of epitopes and on the relative avidity of different antibodies. It is not possible to distinguish between the reaction with a single epitope or the reaction with spatially closely related epitopes.

DISCUSSION

The results presented here show clearly that the observed specificity of a Mab depends both on the characteristics of its antigen-binding site and on the expression of the relevant epitope on the antigen(s) used for testing. Although this conclusion appears obvious, the phenomena leading to the conclusion could only be evaluated in somewhat more detail when a series of Mabs directed to a well-defined antigen cluster (such as the human Igs) was studied. Seemingly trivial changes in assay conditions may lead to highly selective changes at the epitope level; epitopes may appear or disappear without logical physico-chemical explanation.

Epitopes may be divided broadly into two groups: on the one hand, continuous epitopes that are formed by a linear array of adjacent amino acids (protein antigens) from one polypeptide chain and, on the other hand, discontinuous or topographical epitopes which are formed by residues from different chains (or non-adjacent residues from one chain) brought together by the quaternary structure of the total protein molecule. The quaternary structure of (large) proteins can easily be disturbed. It depends largely on interaction between the molecule and its solute, on physical adsorption forces and on conditions in general that interfere with the normal (free in solution) intra-molecular equilibrium. Changes in quaternary structure result in changes in epitopes. The 'assay specificity' of a number of our Mabs may be explained by the presence or absence of a particular epitope under different assay conditions. It appears likely that immunization with complete antigen molecules will prefer-entially lead to antibodies directed against discontinuous epitopes, since these will be located mostly on the surface of the molecule. Several points, however, should be made in this respect.

(a) The distinction between continuous and discontinuous epitopes is arti-ficial; also, continuous epitopes are recognized by their space-filling form and charge distribution. The dimensions of continuous epitopes may also change under different conditions.

(b) There is no satisfactory explanation as to why discontinuous epitopes at the surface of a molecule should be more immunogenic than continuous epitopes similarly exposed.

(c) Before an effective immune response can take place, the antigen should be processed by antigen-presenting cells. One would expect that preservation of discontinuous epitopes after antigen processing would be the exception rather than the rule.

The fraction of antibodies that react with discontinuous epitopes after immunization with complete antigen molecules varies considerably (Arnon, 1973). Atassi (1975) studied myoglobin and found that 65% of antibody activity in a conventional antiserum could be removed by five cyanogenbromide frag-ments. These antibodies were shown to react with five epitopes consisting of linear sequences of amino acids. The remaining 35% of the anti-myoglobin anti-serum reacted only with complete molecules. Atassi attributed the antigenicity of the linear epitopes to their chemical nature *per se*. Lerner and co-workers (Lerner, 1982; Lerner, 1984) took a different approach. They studied a large series of Mabs against complete influenza virus haemagglutinin and found that the Mabs could be grouped into a small number of clusters corresponding to antigenic sites. However, when they prepared synthetic peptides corresponding in amino acid sequence with 'non-immunogenic' parts of the haemagglutinin molecule, these peptides yielded antisera that reacted with the complete antigen molecule.

From the Atassi and Lerner studies one might conclude that the composition of an antiserum in terms of antibodies directed against continuous or discon-tinuous epitopes depends on the antigen itself, the mode of its presentation, and the animal used for immunization. The composition cannot easily be predicted for a new antigen.

Determination of the nature of an epitope recognized by a given Mab is only possible in exceptional cases. If the amino acid sequence of an antigen is known, it is possible to synthesize a large number of small peptides with overlapping sequences and to test a given antibody to the antigen for reactivity. With this technique, Geysen *et al.* (1985) were able to localize two antigenic epitopes on VP1, a capsid glycoprotein of foot and mouth disease virus. It is questionable whether this method is also applicable to larger proteins.

The specificity of Mabs for their corresponding epitopes can be extreme. One of the best examples are Mabs against idiotypic determinants of Igs. These reagents combine only efficiently with, for example, one molecular species within an excess of 10^7 similar molecules. The molecular difference between the Igs can be only a few amino acid substitutions.

On the other side of the spectrum are Mabs which will combine with antigens possessing seemingly very distinct structures. The avidity of the reactions can be considerable. The admissible variations in epitope structure allowing a Mab to bind depend on the individual characteristics of the antigen-binding site. In addition, secondary factors such as hydrophobic regions bordering the epitope that will expel Mab molecules via structures outside the variable region and steric influences which can limit the access of Mab to the epitope also play a role.

Assay specificity is a phenomenon that arises if there is incongruency between epitope presentation during antiserum preparation and epitope presentation in the test situation (Milstein *et al.*, 1983). Too little is known about the general principles that determine exactly what antibodies are made by a given individual under a variety of conditions. It appears, therefore, not very rewarding to attempt to mimic antigens, as presented in the assay, during the immunization procedure. Rather, one selects those Mabs from a fusion experiment that perform in the eventual test to be used. If Mabs are intended for use in immunochemistry for example, it may be necessary to screen all primary supernatants of histological specimens and to select those that give an expected staining pattern (Naiem *et al.*, 1982).

Although this approach is theoretically correct, many problems may arise in practice. The most notable is the fact that, for many antigens, there will not yet be 'an expected staining pattern'. If nothing had been known about the distribution of C-IgA cells in the duodenum, it would have been impossible to decide which of the two staining patterns illustrated in figure 5 was the correct one. Is Mab 194–7.1 (a-A) deficient or is Mab 184–6.1 (a-A) non-specific? In the case of IgA, use could be made of polyclonal antisera which served as references. It should be appreciated that the reasoning is inherently circular.

If the conclusion is reached that Mab quality is intimately related to epitope presentation in a particular assay (Kammer, 1983), the quality can only be evaluated in that assay by performance testing.

Performance testing in ELISA does not present too many problems if the following considerations are taken into account.

(a) Conclusions with regard to the specificity of a Mab are clearly limited by the selection of antigens used. See, for example, the result with our anti-IgG3 which proved to be anti-IgG3m(U).

(b) Antigen–antibody interactions are strongly concentration dependent. If the concentration of an antibody is increased sufficiently, it will bind to any antigen with electrostatic forces. It is, therefore, obligatory to do a complete titration of a given Mab with all available relevant antigens.

(c) Some epitopes may disappear on adsorption of an antigen to a plastic surface, and new epitopes may appear (Friguet *et al.*, 1984; Mierendorf and Dimond, 1983). An ELISA with plate-bound antigens should be complemented, preferably with a competition design in which the Mab under test is coated on to the plate and reacted with labelled antigen in the presence of various concentrations of unlabelled antigens. An example of a very special case of an adsorption-induced epitope is the specific binding of Mab 214-2.1 (a-K) to one lambda-IgG1. The possible induction of neo-epitopes may cause serious disappointment if the ELISA is used as the primary screen for detecting positive supernatants in a fusion experiment. If the right checks are not made at an early stage of the clone selection process, much effort may be wasted.

(d) The concentration and spatial arrangement of antigen molecules adsorbed to a plastic plate, together with the epitope density per antigen molecule (Lew, 1984; Nimmo *et al.*, 1984; Steward and Lew, 1985; Koertge and Butler, 1985), determine whether antibody molecules are able to bind with only one binding site or with both binding sites. The kinetics of a dual-binding system suggest a much higher avidity than a single-bond system. The titration curves are steeper, and the same amount of antibody complex is formed at a lower concentration of antibody. It should be established that all target antigens are coated to the same actual density for proper evaluation of antisera in ELISA.

Performance testing of anti-Ig reagents using cytoplasmic immunofluorescence and human bone marrow cells has been described in detail for polyclonal antisera (Hijams *et al.*, 1971). Recently, this technique was extended to pokeweed mitogen stimulated peripheral blood cells (Lobo, 1983).

The greatest advantage of the c-IF technique is most probably the relative ease with which double staining can be performed (Hijmans *et al.*, 1971; Hijmans *et al.*, 1981). The binding of fluorescein and rhodamine conjugates can be visualized within the same cell by sequential illumination. The amount of intracytoplasmic Ig is sufficiently large to accommodate two or more antibodies, even if they are directed against the same epitope; it is very difficult to show competition between Mabs with bone marrow cells as the substrate. Double staining offers a unique possibility of comparing and contrasting the reactivities of various Mabs. A drawback is the near necessity of purifying and labelling each Mab separately. Indirect techniques with two different anti-mouse Ig reagents are applicable in exceptional cases; however, adequate attention should be given to unexpected cross-reactivity patterns.

Acid–ethanol preserves the epitopic structure of Igs quite well. Very few discrepancies have been found between the specificity spectrum in c-IF as compared with ELISA. Those that were found could probably be attributed to the presence of an unusual epitope on the antigen used for immunization and to damage of Mab caused by fluorochrome labelling. The epitope preservation with acid–ethanol was confirmed in ELISA studies (unpublished results). Antigens were coated on to plastic plates and fixed for 15 min at $-20°$ with acid–ethanol: no decrease in Mab binding was observed.

The formalin in the FAM fixative is a cross-linking agent. This may explain the deleterious effect of formalin fixation on a number of epitopes. Tainer *et al.* (1984) and Westhof *et al.* (1984) showed, almost simultaneously, that a certain degree of intramolecular flexibility is needed for optimal antigen–antibody interaction. It is not unlikely that cross-linking disturbs the normal flexibility.

The most significant finding, however, is the specificity of the fixation artifacts: epitopes which are spatially very closely linked may be affected very differently. This is true not only for Igs but also for cell surface (glyco) proteins (Ewijk *et al.*, 1980; Walker *et al.*, 1984).

Histomorphological information is retained in the c-PO technique. This constitutes an important asset over, for example, the c-IF technique with cytocentrifuge slides. Mabs make it possible to determine the localization of cells containing various Ig classes and subclasses within different lymphoid tissues. Little is known about the differences in biological function of Ig subclasses. The immunobiology of the C-Ig cells may give clues in this respect.

An indirect technique with unlabelled Mab and a peroxidase-labelled polyclonal anti-mouse Ig reagent was favoured for routine purposes. Although direct enzyme labelling of Mabs is quite possible (Boorsma, 1984), we ourselves consistently lose a large proportion of antibody activity.

More elaborate indirect techniques such as staining with PAP complexes or the use of ABC (avidin–biotin complexes) (Hsu *et al.*, 1981; Wilchek and Bayer, 1984) do not appear to have significant advantages in our experience over the anti-Ig method in studying C-Ig cells (Haaijman and Slingerland-Teunissen, 1978). The amount of intracellular Ig is large enough to compensate for a possible difference in sensitivity by increasing the antibody concentration.

Double staining experiments are less easily performed in the c-PO than in the c-IF technique. The admixture of a small amount of one colour to an excess of the other colour is difficult to detect with absorption colours. The double direct method in which two Mabs are conjugated with, for example, peroxidase and alkaline phosphatase is the most straightforward technique (Boorsma, 1984). The loss of antibody activity after conjugation, however, makes this method less suitable in routine experimentation. An alternative is the double anti-Ig technique of Hsu and Soban (1982), in which a first cycle of Mab and anti-Ig/PO is developed with DAB in the presence of cobalt chloride. This results in a black precipitate. The next cycle, with a second Mab and anti-Ig/PO, is then developed with AEC, which gives a red precipitate. The technique performs quite well with selected pairs of Mabs but is not generally applicable. Cells which stain double with the two Mabs cannot be evaluated. A third alternative provides the hapten sandwich systems first described by Wofsy *et al.* (1974). By judicious choice of haptens and anti-hapten antibodies, it appears possible to devise a generally applicable double staining system with peroxidase and alkaline phosphatase (unpublished results). Cells containing both epitopes recognized by either Mab can be distinguished within certain limits (e.g. heavy and light chain determinants).

All immunological assays pose different requirements to Mab characteristics. This is true not only for the assays described above in detail but also for membrane immunofluorescence, haemagglutination (inhibition), precipitation and other methods. As was shown above, the characteristics cannot easily be described with a single parameter such as avidity. To set general guidelines for required avidities in different assays (Péterfy *et al.*, 1983), therefore, appears impossible.

Because there are no general guidelines for predicting epitope preservation, Mabs should be tested separately for performance in each assay (Reimer *et al.*, 1984; Jefferis *et al.*, 1985). On the one hand, the assay specificity of Mabs appears as a disadvantage compared with polyclonal antibodies (Pabs); on the other hand, it is possible with the Mab technique to select reagents with optimal qualities for a given assay. The future for more general-purpose monospecific reagents, we believe, lies with standardized mixtures of Mabs with desired assay characteristics (Jefferis *et al.*, 1985; Ehrlich *et al.*, 1982), thus combining in these oligoclonal reagents (Oabs) constant quality with broad applicability. This is not meant to indicate that Pabs will become outdated. Especially for broadly specific antisera, it is hard to conceive that Mabs will ever replace Pabs.

In any case, manufacturers of Mabs, Oabs and Pabs will be increasingly required to specify, in great detail, the reactivity patterns of their reagents. Also, the many diverse efforts to arrive at central data bases for a more rapid exchange of information and materials should take the assay characteristics more into account. To know that a Mab exists is a step forward; to know for what purposes it can be used is two steps forward.

SUMMARY

Mabs were prepared against human Igs, light chains and the J-chain. They were applied in a variety of immunoassays: ELISA, c-IF of bone marrow cells, immunoperoxidase staining of histological specimens of lymphoid tissue, m-IF, haemagglutination, and precipitation. Each assay appears to pose different requirements of the Mabs for optimal performance, and very few Mabs perform equally well in the various assay systems. This form of assay specificity is explained by assuming, on the one hand, changes in epitope expression under various assay conditions and, on the other hand, variations in the properties of the constant domains of individual antibodies.

The criteria for performance are discussed for each immunoassay, together with the pitfalls which may be encountered specifically with Mabs.

It is concluded that general purpose reagents for the detection of human immunoglobulins can only be constructed by mixing two or more well-defined Mabs. These oligoclonal mixtures (Oabs) should be rigorously tested for performance and, if marketed commercially, should be accompanied by a detailed description of the assay in which they can be applied successfully and in what assay they are inactive or suboptimal.

ACKNOWLEDGEMENTS

We sincerely thank Dr. W. Hijmans and Mrs. H. R. E. Schuit for their discussions and critical reading of the manuscript, Dr. F. Skvaril for donating the purified IgG subclass preparations, Dr. J. Mestecky for supplying the J-chain protein, Mrs. E. Jol-van der Zijde for the monomer (7S) IgM and Dr. G. de Lange for evaluating a number of our Mabs in the haemagglutination assay.

Part of this study was made possible by a grant from Nordic Immunological Laboratories, Tilburg, The Netherlands.

REFERENCES

Arnon, R. (1973). Immunochemistry of enzymes. In Sela, M. (ed.), *The antigens*, Academic Press, New York, 87–159

Atassi, M. Z. (1975). Antigenic structure of myoglobin. The complete immuno-chemical anatomy of a protein and conclusions relating to antigenic structures of proteins. *Immunochemistry*, **12**, 423–438

Bergquist, N. R. and Nilsson, P. (1974). The conjugation of immunoglobulins with tetramethyl rhodamine isothiocyanate by utilisation of dimethylsulphoxide (DMSO) as a solvent. *J. Immunol. Methods*, **5**, 189–198

Bloemmen, F. J., Radl, J., Haaijman, J. J., Berg, P. van der, Schuit, H. R. E. and Hijmans, W. (1976). Microfluorometric evaluation of the specificity of fluorescent antisera against mouse immunoglobulins with the defined antigen substrate spheres (DASS) system. *J. Immunol. Methods*, **10**, 337–355

Boorsma, D. M. (1984). Direct immunoenzyme double staining applicable for monoclonal antibodies. *Histochemistry*, **80**, 103–106

Bosman, F. T.; Lindeman, J., Kuiper, G., Wal, A. van der and Kreunig, J. (1977). The influence of fixation on immunoperoxidase staining of plasma cells in paraffin sections of intestinal biopsy specimens. *Histochemistry*, **53**, 57–62

Bruin, G., Musters, W. and Biewenga, J. (1983). Production and characterization of antibodies specific for domains of human IgM. *J. Immunol. Methods*, **60**, 319–328

De Blas, A. L., Ratnaparkhi, M. V. and Mosimann, J. E. (1981). Estimation of the number of monoclonal hybridomas in a cell fusion experiment. Effect of post-fusion cell dilution on hybridoma survival. *J. Immunol. Methods*, **45**, 109–115

Ehrlich, P. H., Moyle, W. R., Moustafa, Z. A. and Canfield, R. E. (1982). Mixing two monoclonal antibodies yields enhanced affinity for antigen. *J. Immunol.*, **128**, 2709–2713

Ehrlich, P. H. and Moyle, W. R. (1983). Cooperative immunoassays: ultrasensitive assays with mixed monoclonal antibodies. *Science*, **221**, 279–281

Ewijk, W. van, Coffman, R. C. and Weissman, I. L. (1980). Immunoelectron microscopy of cell surface antigens: a quantitative analysis of antibody binding after different fixation protocols. *Histochemical J.*, **12**, 349–361

Ey, P. L., Prowse, S. J. and Jenkin, C. R. (1978). Isolation of pure IgG1, IgG2a and IgG2b immunoglobulins from mouse serum using protein-A Sepharose. *Immunochemistry*, **15**, 429–436

Fazekas de St. Groth, S. and Scheidegger, D. (1980). Production of monoclonal antibodies: strategy and tactics. *J. Immunol. Methods*, **35**, 1–21

Friguet, B., Djavadi-Ohaniance, L. and Goldberg, M. E. (1984). Some monoclonal antibodies raised with a native protein bind preferentially to the denatured antigen. *Molecular Immunol.*, **21**, 673–677

Geysen, H. M., Barteling, S. J. and Meloen, R. H. (1985). Small peptides induce antibodies with sequence and structural requirement for binding antigen comparable to antibodies raised against the native protein. *Proc. Natl. Acad. Sci. USA*, **82**, 178–182

Giessen, M. van der, Lange, B. de and Lee, B. van der (1974). The production of precipitating antiglobulin reagents specific for the subclasses of human IgG. *Immunology*, **27**, 655–663

Graham, R. C. and Karnovsky, N. J. (1966). The early stages of absorption of injected horseradish peroxidase in the proximal tubules of mouse kidney: ultrastructural cytochemistry by a new technique. *J. Histochem. Cytochem.*, **14**, 291–302

Graham, R. C., Lundholm, U. and Karnovsky, N. J. (1965). Cytochemical demonstration of peroxidase activity with 3-amino-9-ethylcarbazole. *J. Histochem. Cytochem.*, **13**, 150–155

Haaijman, J. J. (1977). Quantitative immunofluorescence microscopy; methods and applications. *Thesis*, Leiden, The Netherlands

Haaijman, J. J. (1982). Production of monoclonal antibodies for the analysis of the ontogeny of the murine lymphoid system by flow cytometry. In Wick, G., Traill, K. N. and Schauenstein, K. (eds.), *Immunofluorescence technology*, Elsevier Biomedical Press, Amsterdam, 129–151

Haaijman, J. J. and Slingerland-Teunissen, J. (1978). Equipment and preparative procedures in immunofluorescence microscopy; quantitative studies. In Knapp, W., Holubar, K. and Wick, G. (eds.), *Immunofluorescence and related staining techniques*, Elsevier Biomedical Press, Amsterdam, 11–29

Haaijman, J. J., Deen, C., Kröse, C. J. M., Zijlstra, J. J., Coolen, J. and Radl, J. (1984a). Monoclonal antibodies in immunocytology; a jungle full of pitfalls. *Immunology Today*, **5**, 56–58

Haaijman, J. J., Bast, E. J. E. G. and Radl, J. (1984b). The evaluation of monoclonal antibodies for application in immunohistology. In De Weck, A. L. (ed.), *Lymphoid cell functions in aging*, Eurage Vol. III, 89–94

Halpern, M. S. and Koshland, M. E. (1970). Novel subunit in secretory IgA. *Nature*, **228**, 1276–1278

Hijmans, W., Haaijman, J. J. and Schuit, H. R. E. (1981). Immunofluorescence. In Adler, W. H. and Nordin, A. A. (eds.), *Immunological techniques applied to aging research*, CRC Press, Boca Raton, Fla, 141–163

Hijmans, W., Schuit, H. R. E. and Hulsing-Hesselink, E. (1971). An immunofluorescence study on intracellular immunoglobulins in human bone marrow cells. *Ann. NY Acad. Sci.*, **177**, 290–305

Hijmans, W., Schuit, H. R. E. and Klein, F. (1969). An immunofluorescence procedure for the detection of intracellular immunoglobulins. *Clin. Exp. Immunol.*, **4**, 457–472

Hsu, S. M., Raine, L. and Fanger, H. (1981). Use of avidin–biotin–peroxidase complex (ABC) in immunoperoxidase techniques. A comparison between ABC and unlabelled anitbody (PAP) procedures. *J. Histochem. Cytochem.*, **29**, 577–580

Hsu, S. M. and Soban, E. (1982). Colour modification of diaminobenzidine (DAB) precipitation by metallic ions and its application for double immuno-histochemistry. *J. Histochem. Cytochem.*, **30**, 1079–1082

Jefferis, R., Lowe, J., Ling, N. R., Porter, P. and Senior, S. (1982). Immunogenic and antigenic epitopes of immunoglobulins. I. Crossreactivity of murine monoclonal antibodies to human IgG with the immunoglobulins of certain animal species. *Immunology*, **45**, 71–77

Jefferis, R., Reimer, C. B., Skvaril, F., *et al.* (1985). Evaluation of monoclonal antibodies having specificity for human IgG subclasses: results of an IUIS/WHO collaborative study. *Immunol. Letters*, **10**, 223–252

Jol-van der Zijde, C. M., Vossen, J. M., Weijden-Ragas, R. van der and Radl, J. (1983). Low molecular weight IgM in sera of children following bone marrow transplantation for severe aplastic anaemia and acute leukaemia. *Clin. Exp. Immunol.*, **53**, 151–158

Kammer, K. (1983). Monoclonal antibodies to influenza A virus FM1 (H1N1) proteins require individual conditions for optimal reactivity in binding assays. *Immunology*, **48**, 799–808

Koertge, T. E. and Butler, J. E. (1985). The relationship between the binding of primary antibody to solid-phase antigen in microtitration plates and its detection by ELISA. *J. Immunol. Methods*, **83**, 283–299

Köhler, G. and Milstein, C. (1975). Continuous cultures of fused cells secreting antibody of predefined specificity. *Nature*, **256**, 495–497

Lerner, R. A. (1982). Tapping the immunological repertoire to produce antibodies of predetermined specificity. *Nature*, **299**, 592–596

Lerner, R. A. (1984). Antibodies of predetermined specificity in biology and medicine. *Adv. Immunol.*, **36**, 1–44

Lew, A. M. (1984). The effect of epitope density and antibody affinity on the ELISA as analysed by monoclonal antibodies. *J. Immunol. Methods*, **72**, 171–176

Lobo, P. I. (1983). Double immunofluorescence staining of pokeweed mitogen differentiated plasma cells – a sensitive assay to ascertain purity of anti-human Ig reagents as each cell produces only one isotype. *J. Immunol. Methods*, **65**, 383–387

Loghem, E. van and Biewenga, J. (1983). Allotypic and isotypic aspects of human immunoglobulin A. *Molecular Immunol.*, **20**, 1001–1007

Markwell, M. A. K. (1982). A new solid-state reagent to iodinate proteins. *Anal. Biochem.*, **125**, 427–432

McCune, J. M., Lingappa, V. R., Fu, S. M., Blobel, G. and Kunkel, H. G. (1980). Biogenesis of membrane-bound and secreted immunoglobulins. I. Two distinct translation products of human u-chain with identical N-termini and different C-termini. *J. Exp. Med.*, **152**, 463–468

Mestecky, J., Zikan, J. and Butler, W. J. (1971). Immunoglobulin M and secretory immunoglobulin A: presence of a common polypeptide different from light chains. *Science*, **171**, 1163–1165

Mestecky, J., Zikan, J., Butler, W. T. and Kulhavy, R. (1972). Studies on human secretory immunoglobulin A. III. J chain. *Immunochemistry*, **9**, 883–900

Mierendorf, R. C. and Dimond, R. L. (1983). Functional heterogeneity of monoclonal antibodies obtained using different screening assays. *Anal. Biochem.*, **135**, 221–229

Milstein, C., Wright, B. and Cuello, A. C. (1983). The discrepancy between the cross-reactivity of a monoclonal antibody to serotonin and its immunohisto-chemical specificity. *Molecular Immunol.*, **20**, 113–123

Moudallal, Z. A., Atlschuh, D., Briand, J. P. and Regenmortel, M. H. V. van (1984). Comparative sensitivity of different ELISA procedures for detecting monoclonal antibodies. *J. Immunol. Methods*, **68**, 35–43

Naiem, M., Gerdes, J., Abdulaziz, Z., Sunderland, C. A., Allington, M. J., Stein, H. and Mason, D. Y. (1982). The value of immunohistological screening in the production of monoclonal antibodies. *J. Immunol. Methods*, **50**, 145–160

Nimmo, G. R., Lew, A. M., Stanley, C. M. and Steward, M. W. (1984). Influence of antibody affinity on the performance of different antibody assays. *J. Immunol. Methods*, **72**, 177–187

Oi, V. T., Bryan, V. M., Herzenberg, L. A. and Herzenberg, L. A. (1980). Lymphocyte membrane IgG and secreted IgG are structurally and allotypically distinct. *J. Exp. Med.*, **151**, 1260–1274

Oi, V. T. and Herzenberg, L. A. (1981). Immunoglobulin producing hybrid cell lines. In Mishell, B. B. and Shiigi, S. M. (eds.), *Selected methods in cellular immunology*, W. H. Freeman and Co., San Francisco, 371–372

Partridge, L. J., Lowe, J., Hardie, D. L., Ling, N. R. and Jefferis, R. (1982). Immunogenic and antigenic epitopes of immunoglobulins. II. Antigenic differences between secreted and membrane IgG demonstrated using monoclonal antibodies. *J. Immunol.*, **128**, 1–6

Péterfy, F., Kuusela, P. and Mäkelä, O. (1983). Affinity requirements for antibody assays mapped by monoclonal antibodies. *J. Immunol.*, **130**, 1809–1813

Reimer, C. B., Phillips, D. J., Aloisio, C. H., Moore, B. D., Galland, G. G., Wells, T. W., Black, C. M. and McDougal, J. S. (1984). Evaluation of thirty-one mouse monoclonal antibodies to human IgG epitopes. *Hybridoma*, **3**, 263–275

Schönherr, O. T. and Roelofs, H. (1982). Monoclonal antibodies for diagnostic tests and affinity chromatography: a first step to antibody engineering. *Develop. Biol. Standard*, **50**, 235–242

Schuit, H. R. E., Hijmans, W. and Asma, G. E. M. (1980). Identification of mononuclear cells in human blood. I. Qualitative and quantitative data on surface markers after formaldehyde fixation of the cells. *Clin. Exp. Immunol.*, **41**, 559–566

Schuit, H. R. E., Hijmans, W. and Jansen, J. (1984). Surface bound or cytoplasmic immunoglobulins: interpretation of the immunofluorescence observed in cytocentrifuge slides of human lymphocytes. *Clin. Exp. Immunol.*, **56**, 694–700

Shulman, M., Wilde, C. D. and Köhler, G. (1978). A better cell line for making hybridomas secreting specific antibodies. *Nature*, **276**, 269–270

Singer, P. A. and Williamson, A. R. (1980). Cell surface immunoglobulins u and chains of human lymphoid cells are of higher apparent molecular weight than their secreted counterparts. *Eur. J. Immunol.*, **10**, 180–186

Sinigaglia, F., Scheidegger, D., Talmadge, K. and Garotta, G. (1985). A sensitive and quantitative micro assay for the detection of mycoplasma contamination: inhibition of IL-2 dependent cell line proliferation. *J. Immunol. Methods*, **76**, 85–92

Skvaril, F. and Schilt, U. (1984). Characterization of the subclasses and light chain types of IgG antibodies to rubella. *Clin. Exp. Immunol.*, **55**, 671–676

Steward, M. W. and Lew, A. M. (1985). The importance of antibody affinity in the performance of immunoassays for antibody. *J. Immunol. Methods*, **78**, 173–190

Swaab, D. F., Pool, C. W. and Leeuwen, F. W. van (1977). Can specificity ever be proved in immunocytochemical staining? *J. Histochem. Cytochem.*, **25**, 388–396

Tainer, J. A., Getzoff, E. D., Alexander, H., Houghten, R. A., Olson, A. J. and Lerner, R. A. (1984). The reactivity of anti-peptide antibodies is a function of the atomic mobility of sites in a protein. *Nature*, **312**, 127–134

Tsu, T. T. and Herzenberg, L. A. (1980). Solid-phase radioimmune assays. In Mishell, B. B. and Shiigi, S. M. (eds.), *Selected methods in cellular immunology*, W. H. Freeman & Co., San Francisco, 373–397

Vassalli, P., Tedghi, R., Lisowska-Bernstein, B., Tartakoff, A. and Jaton, J. C. (1979). Evidence for hydrophobic region within heavy chains of mouse B lymphocyte membrane-bound IgM. *Proc. Natl. Acad. Sci. USA*, **76**, 5515–5519

Walker, W. S., Beelen, R. H. J., Buckley, P. J., Melvin, S. L. and Shing-Erh, Y. (1984). Some fixation reagents reduce or abolish the detectability of Ia-antigen and HLA-DR on cells. *J. Immunol. Methods*, **67**, 89–99

Westhof, E., Altschuh, D., Moras, D., Bloomer, A. C., Mondragon, A., Klug, A. and Regenwortel, M. H. V. van (1984). Correlation between segmental mobility and the location of antigenic determinants in proteins. *Nature*, **311**, 123–126

Wilchek, M. and Bayer, E. A. (1984). The avidin–biotin complex in immunology. *Immunol. Today*, **5**, 39–43

Wofsy, L., Baker, P. C., Thompson, K., Goodman, J., Kimura, J. and Henry, C. (1974). Hapten-sandwich labelling. I. A general procedure for simultaneous labelling of multiple cell surface antigens for fluorescence and electromicroscopy. *J. Exp. Med.*, **140**, 523–537

ABBREVIATIONS USED

AEC	3-amino-9-ethylcarbazole
BHS	Biotinyl hydroxysuccinimide
BSA	Bovine serum albumin
c-IF	Cytoplasmic immunofluorescence test on bone marrow cells
C-Ig cells	Cytoplasmic immunoglobulin containing cells
c-PO	Detection of cytoplasmic immunoglobulin in FAM-fixed cells using peroxidase labelled anti-Ig reagents
DAB	3,3$'$-diaminobenzidine
DMEM	Dulbecco's modification of minimal essential medium
DMSO	Dimethyl sulphoxide
ELISA	Enzyme-linked immunosorbent assay
FAM fixative	Formalin–acetic acid–mercury chloride fixative
FCS	Foetal calf serum
FITC	Fluorescein isothiocyanate
GAM/Ig/FITC	Fluorescein-labelled goat antiserum directed against mouse Igs
GAM/PO	Peroxidase-labelled goat antiserum directed against mouse Igs
HAT	Hypoxanthine-, aminopterin- and thymidine-containing medium
Ig	Immunoglobulin
Mab	Monoclonal antibody
MEMS	Minimal essential medium for spinner cultures
m-IF	Membrane immunofluorescence test on MNCs
m-Ig	Membrane-bound immunoglobulin
MNC	Mononuclear cells
MW	Molecular weight

Oab	Oligoclonal antibodies, i.e. mixture of two or more Mabs
OPD	Ortho-Phenylenediamine Dihydrochloride
Pab	Polyclonal antibodies, i.e. conventional antiserum
PBS	Phosphate-buffered saline
PEG	Polyethylene glycol
RAM/PO	Peroxidase-labelled rabbit antiserum directed against mouse Igs
RIA	Radioimmunoassay
RT	Room temperature
SPF	Specific pathogen free
TRITC	Tetramethyl rhodamine isothiocyanate

4. Conjugation of Haptens and Macromolecules to Phycobiliprotein for Application in Fluorescence Immunoassay

N. MONJI AND A. CASTRO

INTRODUCTION

Phycobiliproteins are large proteins made by red algae and cyanobacteria as part of their photosystem II high harvesting system (Glazer, 1977; Gantt and Lipschultz (1973); Lipschultz and Gantt, 1981). *R*-phycoerythrin (PE) is a phycobiliprotein composed of three non-covalently associated subunits, each of which contains fluorescent bilin groups.

PE has been increasingly used for immunoassay in recent years as a fluorescence probe. The basic advantages of using phycobiliproteins as compared with other fluorophores are due to their following properties: (a) they contain multiple bilin chromophores and hence have extremely high absorbance coefficients over a wide spectrum range; (b) excitation and emission is at the red end of the spectrum (non-specific fluorescence from biological materials tends to be less); (c) there is high solubility in an aqueous environment, so that non-specific binding effects are minimal; (d) interference for Rayleigh and Raman scatter is less significant or non-existent because of a large Stokes shift; (e) quantum yields are constant over a broad pH range; (f) on account of the protein content, it is easy to carry out protein–protein conjugation reactions using homo- or hetero-bifunctional reagents (Ledbetter *et al.*, 1984; Oi *et al.*, 1982; Kronick and Grossman, 1983).

We describe here the methods for conjugating antibody to PE, as an example of conjugation of macromolecular protein to PE, and digoxin analogues to PE as an example of conjugating haptens to PE.

CONJUGATION OF ANTIBODY (Ab) TO PE

For application in fluorescence immunoassay, PE has been conjugated to Ab by several procedures. For non-covalent conjugation methods, avidin–biotin (Oi *et al.*, 1982; Kronick and Grossman, 1983) and protein A (Kronick and Grossman, 1983) systems have been used. For the covalent linkage method, various hetero-bifunctional reagents such as *N*-succinimidyl 3-(2-pyridylthio)propionate (SPDP), succinimidyl *m*-maleimidobenzoate (MBS) and succinimidyl trans-4-(*N*-maleimidylmethyl)cyclohexane-1-carboxylate (SMCC) have been commonly used. Since the covalent linkages are much more stable and precise in terms of molar requirement, we have been using the covalent linkage method to conjugate monoclonal Ab (McAb) to PE.

Using one of the methods developed for Ab–enzyme conjugation (Ishikawa, 1983), we conjugated McAb to PE with a slightly different procedure. The sulphhydryl groups were introduced to McAb through the use of *S*-acetylmercaptosuccinic anhydride (SAMSA). PE was conjugated with SMCC. Thioether linkage was then used to conjugate the two proteins. In this section, we describe briefly the two existing methods for conjugating McAb to PE, namely SPDP–SPDP (disulphide linkage) and SMCC–SPDP (thioether linkage) methods and, in more detail, our new SMCC–SAMSA (thioether linkage) method.

SPDP–SPDP Method (Disulphide Linkage) (Figure 1)

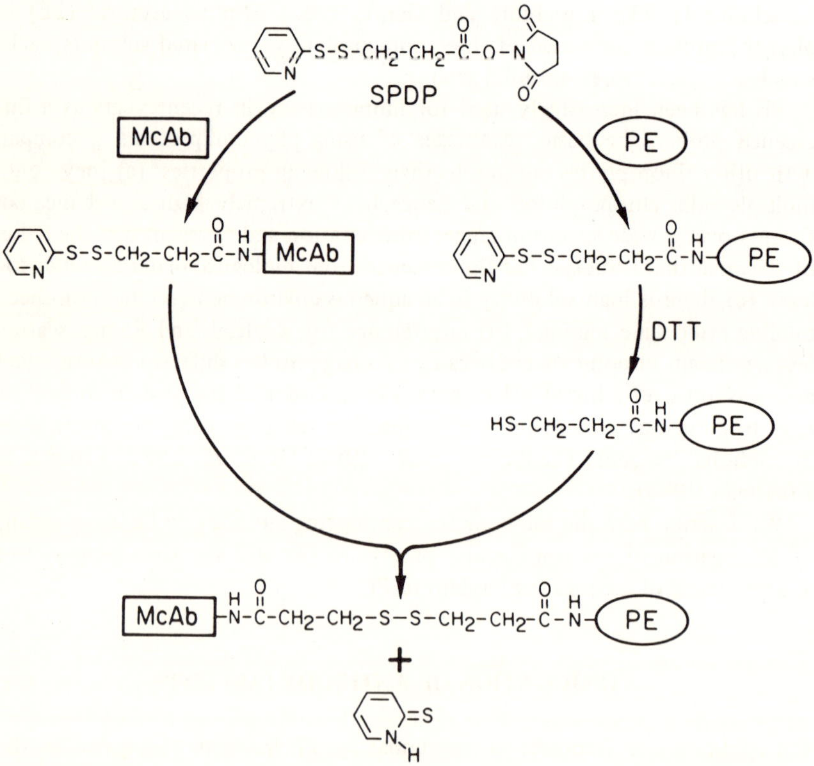

Figure 1   Conjugation of monoclonal antibody (McAb) to *R*-phycoerythrin (PE) by the SPDP–SPDP method. Abbreviations: SPDP, *N*-succinimidyl 3-(2-pyridylthio)propionate; DTT, dithiothreitol.

This method has been adapted most widely for Ab–PE conjugation (Ledbetter *et al.*, 1984; Oi *et al.*, 1982; Kronick and Grossman, 1983). Briefly, SPDP was conjugated to lysine residues of the Ab, and then another SPDP was conjugated to PE. The pyridylthiol group of PE conjugated to SPDP was then removed by addition of dithiothreitol. Thiolated phycoerythrin was then mixed with SPDP-conjugated Ab, resulting in conjugation of Ab to PE through a disulphide linkage. This method has been under some criticism for the following reasons: (1) the conjugation procedure requires rather a lengthy incubation time (at least 24 h for disulphide conjugation); (2) disulphide linkage may not be very stable at physiological pH.

SMCC–SPDP Method (Thioether Linkage) (Figure 2)

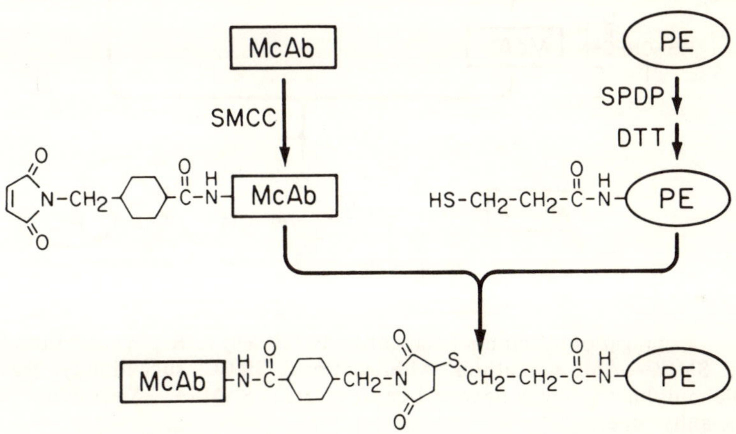

Figure 2   Conjugation of monoclonal antibody (McAb) to *R*-phycoerythrin (PE) by the SMCC–SPDP method. Abbreviations: SPDP, *N*-succinimidyl 3-(2-pyridyl-thio)propionate; DTT, dithiothreitol; SMCC, succinimidyl *trans*-4-(*N*-maleimidyl-methyl)cyclohexane-1-carboxylate.

This procedure involves conjugation of Ab with SMCC; the SMCC-conjugated Ab was then mixed with the thiolated PE (which was described in the SPDP–SPDP method (Ishikawa, 1983). The thioether linkage was formed through the maleimide group of SMCC and the thiol group of SPDP. This procedure must be regarded cautiously from two different aspects: (1) conjugation of SMCC to Ab results in a rather hydrophobic Ab conjugate; (2) over-conjugation of SPDP to PE may result in dimerization of PE through disulphide linkages.

SMCC–SAMSA Method (Thioether Linkage) (Figure 3)

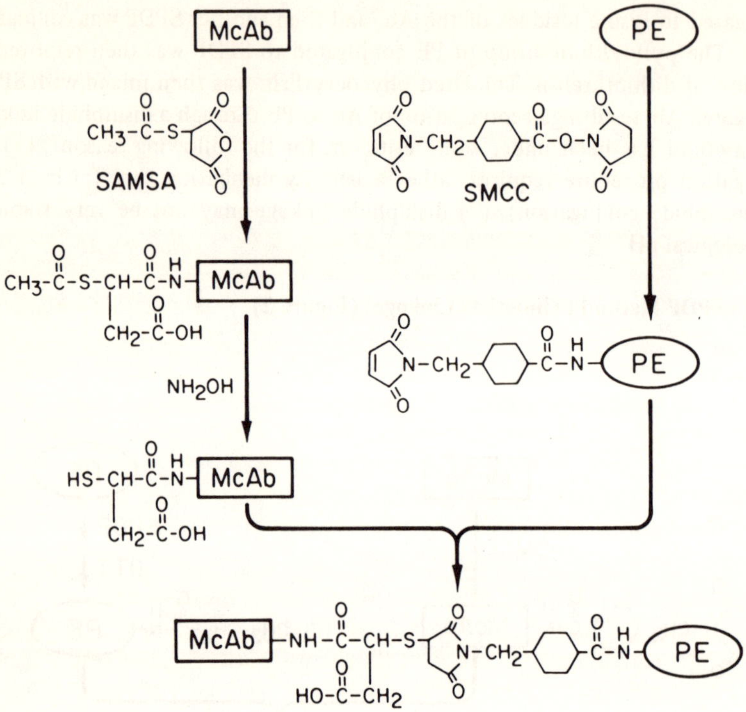

Figure 3   Conjugation of monoclonal antibody (McAb) to *R*-phycoerythrin (PE) by the SMCC–SAMSA method. Abbreviations: SMCC, succinimidyl *trans*-4-(*N*-maleimidylmethyl)cyclohexane-1-carboxylate; SAMSA, *S*-acetylmercapto-succinic anhydride.

We use this reaction to conjugate Ab to PE because of the following advantages: (1) SAMSA is a small molecule and, after conjugation, the resulting Ab conjugate is charged because of the introduction of a free carboxyl group making still hydrophilic Ab; (2) since SMCC is introduced into PE, no dimerization of PE may result. We have modified the procedure used for conjugation of horseradish peroxidase to Ab (Ishikawa, 1983). The detailed procedure is described as follows.

Introduction of Thiol Groups into IgG Using S-acetylmercaptosuccinic Anhydride (SAMSA)

Two and a half milligrams (15.6 nmol) of IgG was dissolved in 0.5 ml PBS. Then, 5 μl (1.72 μmol) of SAMSA dissolved in dimethylformamide (DMF) at a concentration of 60 mg/ml was added. The reaction mixture was incubated for 30 min with continuous stirring. After the incubation, 0.05 ml of 0.1 M Tris HCl, pH 7.0, containing 0.1 M ethylenediaminetetraacetic acid (EDTA) and 0.05 ml of 1 M hydroxylamine, pH 7.0, were added. The reaction mixture was again incubated for 10 min at room temperature. Then the mixture was applied to Sephadex G-25 columns (1.0 cm × 45 cm) equilibrated with 0.02 M phosphate buffer, pH 6.0, containing 5 mM EDTA. The column was eluted with the same buffer and the fractions containing the highest IgG concentration were collected. About eight thiol groups were introduced per IgG molecule by this method after examination of the number of thiol groups introduced into IgG by the 2,2′-dithiodipyridine method (Grassetti and Murray, 1960).

Introduction of Maleimide Groups (SMCC) into PE

One milligram (4.2 nmol) of PE was dissolved in 1.0 ml of 0.1 M phosphate buffer, pH 7.0. To that solution, 25 μl (68 nmol) of SMCC dissolved in DMF at a concentration of 0.9 mg/ml was added. The reaction mixture was incubated at 30°C for 30 min and applied to a Sephadex G-25 column (1.0 cm × 45 cm) equilibrated with 0.1 M phosphate buffer, pH 6.5. The column was eluted with the same buffer and the fractions containing the highest PE concentration were collected and examined for the number of maleimide groups by the cysteine-2,2′-dithiodipyridine method (Grassetti and Murray, 1960).

Conjugation of the Thiolated IgG to the Maleimide Derivative of PE

Seven tenths of a milligram (3 nmol) of PE was dissolved in 1.0 ml of 0.1 M phosphate buffer, pH 6.5. To that PE solution, 1.5 mg (10 nmol) of the thiolated IgG in 0.5 ml of 0.02 M phosphate buffer, pH 6.0, containing 5 mM EDTA, was added, and the reaction mixture was incubated for 2 h at room temperature. Then, 50 μl of 0.1 M *N*-ethylmaleimide dissolved in DMF was added at the end of incubation to react with unreacted thiol groups in the IgG molecules. After 10 min of incubation at room temperature, the reaction mixture was applied to a Sephacryl S-300 column (1.5 cm × 110 cm) equilibrated with phosphate-buffered saline containing 0.1% NaN_3 (PBS–NaN_3). The column was eluted with the same PBS–NaN_3 buffer. The elution profile was monitored for PE at 545 nm and for total protein at 280 nm.

Sephacryl S-300 Chromatographic Profiles

The typical separation of McAb–PE conjugate from unconjugated McAb and PE is shown in figure 4. It was found that the efficiency of conjugation was different depending on the kind of McAb which had been used. With more hydrophilic McAb, such as McAb (3F6), the yield of McAb–PE conjugate with the first peak was much higher than the more acidic McAbs, such as McAb (2C3) and McAb (G17-2). For the binding ratio between McAb and PE, we found that about 1.0–1.5 molecules McAb were conjugated to one PE molecule.

When the affinity-purified polyclonal Ab was conjugated, the Sephacryl S-300 chromatographic profile was little different; three distinct peaks appeared

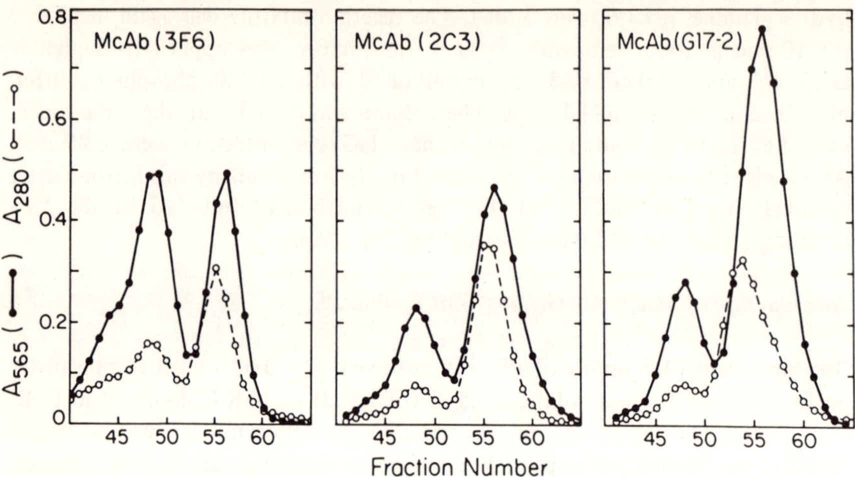

Figure 4 Sephacryl S-300 gel filtration chromatographic profiles of monoclonal antibody (McAb)–*R*-phycoerythrin (PE) conjugation reaction mixtures.

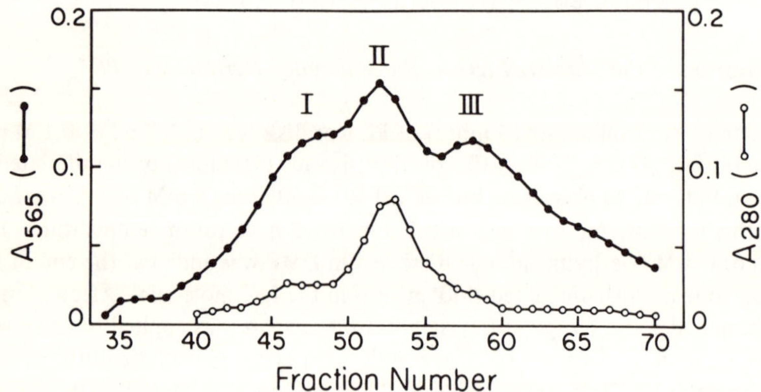

Figure 5 Sephacryl S-300 gel filtration chromatographic profile of polyclonal antibody (affinity purified)–*R*-phycoerythrin (PE) conjugation reaction mixture.

(figure 5). The first peak (P-I) was found to be the Ab–PE conjugate. The second peak appeared to be due to the contaminated proteins conjugated to PE, since this peak showed little antibody activity as examined by immunoassay. The third peak is that of unconjugated PE.

Concentration of Ab-PE Conjugate Isolated on Sephacryl S-300
Chromatography by Biotin-Agarose Column

During the course of investigation, we found that both PE alone and Ab–PE conjugate bound strongly to the biotin-agarose column even though they were

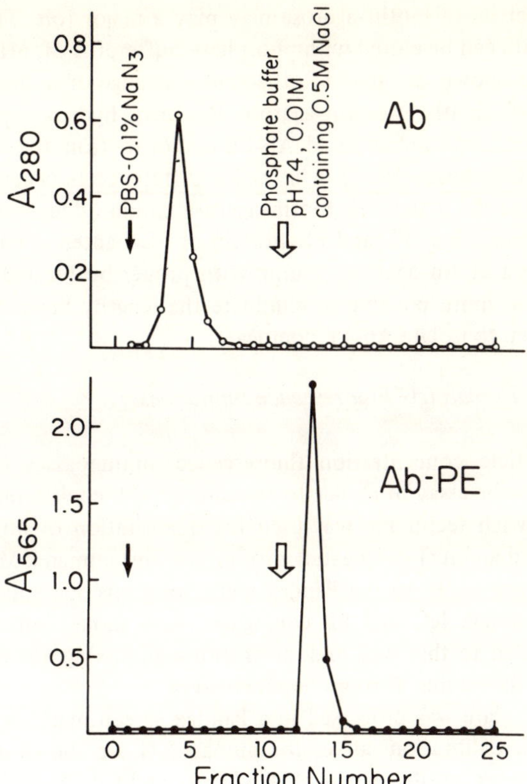

Figure 6   Elution profiles of antibody (Ab) alone and Ab–*R*-phycoerythrin conjugate on a biotin–diaminodipropylamine (DADPA) – agarose column.

dissolved in PBS–NaN$_3$ (figure 6). Ab alone did not bind to the biotin–agarose column. The exact mechanism for binding is not known; however, some ion

Table 1   Binding of PE to various gels

Gel	Percentage PE recovered after elution with PBS–0.1% NaN$_3$	Percentage PE recovered after elution with 0.01 M phosphate buffer, pH 7.4, containing 0.5 M NaCl
Biotin–DADPA–agarose[a]	0.5	89
DADPA–agarose	99	0
Cholesteryl–DADPA–agarose	0	0
Phenyl Sepharose 4B	75	15
Octyl Sepharose 4B	60	0
DEAE Sepharose 6BCl	85	10
DEAE Affigel blue	82	7

[a] (1) Preincubation of PE with biotin did not prevent the binding of PE to the gel; (2) DADPA, diaminodipropylamine.

exchange properties of biotin–agarose may play a major role. The bound PE or Ab–PE conjugate can be eluted with phosphate buffer, 0.1 M, pH 7.4, containing 0.5 M NaCl. As shown in table 1, other ion exchange or hydrophobic gels did not bind PE as efficiently as biotin–agarose. Recently, hydroxylapatite chromatography has been used to separate McAb–PE conjugate from the reaction mixture (Kronick and Grossman, 1983). The major difference between biotin–agarose and hydroxylapatite is that the biotin–agarose column does not bind immunoglobulins and only binds PE and PE–protein or PE–hapten conjugate. With one step, and using a biotin–agarose column with proper buffer and salt concentrations, it may be quite possible to eliminate the lengthy Sephacryl S-300 chromatographic step to isolate Ab–PE conjugate.

Application to Human IgG Fluorescence Immunoassay

We chose particle concentration fluorescence immunoassay (PCFIA) (Jolley *et al.*, 1984) as the assay of choice to examine Ab–PE conjugate, and the double antibody sandwich technique was used for quantitation of human IgG. Latex beads (0.8 μm diameter) conjugated with mouse anti-human k McAb, suspended in 1% BSA, were added to the Pandex well. Solutions containing both defined quantities of human IgG and PE conjugated with mouse anti-human γ McAb (3F6) were added to that well and, after thorough mixing, the reaction mixture was incubated for 60 min at room temperature.

The Pandex plate was processed in a Pandex screen machine with two 5 min washing cycles. Calibration curves for human IgG are shown in figure 7 using both (a) PE–mouse antihuman γ McAb (3F6) and (b) PE–rabbit antihuman γ polyclonal Ab (affinity purified). Because of the high affinity of the Ab, the

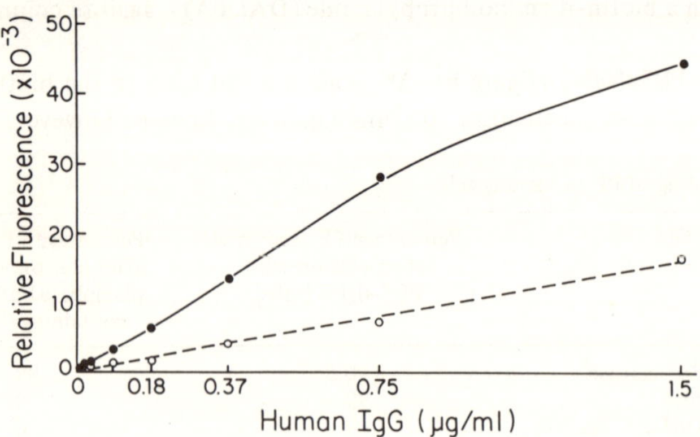

Figure 7 Calibration curves for human IgG in particle concentration fluorescence immunoassay (PCFIA) using either mouse anti-human γ McAb (3F6) – *R*-phycoerythrin (PE) conjugate (○---○) or rabbit anti-human γ antibody (affinity purified)–PE conjugate (●——●).

sensitivity of the assay using PE–polyclonal Ab was about four times higher (2 ng/assay) than that of the assay using PE–McAb (3F6) conjugate (8 ng/assay).

CONJUGATION OF HAPTEN TO PE: APPLICATION TO DIGOXIN FLUORESCENCE IMMUNOASSAY

We selected digoxin fluorescence immunoassay as an assay of choice because the assay for detection of serum digoxin levels requires a high sensitivity (0.4 ng/ml). The methods used for conjugation of digoxin or digoxin analogues to PE are similar to those used for conjugating them to enzyme, except that the reaction must be free from inactivation of PE chromophore groups. We describe here three different procedures for conjugating a small hapten to PE (i.e. periodate, mixed acid anhydride and carbodimide methods) together with sensitivity and specificity studies on these prepared conjugates.

Synthesis of Digoxigenin(12-OH)-3-*o*-Succinate and Digoxigenin(12-OAc)-3-*o*-Succinate (Figure 8)

Digoxigenin(12-OH)-3-*o*-succinate and digoxigenin(12-OAc)-3-*o*-succinate were synthesized by the published procedure (Rutner *et al.*, 1974). The prepared compound was purified by silica gel thin layer chromatography (ethyl acetate:methanol, 95:5) and gave the melting point quoted in the literature.

Conjugation of either Digoxigenin(12-OH)-3-*o*-Succinate or Digoxigenin (12-OAc)-3-*o*-Succinate to PE by a Mixed Acid Anhydride Method (Figure 9)

Seven milligrams of either digoxigenin(12-OH)-3-*o*-succinate or digoxigenin-(12-OAc)-3-*o*-succinate was dissolved in 284 μl of dry dioxane. To that solution, 9 μl of tributylamine was added and the solution was cooled to 10–12°C. Seven microlitres of isobutylchloroformate was then added and the reaction mixture was stirred for 20 min while maintaining the temperature at 10–12°C. Ten microlitres of the above mixed anhydride solution was added to the cooled solution of PE in water (1 mg/ml). The reaction mixture was stirred overnight at 4°C and then applied to a Sephadex G-25 column (1 cm × 35 cm). The column was eluted with PBS containing 0.1% NaN$_3$. The fractions containing the major portion of PE were pooled and stored at 4°C until further use.

Conjugation of either Digoxigenin(12-OH)-3-*o*-Succinate or Digoxigenin(12-OAc)-3-*o*-Succinate to PE by the Carbodiimide Method (Figure 10)

To 1 ml H$_2$O containing 1 mg of PE, 50 μl of DMF (containing 0.25 mg of digoxin analogues) was added dropwise and stirred at room temperature. To that

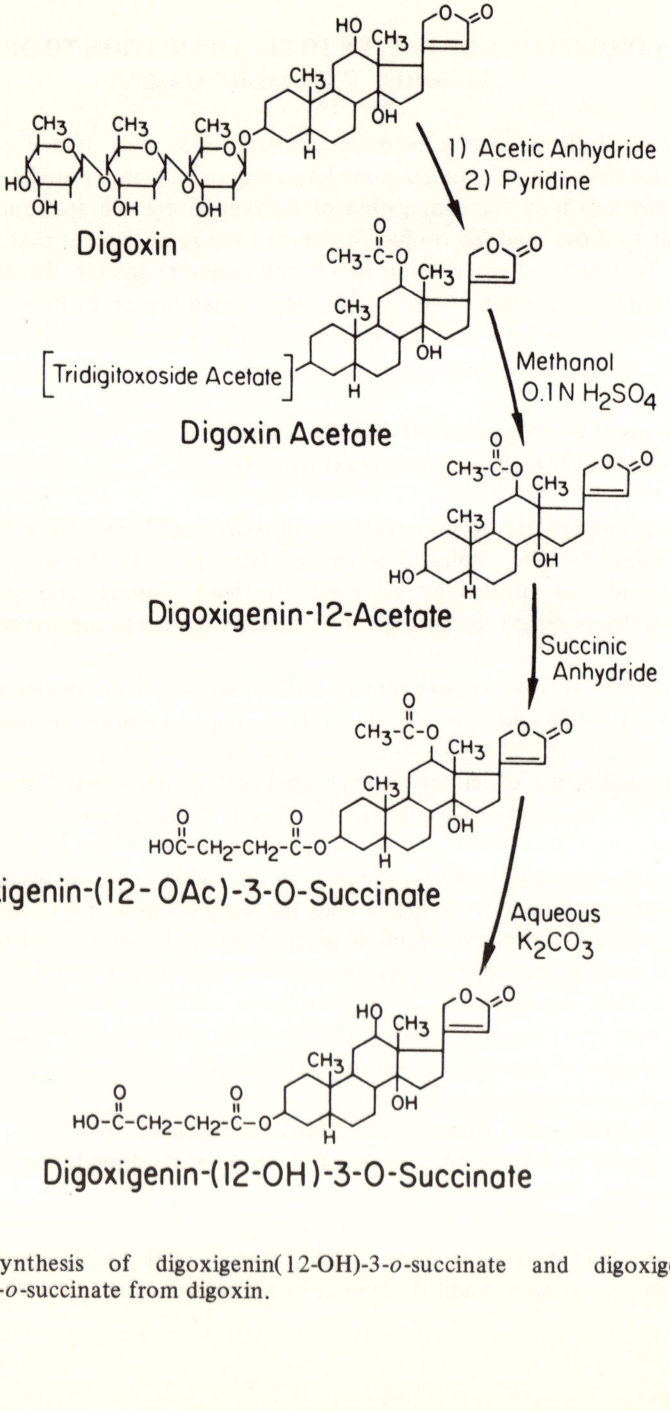

Figure 8 Synthesis of digoxigenin(12-OH)-3-*o*-succinate and digoxigenin-(12-OAc)-3-*o*-succinate from digoxin.

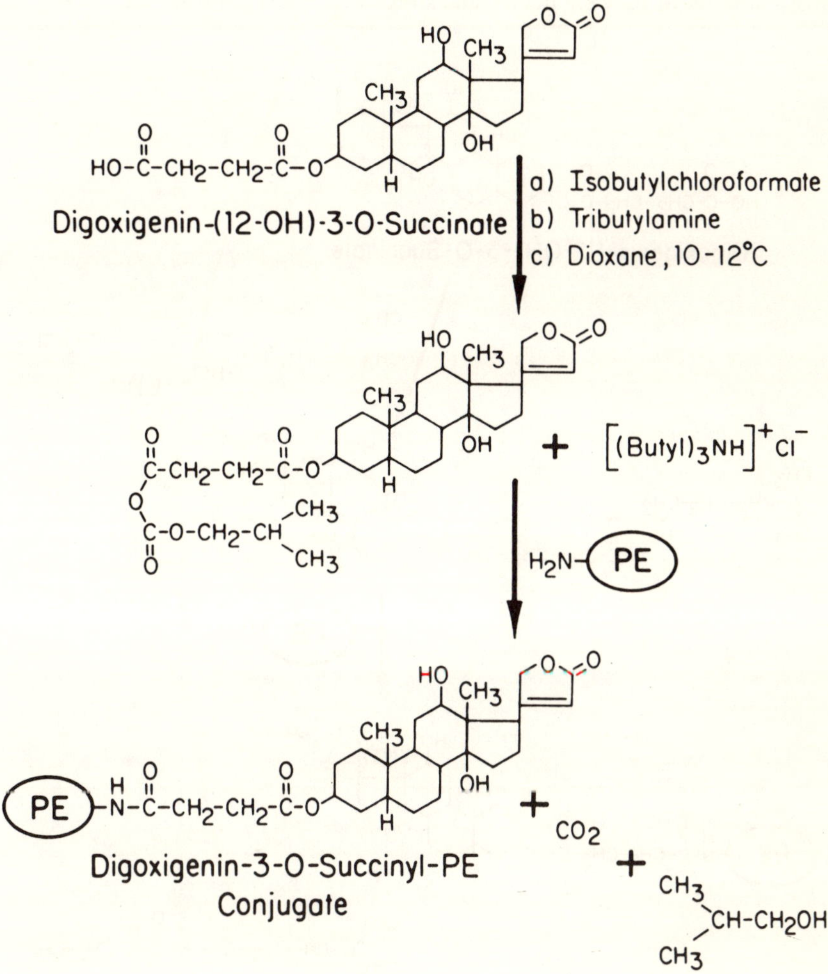

Figure 9   Conjugation of digoxigenin(12-OH)-3-*o*-succinate to *R*-phycoerythrin (PE) by a mixed acid anhydride method.

mixture, 25 μl of water containing 0.5 mg of 1-ethyl-3-(3-dimethylaminopropyl)-carbodiimide-HCl (EDC) was added and stirring was continued. Ten minutes later, another 12.5 μl of EDC solution was added. The reaction mixture was stirred at room temperature for 18 h and then applied to a Sephadex G-25 column (1 cm × 30 cm) equilibrated and eluted with PBS–NaN_3. The fractions containing the largest amount of PE were pooled and stored at 4°C until further use.

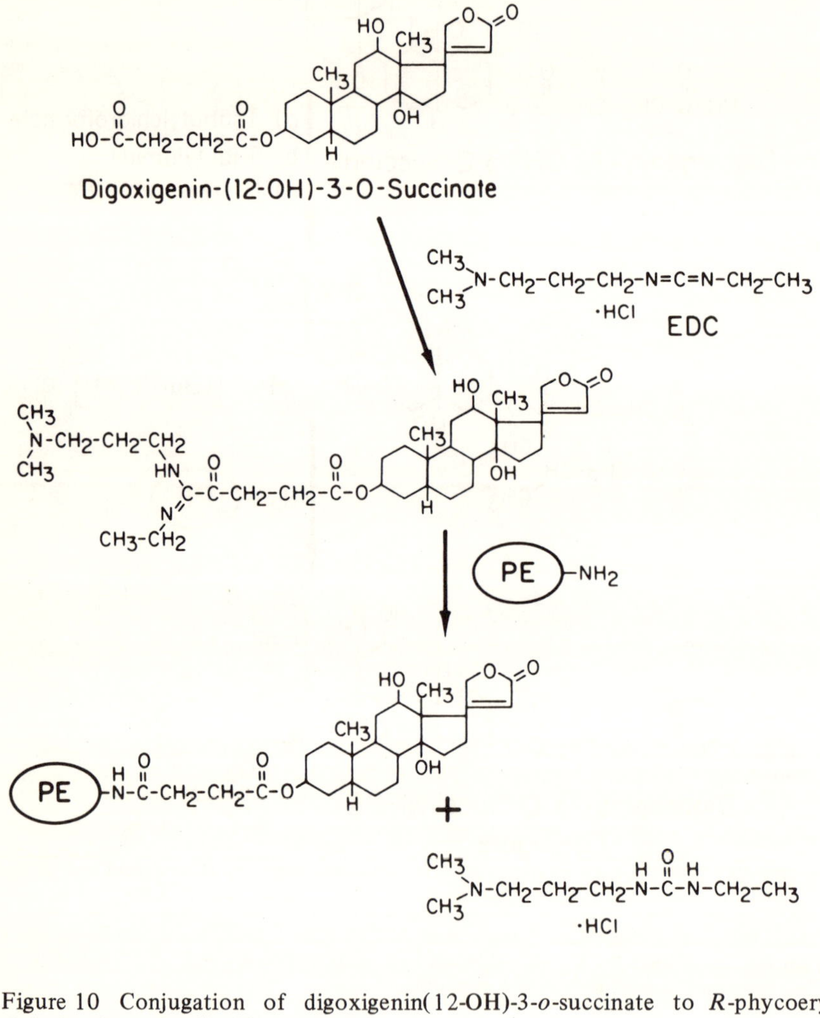

Figure 10 Conjugation of digoxigenin(12-OH)-3-*o*-succinate to *R*-phycoerythrin by the carbodiimide method.

Conjugation of Digoxin or Ouabain to PE by the Periodate Method (Figure 11)

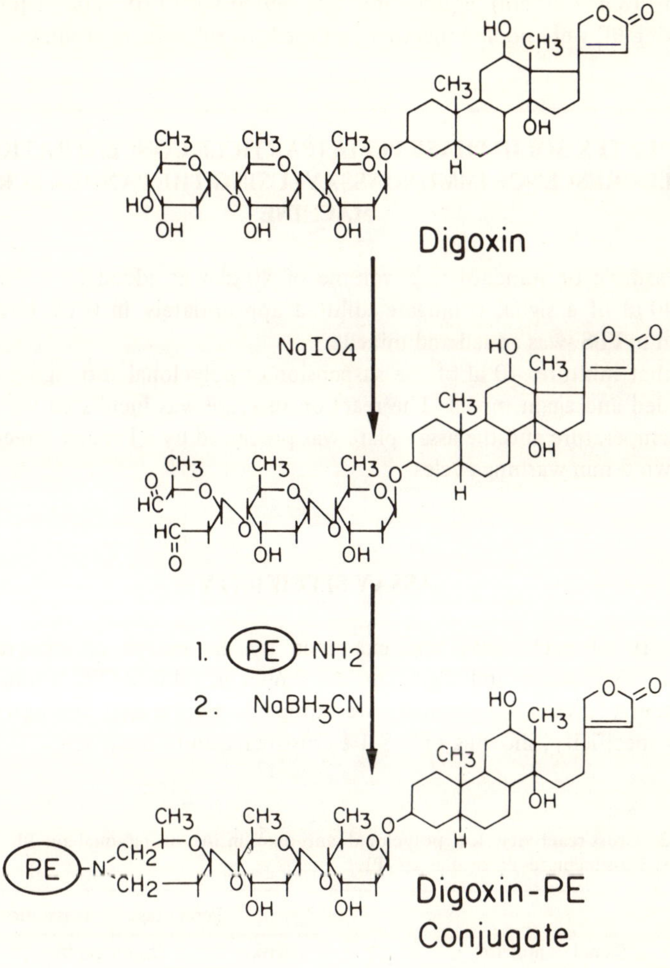

Figure 11   Conjugation of digoxin to *R*-phycoerythrin by the periodate method.

Either digoxin or ouabain in an amount of 20 mg (0.0256 nmol) was dissolved in 1 ml absolute ethanol. To that solution, 1 ml of 0.1 M Na_2IO_4 was added. After brief mixing, the mixture was incubated for 30 min at room temperature. At the end of incubation, 30 μl of 1 M ethylene glycol was added and incubated for 5 min; 20 μl of the above reaction mixture were then added to 0.55 ml of PBS containing 0.6 mg (2.5 nmol) of PE. The reaction mixture was incubated for 1 h at 25°C. A freshly prepared solution of $NaBH_3CN$ in PBS (10 mg/ml) in a volume of 22 μl (0.22 mg, 0.0035 mmol) was then added and incubated further for 48 h at 25°C (use of $NaBH_4$ instead of $NaBH_3CN$ resulted in inactivation of PE chromophores). The reaction mixture was then applied to a Sephadex G-25 column (1 cm × 20 cm), equilibrated and eluted with PBS. The major fractions containing PE were pooled together and used for subsequent studies.

LATEX SOLID PHASE PCFIA (PARTICLE CONCENTRATION FLUORESCENCE IMMUNOASSAY) USING THE PANDEX SCREEN MACHINE

Either sample or standard in a volume of 40 μl was added to a Pandex well. Then 40 μl of a signal conjugate, diluted appropriately in 0.1% bovine serum albumin in PBS, was added and mixed.

To that mixture, 40 μl of the suspension of polyclonal anti-digoxin antibody was added and again mixed. The reaction mixture was incubated for 10 min at room temperature and the assay plate was processed by a Pandex screen machine using two 5 min washing cycles.

ASSAY SPECIFICITY

Specificity of each assay was examined by the extent of cross-reaction to digoxin, digoxigenin and digitoxin. As shown in table 2, PE conjugated with digoxigenin(12-OH)-3-*o*-succinate was found to be the best conjugate with the highest specificity, showing only 9.1% cross-reaction to digitoxin.

Table 2 Cross-reactivity for polyclonal anti-digoxin Ab using ouabain–PE, digoxigenin-(12-OH)-3-*o*-succinate–PE or digoxin–PE

	Percentage cross-reaction to		
Signal conjugate	Digoxin	Digoxigenin	Digitoxin
Ouabain–PE	100	55.3	20.7
Digoxigenin(12-OH)-3-*o*-succinate–PE	100	80.0	9.1
Digoxin–PE	100	88.3	16.8

ASSAY SENSITIVITY

The sensitivity of the assay was examined by displacement of signal at various digoxin concentrations. The highest sensitivity in the assay was achieved by ouabain-conjugated PE (15 pg/assay), followed by digoxigenin(12-OH)-3-*o*-succinate-conjugated PE (30 pg/assay) and digoxin-conjugated PE (60 pg/assay).

For the final, optimized assay, we used ouabain-conjugated PE. The assay had a maximum sensitivity of 0.4 ng/ml using a 40 μl sample size and had an overall CV of 7.2%. The calibration curve for digoxin in serum is shown in figure 12.

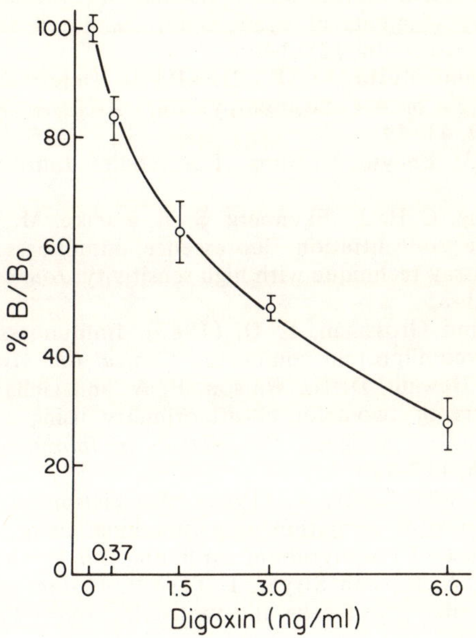

Figure 12 Calibration curve for digoxin in serum by particle concentration fluorescence immunoassay (PCFIA). Symbols: B, antibody-bound signal conjugate at the added amount of digoxin standard; B_0, antibody-bound signal conjugate at zero addition of digoxin standard.

DISCUSSION

We have demonstrated here that macromolecules, such as monoclonal and polyclonal immunoglobulins, and haptens, such as digoxin, ouabain, and digoxin analogues, can be readily conjugated to PE by a variety of methods. One must choose the best procedure, depending on the kind of molecules selected for conjugation. Information about the physicochemical properties of the molecules should be collected and examined in detail before attempting the conjugation reaction.

We have used R-phycoerythrin because it has many interesting properties, as referred to in the introduction. Use of phycoerythrins in immunoassay will increase substantially in the next few years, as the limitation of enzyme immunoassay technology currently employed is increasingly realized.

REFERENCES

Gantt, E. and Lipschultz, C. A. (1973). Energy transfer in phycobilisomes from phycoerythrin to allophycocanin. *Biochimica et Biophysica Acta*, **292**, 858–861

Glazer, A. N. (1977). Structure and molecular organization of the photosynthetic accessory pigments of cyanobacteria and red algae. *Molecular and Cellular Biochemistry*, **18**, 125–140

Grassetti, D. R. and Murray, J. F., Jr. (1960). Determination of sulfhydryl groups with 2,2′- or 4,4′-diothiodipyridine. *Archives of Biochemistry and Biophysics*, **119**, 41–49

Ishikawa, E. (1983). Enzyme-labelling of antibodies. *Journal of Immunoassays*, **4**, 208–327

Jolley, M. E. Wang, C.-H. J., Ekenberg, S. J., Zuelke, M. S. and Kelso, D. M. (1984). Particle concentration fluorescence immunoassay (PCFIA): a new rapid immunoassay technique with high sensitivity. *Journal of Immunological Methods*, **67**, 21–35

Kronick, M. N. and Grossman, P. D. (1983). Immunoassay techniques with fluorescent phycobiliprotein conjugates. *Clinical Chemistry*, **29**, 1582–1586

Ledbetter, J. A., Hewgill, D. H., Watson, B. A. and Gallagher, M. S. (1984). Practical aspects of two-color cytofluorimetry using a single argon laser. Lymphocyte surface antigens. *Perspectives in Immunogenetics and Histocompatibility*, **6**, 119–129

Lipschultz, C. A. and Gantt, E. (1981). Association of phycoerythrin and phycocyanin: in vitro formation of a functional energy transferring phycobilisome complex of Porphyridium sordidum. *Biochemistry*, **20**, 3371–3381

Oi, V. T., Glazer, A. N., and Stryer, L. (1982). Fluorescent phycobiliprotein conjugates for analyses of cells and molecules. *Journal of Cell Biology*, **93**, 981–986

Rutner, H., Rapum, R. and Lewis, N. (1974). Derivative of digoxigenin. *U.S. Patent 3,855,208*

BIBLIOGRAPHY

Molecular Probes (1984). *Conjugations of Phycobiliproteins to Biological Molecules*, Molecular Probes Inc., 24750 Lawrence Road, Junction City, OR 97448, U.S.A.

5. Nicotine Enzyme Immunoassay

A. CASTRO AND N. MONJI

Numerous procedures for the determination of levels of nicotine in body fluids have been developed in recent years, all of which have certain disadvantages. Radioimmunoassay and related procedures have proved to have unique advantages, however, with small samples and in circumstances of low nicotine concentration, 2- and 6-aminonicotine have been found not to be suitable functionalized nicotine haptens for various reasons. In the present study on the use of racemic aminonicotine as a functionalized hapten, nicotine antibodies suitable for use in nicotine determinations have been produced from antigens in which both 'flexible' and 'semi-rigid' chains serve to couple racemic 6-aminonicotine to bovine serum albumin.

Nicotine enzyme immunoassay has been developed for the first time using antibodies produced against 6-(ϵ-aminocapramido)-DL-nicotine and β-galactosidase nicotine enzyme. The assay is a double antibody method which requires 60 and 15 min incubation respectively. The correlation of nicotine-pooled plasma with controls was found to be 0.994 with very good precision and accuracy. The sensitivity, defined as the concentration of nicotine measured at a free-to-bound ratio $\Delta F/\Delta F_0 = 90\%$, was found to be 10 μg/l. Samples of human smokers ($N = 9$) after one cigarette at 3 min were 50–100 μg/l and at 15 min were 30–60 μg/l.

INTRODUCTION

The appearance of nicotine in the blood and urine after use of tobacco or other nicotine-containing products has led to increasing interest in precise methods for its measurement in these body fluids. Procedures include thin-layer chromatographic methods dependent on measurement of the radioactivity of administered isotopic nicotine labelled with ^{14}C or tritium (McKennis, 1965; McNiven *et al.*, 1965; Pilotti *et al.*, 1976), liquid and gas chromatography (Horning *et al.*, 1973; Turner, 1969) and competitive binding (radioimmunoassay) procedures (Horning *et al.*, 1973; Langone, 1973; Castro and Prieto, 1975; Castro *et al.*, 1979; Castro *et al.*, 1980). These methods have limited reproducibility and/or limited validation. In some applications of thin-layer chromatography, for example, possible quantitative significance of the methyl exchange, where radioactivity of nicotine ^{14}C-methyl was used as an indicator of nicotine concentration, was not investigated (Matsukura *et al.*, 1974; Haines *et al.*, 1974).

Some gas chromatographic procedures for measurement of small amounts of nicotine underestimate nicotine levels because of the volatility of nicotine (Pilotti, 1975), although a proper choice of internal standard will diminish or eliminate this problem (Chichibabin and Kirssanov, 1924). Also, some gas chromatographic methods apply lidocaine as an internal standard (Pilotti, 1975), which is used in the treatment of cardiac arrhythmias and other conditions. Other disadvantages regarding the use of therapeutic agents as internal standards may also be cited (Turner, 1969).

With small samples and low concentrations of nicotine, radioimmunoassays and related procedures have unique advantages. These have been previously discussed (Abraham, 1969) and include automation, which provides for rapid determination of several hundred samples in a day.

Nicotine is an alkaloid present in the leaves of *Nicotiana tabacum* and *n. rustica* in amounts of about 2-8%. In recent years, interest in nicotine metabolism has been stimulated by increased consideration of the possible role of nicotine as a reinforcer in the habitual use of tobacco (Jarwick, 1977) and by many studies on the short half-life of nicotine in human blood plasma (Langone *et al.*, 1973; Isaac and Rand, 1972; Armitage, 1975). Also, some of the nicotine metabolites appear physiologically to oppose or enhance the effects of nicotine (McKennis, 1965; von Euler *et al.*, 1970; Wilson *et al.*, 1976). These and other considerations have contributed to the development of effective methods for the measurement of nicotine in biological fluids.

Limitations and advantages of gas chromatography and combined gas chromatography–mass spectrometry methods have been previously reviewed (Pilotti *et al.*, 1976; Pilotti, 1975). Because of the specificity and sensitivity of these assays, several groups of workers have studied various immunological techniques for the rapid determination of nicotine. Radioimmunoassay of nicotine has been developed; (Castro and Prieto, 1975; Castro *et al.*, 1985); however, commercial preparations of [3]H- or ^{14}C-labelled nicotine of high specific activity have become increasingly scarce. ^{125}I-labelled nicotine of high specific activity has been prepared (Castro and Prieto, 1975), but it has a short shelf-life, and there is considerable batch-to-batch variation in the material. The nicotine enzyme immunoassay (EIA) described here avoids such RIA disadvantages as high cost of tracer, short shelf-life and potential radiation hazard together with waste disposal problems. EIA is as sensitive, fast and efficient as RIA.

MATERIALS AND METHODS

Compounds

(S)-nicotine, *N*-methylpyrrolidine and *p*-aminobenzoic acid were obtained from the Aldrich Chemical Company. (R,S)-6-aminonicotine and (R,S)-2-aminonicotine were synthesized by a previously reported method (Chichibabin and Kirssanov, 1924). (R)-nicotine di-(*d*)-tartrate was prepared from racemic nicotine. (S)-*N'*-nitrosonornicotine was a gift from Dr. Richard Manning of the U.S. Tobacco Company.

Preparation of Immunogens

The conjugate of (R,S)-6-(ε-aminocapramido)-nicotine with bovine serum albumin was prepared as previously described (Castro *et al.*, 1979). (R,S)-6-(*p*-aminobenzamido)-nicotine and (R,S)-2-(*p*-aminobenzamido)-nicotine conjugates with bovine serum albumin were prepared according to the procedures described by Castro *et al.* (1980) (for compounds, see table 1). For preparation of the conjugate of bovine serum albumin with 6-aminonicotine, a solution of 200 mg of 6-aminonicotine in 10 ml of distilled water was stirred with bovine serum albumin (200 mg) until the protein was completely dissolved. The pH was adjusted to 5.0 with dilute HCl. One millilitre of 1 M ethyl-(ε-dimethylaminopropyl)-carbodiimide hydrochloride was added; the reaction mixture was allowed to stand at room temperature for 2 h and then at 4°C overnight. The mixture was then dialysed against 3 l of 0.05 M sodium phosphate buffer (pH 7.0) for 3 days with three buffer changes. Immunogen was freeze dried and then stored at 4°C.

Functionalized Hapten

6-aminonicotine was prepared by the previously described method (Jarwick, 1977) and converted to the *N-p*-aminobenzoyl derivative (Matsukura *et al.*, 1974). For a 'semi-rigid' coupling, the aminobenzoyl compound was diazotized and coupled to bovine serum albumin essentially (Matsukura *et al.*, 1974). For a 'flexible' coupling chain, racemic 6-(ε-aminocapramido)-nicotine was prepared and coupled to bovine serum albumin (Castro *et al.*, 1979). The resultant antigens contained approximately 25 and 10 mol of aminonicotine per mol of antigen respectively. Comparative data from the corresponding antibodies are given in table 1.

6-Aminonicotine Content of Immunogen

A solution of 50 mg of the conjugate of 6-aminonicotine and bovine serum albumin in 2N HCl was heated at 100°C for 22 h. The solution was then allowed

Table 1   Cross-reactivity studies on nicotine antibodies

Compound[a]	Cross-reactivity (%)	
	Rabbit antibody	Goat antibody
(S)-nicotine	100 (0.17 nmol)[b]	100 (0.62 nmol)[b]
(R,S)-6-aminonicotine	154	3.6
(R,S)-2-aminonicotine	21	0.2
(S)-nicotine-N'-oxide[c]	0.06	0.2
(S)-cotinine	0.1	0.1
4-(3-pyridyl)-4-oxobutyric acid	0.1	0.1
(R,S)-4-(3-pyridyl)-4-aminobutyric acid	0.1	0.1
(R,S)-4-(3-pyridyl)-hydroxybutyric acid	0.1	0.1
(S)-4-(3-pyridyl)-4-methylaminobutyric acid	0.1	0.1
Pyridine	0.1	0.1
(S)-nornicotine	0.8	0.6
Nicotinic acid	0.1	0.1
(S)-cotinine methonium iodide	0.1	0.1
(R,S)-demethylcotinine-N-oxide[c]	0.1	0.1
Allohydroxycotinine	0.1	0.1
(S)-cotinine-N-oxide[c]	0.1	0.1
Nicotinamide	0.1	0.1
2-aminopyridine	0.1	0.1
N-(3-pyridyl) acetylglycine	0.1	0.1
3-acetylpyridine	0.1	0.1
3-pyridylacetic acid	0.1	0.1
Pyrrolidine	0.1	0.1
N-methylpyrrolidine	0.06	0.1
Pyrrolidine-2	0.1	0.1
N-methylpyrrolidine	0.06	0.1
N-methylpyrrolidine-2	0.1	0.1
L-proline	0.1	0.1

[a]Nicotine metabolites, unless otherwise indicated, were natural compounds or synthetic compounds with corresponding chemical and physical properties.
[b]The amount in parentheses is the amount required for 50% binding.
[c]The N-oxides were prepared by the m-chloroperbenzoid acid procedure (Dagne and Castagnoli, 1972).

to cool and was concentrated to dryness on the water bath with the aid of a stream of nitrogen. The dry residue was triturated with 0.5 ml of 0.2 M sodium citrate buffer (pH 2.2). After clarification by centrifugation, an aliquot (20 μl) of the solution was subjected to analysis for 6-aminonicotine by high pressure liquid chromatography on a 25 cm column (4.6 mm ID) using as mobile phase a mixture (pH 5.2) which contained 9 volumes of an aqueous 0.05 N lithium acetate buffer (pH 5.4) and 1 part of acetonitrile. 6-aminonicotine from the hydrolysis emerged at 8 min, with a mobile phase flow rate of 2 ml/min, as a peak distinct from the albumin hydrolysis products which emerged earlier.

The 6-aminonicotine content of the hydrolysates was estimated by means of peak height at 240 nm and/or 294 nm with no essential difference between the two values. Based on an assigned molecular weight of 60 000 for bovine serum albumin, the hydrolysate from the conjugate used in the preparation of the antibodies contained 4.39 mol of 6-aminonicotine per mol of albumin.

Immunogens used were 6-(ε-aminocapramido)-D-(R,S)-L-nicotine–BSA in the goat and 6-(*p*-aminobenzamido)-D ,L-nicotine–BSA in the rabbit. Antiserum used consisted of 0.1 ml/tube of a 40-fold dilution in rabbit antiserum and of a 1000-fold dilution in goat antiserum. Radioimmunoassay was carried out using the charcoal precipitation method as described previously (Castro *et al.*, 1979). When a 1 h incubation time for antibody and antigen interaction was employed, antibody specificities in both species, as examined by the same EIA method and by the automated Centria system which uses Sephadex G-25 for separation of bound and unbound tracer, were similar to the 24 h values. Tracer binding to antibody in the absence of inhibitor in both species with that incubation time was about 20% of the total added.

Immunization

Rabbits were immunized intradermally (in foot pads or in the back), intramuscularly or subcutaneously. A reasonable titre of antibody (1:400) was obtained after 12 weeks.

Preparation of β-Galactosidase Nicotine Conjugate

This method has two parts as described below.

Preparation of M-Maleimidobenzoyl Derivative of 6-(4-Aminobenzamido) Nicotine (II)

Preparations of 3-maleimidobenzoic acid and its carbonyl chloride (**I**) have been described previously (Monji *et al.*, 1978): dissolve 100 mg **I** in 1 ml tetrahydrofuran (THF) and add it to 2 ml THF solution containing 50 mg 6-(4-aminobenzamido)nicotine and a slurry of 10 mg Na_2CO_3; reflux the mixture for 30 min; separate the product by silica-gel chromatography, using chloroform as an eluting solvent.

Conjugation of II with β-Galactosidase

Dissolve 0.5 mg (400 U) β-galactosidase in 1 ml phosphate-buffered saline (Castro and Monji, 1981); add 50 µl THF containing 29 µg **II**; incubate at room temperature for 60 min; dialyse for 24 h at 4°C against the same buffer to remove excess unreacted **II**; apply to a Sephadex G-25 column (10 mm x 400 mm) to remove residual, unreacted **II**; collect the fractions containing the major enzyme activity; add NaN_3 and BSA to 0.1% and, after dividing the solution into 100 µl aliquots, store at −18°C (once a frozen aliquot has been thawed, do not refreeze).

Nicotine Assay

This assay employs competitive binding of nicotine and nicotine–enzyme conjugate to anti-nicotine antiserum. A double antibody method was used for separation of bound from free conjugate. To a polyethylene tube (10 mm × 75 mm) 100 μl of a 100-fold dilution of the peak fraction of nicotine–enzyme conjugate eluted from Sephadex G-25 column was added, followed by addition of 50 μl of the phosphate buffer (pH 7.0, 0.15 M). Fifty millilitres of nicotine standard (0–200 μg/100 ml) was then added and, following brief mixing, 100 μl of 400-fold dilution of rabbit anti-nicotine antiserum was added, vortexed and then incubated for 45 min at room temperature. After incubation, 100 μl of a 20-fold dilution of normal rabbit serum was added, followed by addition of 100 μl of goat anti-rabbit IgG (10-fold dilution). After vortex mixing, the tube was incubated for 15 min in ice and centrifuged for 10 min at 3000 rpm. The pellet was washed twice with phosphate buffer and resuspended in 0.5 ml phosphate buffer–BSA (pH 7.5, 0.05 M, 0.1% BSA). The enzyme activity was assayed using o-nitrophenyl-β-D-galactoside or 4-methylumberlliferyl-β-D-galactoside. The incubation time for the enzyme reaction was 60 min. The amount of o-nitrophenol produced at the end of the incubation time was measured by a Gilford Stasar III spectrophotometer at 420 nm wavelength. In case of umbelliferon being produced, the amount of fluorescent compound is measured by a fluorescence spectrophotometer using 360 nm for excitation and 450 nm for emission.

Calibration Curve

The measuring unit is the change in fluorescence intensity per 60 min, $\Delta F/\Delta t$. If $\Delta F_0/\Delta t$ is obtained at zero nicotine concentration, the ratio $(\Delta F/\Delta t)/(\Delta F_0/\Delta t) = \Delta F/\Delta F_0$ corresponds to the nicotine concentration expressed in μg per litre. Plot $\Delta F/\Delta F_0$ as a percentage *vs.* nicotine concentration.

RESULTS AND DISCUSSION

Suitability of 6-Aminonicotine as a Functionalized Hapten

The present study has provided an opportunity to extend, confirm and/or reject some conclusions reached by previous investigators who employed 6-aminonicotine to produce nicotine antibodies. One group (Langone *et al.*, 1973) considered 2-aminonicotine and 6-aminonicotine, as obtained by a previous method (Chichibabin and Kirssanov, 1924), to be racemic and therefore unsuitable for nicotine antibody production; this has been confirmed (Haines *et al.*, 1974). Others have reported utilization of racemic 6-aminonicotine in antibody production, but with limited information on cross-reactions of the nicotine antibody.

Racemic 6-aminonicotine has been satisfactorily employed as the *p*-aminobenzoyl derivative in production of antisera (Matsushita *et al.*, 1974), which was highly specific for (S)-nicotine, the major nicotine enantiomer in tobacco and tobacco smoke. Cross-reaction to (R)-nicotine was 5%, satisfactory for many practical applications.

The racemic nature of the diazotized *p*-aminobenzoyl 6-aminonicotine (coupled with bovine serum albumin) is also well established (Yi *et al.*, 1977); possible contributions of imino forms of the compound and other structural features are being studied. It appears that the preference of the antibody may result from selective coupling of one of the 6-aminonicotine optical antipodes with bovine serum albumin. This could result in an antigen with a predominant (S)-nicotine configuration. Alternatively, an antigen with (R,S)-nicotine configuration is formed, and the optical specificity of the resultant nicotine is a manifestation of selective biological processes on the resultant intermediate components of the immune system or is derived from the general chirality which characterizes all antibodies to some degree. However, under some conditions of antibody production, with a single optical isomer of 6-aminonicotine as a functionalized hapten, the optical specificity of the nicotine antibody or antibodies could be enhanced. An interesting example of this type of enhancement by utilization of a single antipode is seen in the production of optically stereospecific antibodies for the simultaneous assay of *d*- and *l*-propranolol (Burrows *et al.*, 1970).

Cross-reaction of Nicotine Antibodies

It has been pointed out (Langone *et al.*, 1973) that when nicotine antibodies were prepared with these racemic functionalized nicotine haptens, there was strong cross-reaction with *N*-methylpyrrolidine, a constituent of tobacco smoke. We have prepared nicotine antibodies with racemic forms of both 2-aminonicotine and 6-aminonicotine by coupling bovine serum albumin via a diazonium reaction of the corresponding *p*-aminobenzoyl derivatives; however, only the antibodies from the 6-amino compound have been extensively studied (Table 1). Only a limited cross-reaction with *N*-methylpyrrolidine was noted. In contrast, a 100% value (equal affinity for nicotine and *N*-methylpyrrolidine) has been reported with an antibody derived from antigen prepared by coupling with 2-aminonicotine.

Precision, Accuracy, Detection Limit and Sensitivity

The relative standard deviation (RSD) at each point of the calibration curve, assayed in triplicate, is less than 8%. The between-days RSD is about 9%. In recovery experiments, 20, 30, 40 and 50 µg nicotine per litre of pooled plasma

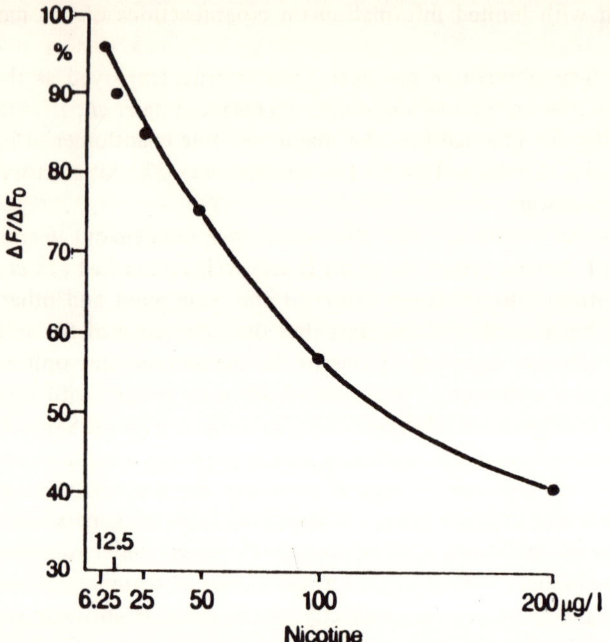

Figure 1   Standard curve of nicotine.

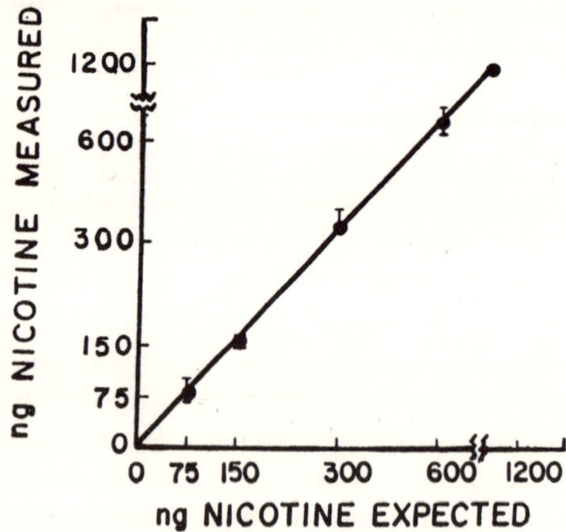

Figure 2   Recovery studies of nicotine in pooled plasma; assays in triplicate.

was prepared and analysed by EIA. The correlation coefficient of found *vs.* expected values was 0.994 (figures 1 and 2). The sensitivity limit, defined as the concentration of nicotine measured at $\Delta F/\Delta F_0 = 90\%$, was found to be 10 µg/l. Since nicotine is a volatile and easily oxidized compound, it is important to process the sample as quickly as possible. Plasma samples must be frozen as quickly as possible so as to ensure the stability of nicotine.

Specificity

Assay specificity is dependent on the antiserum used and the hapten analogue employed for the enzyme–conjugate preparation. In this assay, cross-reactivity (as determined by the same procedure used for nicotine RIA (Castro *et al.*, 1980) was 0.8% for (S)-nornicotine, about 0.1% for (S)-nicotine-N'-oxide, and less than 0.1% for (S)-cotinine, N-methylpyrrolidine and (S)-continine-N-oxide.

The enzyme we chose, β-galactosidase, is not found in human serum. In addition, the coupling procedure is simple and efficient, and conjugate prepared more than 8 months previously continued to remain stable.

Precision studies indicate that good precison can be obtained, both within run (CV = 5.7%) and day to day (CV = 7.9%). Results by our method also correlate well with those by radioimmunoassay. We determined the maximum sensitivity of this assay to be 6 μg/l.

Enzyme activities examined before and after the conjugation step did not show any difference, suggesting full retention of the enzyme functional groups. With the final antiserum dilution of 400-fold, a reproducible nicotine enzyme immunoassay was successfully demonstrated. Incubation times of the assay were 60 and 15 min respectively for competitive binding of nicotine and nicotine antibody enzyme. The highest sensitivity in the assay was observed at 6–25 μg/l. Plasma concentrations of nicotine after smoking vary, depending on whether the subject is a smoker or non-smoker, and inhaler or non-inhaler. Nicotine levels in human smokers (N = 9) after one cigarette range from 50–100 μg/l at 3 min after smoking to 30–60 μg/l at 15 min after smoking.

Blanks and Standard Curve

Blanks

Distilled water and pooled nicotine-free serum from men were used as blanks in tubes not coated with antibody. These blanks showed no detectable enzyme activity.

Standard curve

This standard curve (figure 1) demonstrates the proportional displacement of conjugate by unlabelled nicotine over the concentration range used, 6–200 μg/l.

Analytical Variables

Sensitivity

In the standard curve plotted with each run, the percentage bound for 6 μg/l differed significantly at the 95% confidence level from that for 0.0 mg of nicotine per litre.

Precision

The coefficient of variation for one sample assayed 10 times on the same day was 5.7%, with $\bar{x} = 5.6$ mg/l. The coefficient of variation for nine samples assayed on five different days was 7.9%, the concentration range being from 3.5 to 9.0 mg/l.

Parallelism

We studied parallelism in samples of high nicotine concentration. The samples were diluted 1.5-, 2-, 3-, 6- and 10-fold, in normal nicotine containing serum from men, to study the behaviour of the antibody in comparison with a standard curve. A plot of the observed absorbance *vs*. expected serum concentration paralleled the standard curve. This indicates that the antibody was only binding with nicotine.

We believe this enzyme immunoassay technique represents an improvement over previously reported radioimmunoassay methods.

ACKNOWLEDGEMENTS

This research was supported in part by Grant number 884 from the Council for Tobacco Research, U.S.A., Inc.

Heartfelt thanks go to Richard E. Bailey, M.D., A.C.'s teacher and mentor for many years, for his dedication and patience in supporting his work as a scientist.

REFERENCES

Abraham, G. E. (1969). Solid phase radioimmunoassay of estradiol. *J. Clin. Endocr. & Metab.*, **29**, 866–870

Armitage, A. K. (1975). Nicotine levels in serum after cigar smoking. In *Symposium on Nicotine and Carbon Monoxide*, University of Kentucky, Lexington, KY, 52

Burrows, I. E., Corp, P. J. and Jackson, G. C. (1970). Optical stereospecific antibody production. *Analyst*, **95**, 85–91

Castro, A. and Monji, N. (1981). Steric hindrance enzyme immunoassay (SHEIA) using β-galactosidase as an enzyme label and maleimide derivative of hapten for enzyme coupling. In Langone, J. J. and Vanvenukas, H. (eds.), *Methods of Enzymology*, New York, 523–542

Castro, A., Monji, N., Ali, H., Bowman, E. R. and McKennis, Jr., H. (1985). Comparative studies of procedures for the detection of nicotine in biological material. *Biochem. Arch.*, **1**, 173–177

Castro, A., Monji, N., Ali, H., Vi, J. M., Bowman, E. R. and McKennis, Jr., H. (1980). Nicotine antibodies: comparison of ligand specificities of antibodies produced against two nicotine conjugates. *Eur. J. Biochem.*, **104**, 331–340

Castro, A., Monji, N., Malkus, H., Eisenhart, W., McKennis, Jr., H. and Bowman, E. R. (1979). Automated radioimmunoassay of nicotine. *Clin. Chim. Acta*, **95**, 473–481

Castro, A. and Prieto, I. (1975). Nicotine antibody production: comparison of two nicotine conjugates in different animal species. *Biochem. Biophys. Res. Comm.*, **67**, 583–589

Chichibabin, A. E. and Kirssanov, A. V. (1924). Amination of nicotine with sodium and potassium amide. *Cher. Ber.*, **57B**, 1163–1168

Dagne, E. and Castagnoli, Jr., N. (1972). Cotinine N-oxide, a new metabolite of nicotine. *J. Med. Cher.*, **15**, 840–841

Haines, C. F., Mahajam, D. K., Miljkovic, D., Miljkovic, A. and Vesell, E. S. (1974). Radioimmunoassay of plasma nicotine in habituated and naive smokers. *Clin. Pharm. Therap.*, **16**, 1083–1089

Horning, E. C., Horning, M. G., Carroll, D. I., Stillwell, R. N. and Dzidic, I. (1973). Nicotine in smokers, non-smokers and room air. *Life Sci.*, **13**, 1331–1346

Isaac, P. F. and Rand, M. J. (1972). Cigarette smoking and plasma levels of nicotine. *Nature*, **236**, 308–310

Jarwick, M. E. (1977). Research on smoking behaviour. In Harvich, M., Cullen, J., Britz, E., Vogt, T., West, L. (eds.), *U.S. Government Printing Office Publication 122*, Washington, DC

Langone, J. L., Gjika, H. B. and Van Vunakis, H. (1973). Nicotine and its metabolites. Radioimmunoassays for nicotine and cotinine. *Biochemistry*, **12**, 5025–5030

McKennis, Jr., H. (1965). Nicotine metabolism. In von Euler, U. S. (ed.), *Tobacco Alkaloids and Related Compounds*, Pergamon Press, 98–105

McNiven, N. L., Raisinghani, K. H., Patashnik, S. and Dorfman, R. (1965). Determination of nicotine in smokers' urine by gas chromatography. *Nature*, **208**, 788–789

Matsukura, S., Sakamoto, N., Imura, H., Matsuyoma, H., Tomoda, T., Ishigura, T. and Muranaka, H. (1974). Radioimmunoassay of nicotine. *Biochem. Biophys. Res. Comm.*, **64**, 574–586

Matsushita, H., Noguchi, M. and Tamaki, E. (1974). Conjugate of bovine serum albumin with nicotine. *Biochem. Biophys. Res. Comm.*, **57**, 1006–1010

Monji, N., Malkus, H. and Castro, A. (1978). Maleimide derivative of hapten for coupling to enzyme: a new method in enzyme immunology. *Biochem. Biophys. Res. Comm.*, **85**, 671–675

Pilotti, A. (1975). Nicotine and its metabolites: Analysis by gas chromatography. In *Symposium on Nicotine and Carbon Monoxide*, University of Kentucky, Lexington, KY

Pilotti, A., Enzell, C. R., McKennis, Jr., H., Bowman, E. R., Dutva, E. and Holmstedt, B. (1976). Routes in the metabolism of nicotine. *Beitr. Tabakforsch.*, **6**, 339–344

Turner, D. M. (1969). The metabolism of ^{14}C nicotine in the cat. *Biochem. J.*, **115**, 889–896

von Euler, U. S., Haglid, F., Hedquist, F. and Motelica, I. (1970). Neurotransmitter releasing effects of two quaternary nicotine analogues. *Acta Physiol. Scand.*, **78**, 123–131

Wilson, K. K., Chang, R. S., Bowman, E. R. and McKennis, Jr., H. (1976).

Nicotine-like actions of cis-metanicotine and trans-metanicotine. *J. Pharm. Exp. Ther.*, **196**, 685–695
Yi, J. M., McKennis, J. S., Bowman, E. R. and McKennis, Jr., H. (1977). Diazotization of *p*-aminobenzoyl 6-aminonicotine-BSA. *Va. J. Sci.*, **28**, 85–94

6. Applications of Human Monoclonal Antibodies in Non-isotopic Immunoassays

S. A. GAFFAR AND M. C GLASSY

INTRODUCTION

The specificity of antigen–antibody interaction is the basis for all types of immunoassays (IAs) used in determinations of chemical, biological and pharmaceutical compounds. In all these IAs, a variety of fluorophores (Coons *et al.*, 1941; Soini and Hemmila, 1979), luminescent compounds (Hersh *et al.*, 1979), radioisotopes (Berson and Yalow, 1957), and enzymes (Avrameas, 1969), are chemically conjugated to either antibodies or antigens. The conjugation reaction between the tracer compound and the antibody or the antigen is performed in such a manner that the resulting complex retains the functions of both reactants.

One of the best established detection and diagnostic methods in many clinical and research laboratories is immunofluorescence (Coons *et al.*, 1941); in this technique, a fluorescent dye is conjugated to an antibody, which is then used in tissue staining. However, this assay is laborious and the results are subjective. Highly sensitive and reproducible radioimmunoassays (Berson and Yalow, 1957) are routinely used in many laboratories, but this technology requires costly reagents, complex monitoring equipment and special safety measures in the handling and disposal of radioactive waste. Therefore, many laboratories in both developed and developing countries are unable to perform such assays. An alternative to isotopic IAs, but with a similar high degree of sensitivity, is the enzyme immunoassay (EIA) (Nakane and Pierce, 1967), in which an enzyme is conjugated to either antibody or antigen, which is then used in the assay. Enzymes, among the many available tracer compounds, deserve a special place because of their long shelf life, safety to health and inexpensive instruments required for monitoring their products. All the above-mentioned features of enzymes have contributed to development of numerous EIAs used for the detection and quantitation of a number of biochemical molecules in a variety of samples.

Hybridoma technology (Kohler and Milstein, 1975) has also contributed to the widespread use of EIAs in several laboratories around the world. By mass culturing the hybridomas, large quantities of monoclonal antibodies (MoAbs) can be produced indefinitely. The MoAbs, secreted by the hybridoma cells into the growth medium, are purified and tagged with enzymes for use in the EIAs. Modifications in these assays to increase their sensitivity and suitability have resulted in a variety of EIAs with novel variations. One example is the enzyme immunofiltration assay (EIFA) (Cleveland *et al.*, 1979; Glassy and Cleveland, 1986). A general scheme of these IAs is shown in figure 1. The aims of this Chapter are (a) to provide brief information on the various non-isotopic IAs mentioned in figure 1 and (b) to give a detailed account of those IAs which we use in our own laboratory.

GENERAL ACCOUNT OF IMMUNOASSAYS

IAs are direct or indirect, depending on the type of immune conjugates employed. In the direct IA, a tracer molecule is coupled straight to the test antibody. However, even though the direct IA eliminates the background problem, it is not

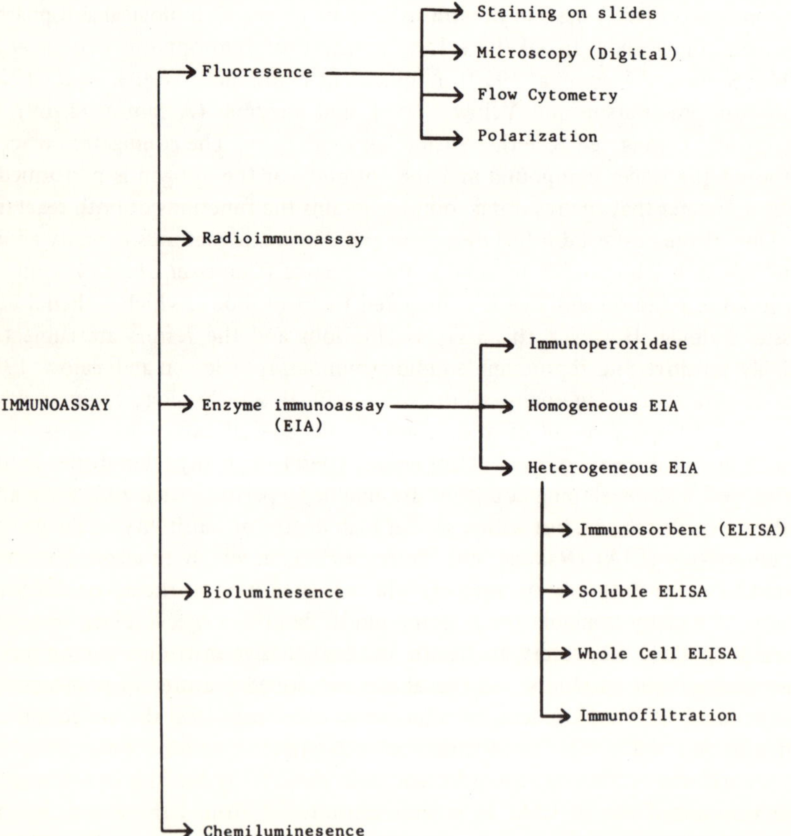

Figure 1   A general scheme of immunoassays.

practical to purify every antibody and tag it with an enzyme or a fluorophore. In the indirect IA, the unaltered test antibody is first reacted with the antigen. This is followed by the addition of an immune conjugate, such as antibody-enzyme or protein A–enzyme, which reacts with the test antibody. The major advantage of the indirect IA is that it permits the testing of crude test antibody preparations.

Fluorescence Polarization

Fluorescence polarization (FP) provides a sensitive means of assessing an antigen concentration in a given test sample. This technique, which is based on the Brownian motion of a molecule in a solution, is simple in procedure but compli-cated in theory (Einstein, 1906; Weber, 1952; Danliker *et al.*, 1980; Spencer, 1973). It is known that at a given temperature and viscosity, a small molecule such as a drug has rapid rotation, while a large molecule such as the antibody has slow free rotation because of the size-dependent frictional drag. However, the small drug molecule, after combining with the antibody, adopts the slow rotation of the large molecule. Therefore, by attaching a small fluorophore molecule such as dansyl chloride (Weber, 1952) or fluorescein isothiocyanate (Weiel and Hershey, 1981) to the drug, the change in the Brownian rotation of the hapten can be precisely and sensitively detected by measuring the depolarization of the light emitted by the fluorophore following excitation with polarized light. This principle of FP is used in many fluoroimmunoassays, where an unlabelled antigen or hapten competes with a fluorophore-labelled antigen or hapten for the binding site of an antibody. In such competition, the FP values drop; this decrease in the values is directly dependent on the amount of unlabelled molecule. Concen-trations of gentamicin (Watson *et al.*, 1976), phenytoin (McGregor *et al.*, 1978), insulin (Spencer *et al.*, 1973) and angiotensin (Maeda *et al.*, 1979) have been determined by this technique, and the results are comparable in sensitivity with those of gas-liquid chromatography.

Digital Fluorescence Microscopy

Digital fluorescence microscopy (DFM), unlike FP, is primarily used for the study of biological phenomena, either on or in living cells, and over extended periods of time. The important point is that DFM experiments can be carried out without disturbing the vital activities of the cells under study (Reynolds, 1972; Plant *et al.*, 1985). In this technique, a data-acquisition system comprising a frame rate video digitizer, a microcomputer and a sensitive video camera, is combined with a fluorescence microscope in order to convert visual information into quantitative image data. In other words, with DFM it is possible to say, not only that point x is brighter than point y but also to state quantitatively how much brighter it is.

One of the useful applications of DFM is for the study of the changing distribution of protein components on the cell membrane (Kaptiza *et al.*, 1985). For example, the distribution of cell membrane proteins changes during the locomotion of a cell (Bretscher, 1984). Using DFM and monoclonal antibodies conjugated with rhodamine, the distribution of a major glycoprotein (GP-80) of the membrane was elucidated during the locomotion of fibroblasts (DiGuiseppi *et al.*, 1985). These studies also showed that the protein GP-80 distributes in a gradient from the leading edge to the trailing edge of the fibroblasts during locomotion; however, this gradient ceases when the cell stops moving. By taking values at different points of the profiles of the original image, and by comparing these values with those generated by theoretical gradients, the concentration gradient of the GP-80 protein on the membrane is thereby expressed.

Flow Cytometry

Flow cytometry generally requires two steps for the detection and quantitation of an antigen or antibody in a given solution. In the first non-immunological step, antigens are adsorbed on to non-fluorescing clear polystyrene microspheres of uniform size (14 or 20 μm) (Bloch *et al.*, 1983). In the second step, these beads (after adsorbing with the protein antigens) are first washed and then reacted with fluorescein-conjugated antibodies. These microspheres, after washing free from the unbound fluorescein–antibody conjugates, are pumped through a fine capillary tube as a jet stream. On its way, this jet stream containing the plastic beads as a string is made to pass through an argon ion laser light beam for the simultaneous measurements of the intensity of the emitted fluorescent light and particle size. These instruments, depending on design and sophistication, can read up to 50 000 microspheres per minute and detect as few as 3000 fluorescein molecules per bead.

A useful additional feature of flow cytometry is the sorting of cells which are phenotypically closely related but functionally different. For the purpose of sorting, the cells are adsorbed first on to the beads and then pumped through the fine capillary tube of the flow cytometer. The resulting microsphere droplets that constitute the jet stream are electrostatically charged either positive or negative. These particles are then passed through a pair of charged deflection plates, which cause the positively or negatively charged droplets to deflect away either to the left or to the right, while the uncharged droplets fall in between. All three kinds of beads are then collected in different beakers for further analysis and clonal expansion of the separated cells.

Chemiluminescent Immunoassays

Chemiluminescent IAs, in contrast to the complexity and novelty of the above-described fluorescein-ligand-based assay methods, are simple and straightforward. These reactions are generally used in spectrophotometric methods to increase the assay sensitivity by a factor of 1000–2500. By combining these luminescence reactions with the EIAs, a similar degree of sensitivity is achieved. Bioluminescence, a natural phenomenon occurring in fireflies and certain bacteria, is a variation of chemiluminescence. All these reactions generally require an enzyme and a luminescent substrate such as luminol, luciferin or lucigenin. Among these compounds, luminol is the most efficient luminescent material. Estimations of IgG (Simpson *et al.*, 1979), biotin (Schroeder *et al.*, 1976) and testosterone (Pratt *et al.*, 1978) have been carried out by using luminol–hapten or luminol–antigen conjugates in a chemiluminescent IA.

Among the chemiluminescent IAs, the bioluminescence reaction of the firefly has been extensively studied (DeLuca, 1978). This particular reaction of the firefly requires luciferin, luciferase, adenosine triphosphate and Mg^{2+}; the reaction is optimally carried out at pH 7.8 in glycine buffer at room temperature. The bacterial bioluminescence reaction (DeLuca, 1978), unlike that of the firefly, requires reduced flavin mononucleotide, molecular oxygen, a long-chain aldehyde and luciferase from the luminescing bacteria. All these bioluminescent EIAs are extremely sensitive; some of these assays have been used for the estimation of steroids (Kohen *et al.*, 1979) present in serum, plasma and urine.

Other Immunoassays

Immunofluorescence, enzyme-linked immunosorbant assay (ELISA) and EIFA are routinely used in our laboratory for the detection of human tumour antigens with human anti-cancer MoAbs. The procedures and results of these IAs, including the methods of human–human hybridoma and MoAbs production, are described below.

HUMAN–HUMAN HYBRIDOMAS

The procedure for generating human–human hybridomas secreting tumour reactive MoAbs has been described in detail elsewhere (Glassy *et al.*, 1983b). In brief, B lymphocytes, isolated from regional-draining lymph nodes of cancerous tissues, were fused with UC 729-6, a diploid, 6-thioguanine resistant human lymphoblastoid B cell line. This cell mixture was gently suspended in a selected growth medium and plated onto 96-well microtitre plates. Supernatants containing immunoglobulins obtained after 2–4 weeks growth of the hybrids were screened for immunoreactivity by a whole-cell ELISA (see below). The hybridomas secreting anti-tumour MoAbs were isolated by limiting dilution and studied for their phenotypic as well as karyotypic characteristics (Glassy *et al.*, 1985). Vulva lymph node (VLN) 5C7, one of the hybridomas used in this study, secretes A431 reactive IgG and non-reactive IgM similar to another hybridoma called VLN3G2 (Glassy, 1987). The VLN5C7 hybridoma, as well as other hybridomas isolated from the same fusion, has been stable for over 1 year in culture.

HUMAN MONOCLONAL ANTIBODIES

Our human hybridomas (e.g. VLN5C7) were grown in RPMI-1640 medium with 10% FCS (GIBCO, Chagrin Falls, OH) and incubated at 37°C in a humidified incubator containing 5% CO_2–95% air. These cultures were harvested by centrifugation after 4 days of continuous growth, and the supernatants containing microgram to milligram quantities of the MoAbs were pooled and concentrated in a dialysis bag surrounded by aquacide. Any insoluble precipitate formed during the concentration of the spent medium was removed by centrifugation and the clear supernatant was fractionated on a Sephadex G-200 gel column. Fractions collected from the column were analyzed by ELISAs for antibody

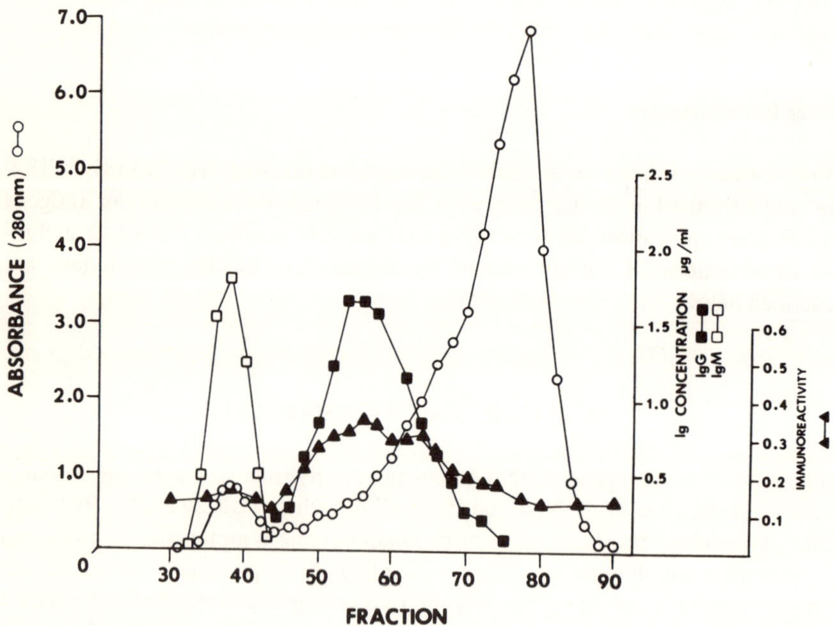

Figure 2   Sephadex G-200 gel column chromatography of VLN5C7 hybridoma supernatant. 200 ml of the culture supernatant were concentrated to 10 ml, loaded onto a column (2.5 cm × 50 cm; void volume 73 ml) and eluted with PBS collecting fractions of 2.3 ml at 4°. These fractions were read for absorbance at 280 nm (○—○), assayed by ELISAs to determine the concentrations of both IgG (■—■) and IgM (□—□), and screened for immunoreactivity of IgG against the target A431 tumour cell line (▲—▲).

concentration and immunoreactivity against the antigens of the target tumour cells (see below). A typical elution profile of the spent medium containing the MoAbs of VLN5C7 is shown in figure 2.

IMMUNOFLUORESCENCE

Immunofluorescence has been widely used for the elucidation of cell surface biology and chemistry. In this technique, successful detection of an antigen, by using its antibody, requires exploration of several parameters, such as stability, availability and nature of the antigen. In direct as well as indirect immuno-fluorescence, antigens bound to the antibodies are easily detected by means of the fluorescence emitted from the antibody–fluorophore conjugates when observed under a fluorescence microscope. A simple and novel technique used in our laboratory for preparing slides prior to the immunofluorescence proce-dure involved in the staining of tumour cell antigens (Glassy and Gaffar, 1987) is described below.

Reagents

(1) *Phosphate-buffered saline (PBS)*: monobasic (1.14 g) and dibasic (2.16 g) sodium phosphate salts and 8.0 g of sodium chloride were dissolved in 1000 ml of distilled water, and the pH was adjusted to 7.4.

(2) *Glycerol*: analytical grade glycerol was dissolved in the PBS (50% v/v).

(3) *FCS buffer*: 10 ml of FCS were mixed with 90 ml of the gelatin buffer containing 0.04% sodium azide.

(4) *Gelatin buffer*: 10 g of gelatin were dissolved in 100 ml of PBS containing 1 g of thiomersal as preservative.

(5) *Human IgG*: purified lyophilized polyclonal human IgG (ICN, Cleveland, OH) was dissolved in PBS at 2 mg/ml concentration and used to stain the control slides.

(6) *Fluorescein–antibody conjugates*: goat anti-human IgG or IgM antibodies conjugated to fluorescein isothiocyanate (Tago, Burlingame, CA) were diluted in FCS buffer before use in immunofluorescence staining.

Tumour Cells

The human cell line A431 (a carcinoma of the vulva) was used as the antigen-positive target cells in this assay. These cells were grown in T-75 culture flasks (Costar, Cambridge, MA), containing RPMI-1640 medium supplied with 10% FCS (v/v), and the culture was incubated for 4 days at 37°C in a humidified incubator containing 5% CO_2 in air.

Preparation of Slides

Antigen positive A431 cells were grown in plastic Petri dishes (Costar) or flat-bottom tissue culture flasks containing RPMI-1640 media. After 4 days of growth, when the cells were in the mid-logarithmic phase, the spent media containing any floating cells were removed and the adherent cells were washed with PBS. Slides with the attached tumour cells were prepared by cutting the bottom of the culture dish or flask into slides of size 4 cm × 2 cm with a heated scalpel. This procedure is shown schematically in figure 3.

Immunofluorescence Staining

After adding the MoAbs to the cells, the slides were incubated for 30 min at 4°C and washed with PBS to remove any of the unreacted proteins. The cells were then combined with 100 μl of a 1:20 diluted goat anti-human IgG conju-

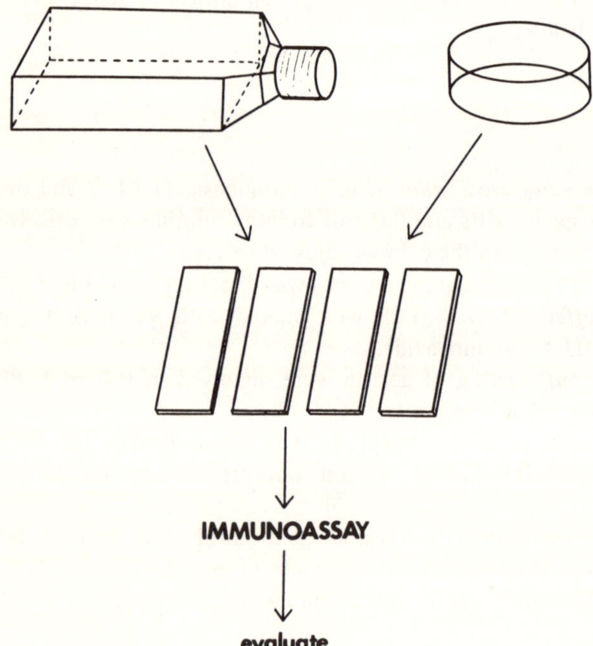

Figure 3   A simple method of preparing slides useful for the immunofluorescence staining of tumour antigens. A431 tumour cells, grown to confluency in either a clear plastic tissue culture flask or a culture dish, were washed with PBS and cut into slides with a heated scalpel. After incubating these cells with VLN5C7 IgG antibodies followed by FITC-goat anti-human IgG antibodies, a coverslip was mounted and the slide was evaluated for immunofluorescence under a fluorescence microscope.

gated to fluorescein isothiocyanate and incubated in the dark for 30 min at 4°C, washed three times with PBS, air dried, and finally mounted with a coverslip and 50% glycerol. Cells treated similarly with an irrelevant human IgG at protein concentrations equivalent to that of MoAbs were used as controls. Immuno-fluorescence of the cells was evaluated under a fluorescence microscope. Shown in figure 4 are immunofluorescence photographs of a human colon tumour grown in an athymic mouse, sectioned, and stained with either VLN5C7 (figure 4A) or an irrelevant IgG control (figure 4B).

ENZYME IMMUNOASSAYS

Enzyme immunoassays, which have made hybridoma technology a practical reality, are broadly divided into homogeneous and heterogeneous assays. Homogeneous EIAs are mostly used for the study of small molecular weight substances such as drugs (Rubenstein *et al.*, 1972). In these assays, a hapten molecule is chemically conjugated to an enzyme in such a manner that the enzyme retains its catalytic activity. However, when the ligand combines with the antibody, the enzyme loses its biological function as a result of either steric hindrance or change in conformation. In such an assay, if the test sample contains a very small amount of the competing hapten, most of the ligand–enzyme complexes bind to the antibodies, resulting in the inactivation of the enzyme molecules. This leaves the substrate of the enzyme in the assay undegraded. If, however, the test material contains a large amount of hapten, most of the ligand–enzyme complexes are displaced from binding to the antibodies, which then convert a disproportionally large amount of the substrate in the assay. Therefore, the essence of these homogeneous EIAs is that they do not require separation of the unbound enzyme–hapten conjugates from those combined with the antibodies.

Although heterogeneous EIAs possess assay principles in common with those of the homogeneous EIAs, they require the separation of free antibody–enzyme conjugates from those combined with the antigens. These heterogeneous EIAs are commonly used in many laboratories for the identification and analysis of antigens. This is facilitated by adsorbing either antigen or antibody onto an insoluble solid phase in such a manner that the immunological reactivity is retained. In our studies of human hybridomas, goat antibodies to human immunoglobulins were adsorbed onto the round-bottom wells of a 96-well micro-titre plate (Glassy *et al.*, 1983a). This type of assay, called soluble ELISA, was used for the quantitation of human IgG and IgM. A second type of assay, termed whole-cell ELISA, was used to determine the immunoreactivity of the anti-tumour human MoAbs (Schroeder *et al.*, 1976). In the whole-cell ELISA the antigen-positive target cells were dried down on the flat-bottom troughs of a 96-well microtitre plate. A general scheme of these two assays is shown in figure 5.

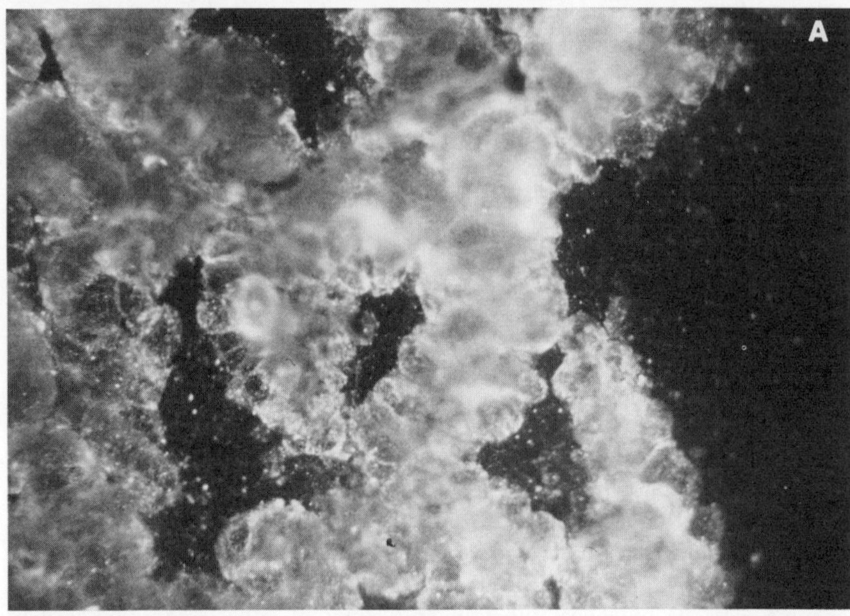

Figure 4 Immunofluorescent staining of human tumour cells with human monoclonal antibody VLN5C7. (A) Adenocarcinoma of the colon grown in an athymic mouse sectioned, and stained with 2 μg/ml VLN5C7. (B) Same as (A) but stained with an irrelevant IgG control.

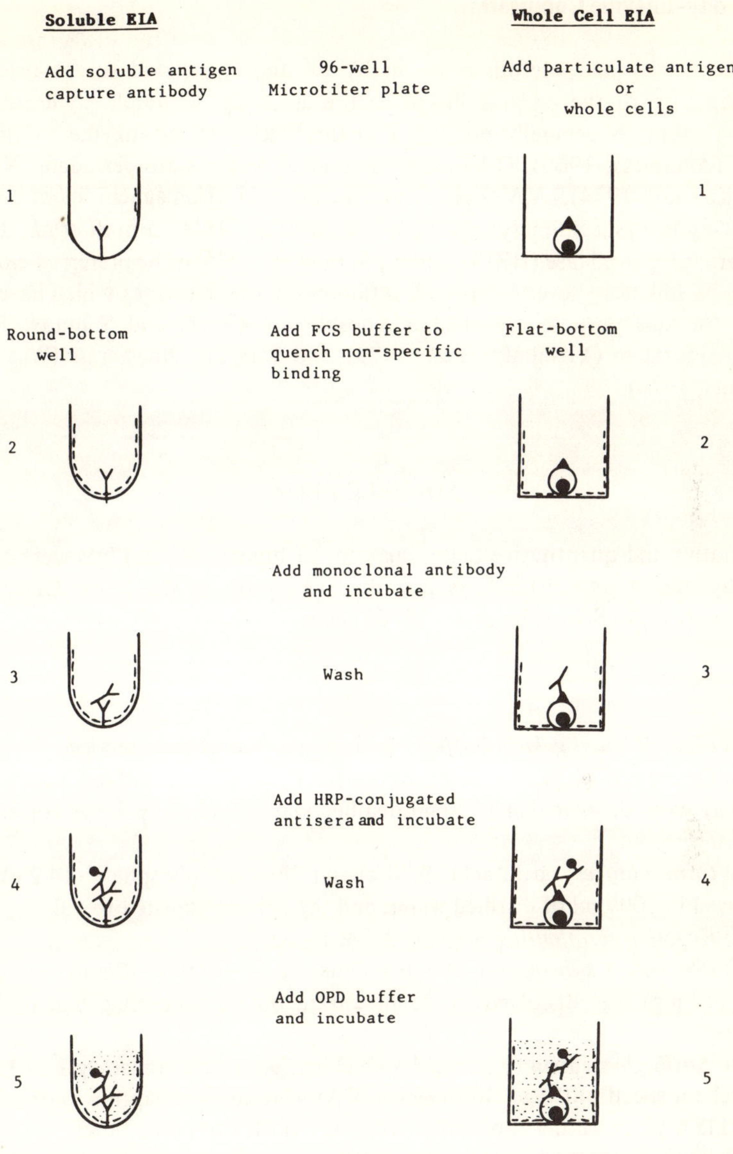

Figure 5 Schematic illustration of soluble and whole-cell ELISAs. In both of these assays, antigens (either soluble or cell bound) were incubated with the immunoreactive VLN5C7 IgG antibodies followed by HRP–goat anti-human IgG antibodies. The assays were then developed by adding the enzyme substrate to the wells of the microtitre plate and the coloured product formed was read at 490 nm.

Antibody–Enzyme Conjugates

The sensitivity and usefulness of an IA are directly related to the reactivity and stability of the enzyme linked to the antibody. Glutaraldehyde, a cross-linking agent, is generally employed in the linking of an enzyme to an antibody (Avrameas, 1969). Other such functional reagents are periodate (Nakane and Kawaoi, 1974), *N,N,O*-phenylenedimaleimide (Hamaguchi *et al.*, 1979) and *N*-hydroxysuccinimidyl ester (Anderson *et al.*, 1960; Smyth *et al.*, 1960). Horseradish peroxidase (HRP) (Voller and Bidwell, 1975) is the preferred enzyme; it can be linked to several types of antibodies. Other enzymes which have been tried for this purpose are alkaline phosphatase (Waart and Schuurs, 1976), β-D-galactosidase (Yoshitake *et al.*, 1979), and acetyl cholinesterase (Waart and Schuurs, 1976).

SOLUBLE ELISA

Qualitative and quantitative determinations of human IgG and IgM were carried out by the soluble ELISA as described (Simpson *et al.*, 1979; Glassy and Cleveland, 1986; Schroeder *et al.*, 1976) below.

Reagents

(1) *PBS, FCS and gelatin buffers*: see Immunofluorescence section.

(2) *Carbonate buffer*: sodium carbonate (1.59 g) and sodium bicarbonate (2.93 g) were dissolved in 1000 ml distilled water, and the pH was adjusted to 9.3.

(3) *Citrate buffer*: citric acid (9.34 g) and disodium phosphate (14.2 g) were dissolved in 1000 ml of distilled water, and the pH was adjusted to 5.0.

(4) *Reaction terminating reagent*: 2.5 M H_2SO_4.

(5) *Peroxidase substrate*: orthophenylene diamine (OPD) (Sigma, St. Louis, MO) (12 mg) was dissolved in 30 ml citrate buffer containing 6 μl of H_2O_2 (Sigma).

(6) *Antibodies*: affinity-purified polyclonal goat anti-human IgG or IgM (γ or μ chain specific) (Tago, Burlingame, CA) were used as capture antibodies in the ELISA after making appropriate dilutions in the carbonate buffer.

(7) *Enzyme–antibody conjugates*: HRP-conjugated goat anti-human IgG or IgM (γ or μ chain specific) (Tago) antibodies were used at calculated dilutions in the ELISAs.

(8) *Human IgG and IgM*: purified polyclonal IgG or IgM (ICN) were serially diluted with the FCS buffer and employed as reference proteins in these assays.

The antibody–enzyme conjugates were stored in concentrated form at 4°C and diluted with the FCS buffer containing no azide immediately before use. The working dilution of the above-mentioned reagent was determined based on the conjugate incubation time and reaction time with the substrate. OPD was prepared as a ten-fold concentrated solution, and 3 ml aliquots of this substrate were frozen in 50 ml tubes. Just prior to use, the required number of tubes containing the frozen OPD were thawed, diluted with citrate buffer and used in the ELISAs.

Preparation of Microtitre Plates

Fifty-microlitre aliquots of a 1:80 diluted goat anti-human IgG or IgM were added to the round bottom troughs of 96-well Immulon I plates (Dynatech, Alexandria, VA) and incubated either overnight at 4°C or for 4 h at 37°C. After incubation, the plates were finger flicked out over a sink to remove the unbound antibodies. This was followed by the addition of 150 μl of FCS buffer per well, and the plates were then reincubated in the cold room, either overnight or until used. For storage up to 30 days, the plates were sealed with plastic sealing devices supplied by the manufacturer.

Assay Procedure

After removing the FCS buffer, 50 μl aliquots of the test samples containing the human IgG and IgM MoAbs, as well as the diluted standard human IgG or IgM, were added to the appropriate wells of capture antibody coated round-bottom microtitre plates and incubated for 30 min at room temperature. These plates were then washed three times with the gelatin buffer. Fifty-microlitre aliquots of the HRP-conjugated antibodies of goat anti-human IgG or IgM, diluted 1:15 000 in the FCS buffer, without azide, were added to the plates and incubated for an additional 30 min. After washing three times with the gelatin buffer, these plates were developed by adding 150 μl of OPD in citrate buffer. The reaction after 30 min of incubation was terminated by the addition of 50 μl of H_2SO_4, and the plates were read at 490 nm. A standard curve was obtained from the titration of human IgG or IgM in the same microtitre plate. Immunoglobulin concentration in the unknown sample was obtained by reading OD_{490} values from the standard curve.

WHOLE-CELL ELISA

A whole-cell solid phase ELISA (Glassy *et al.*, 1983a; Glassy and Cleveland, 1986; Glassy and Surh, 1985) described below was utilized to determine the immunoreactivity of the human MoAbs against the target cell bound antigens.

Reagents

In addition to the reagents described under soluble ELISA, the following reagent is required for the whole-cell ELISA.

(1) *Trypsin solution*: trypsin (Sigma) (0.25 g) and ethylene diamine tetra-acetic acid (Sigma) (0.25 g) were dissolved in PBS, and refrigerated when not used.

Tumour Cells

See Immunofluorescence section.

Cell Preparation

During growth, the A431 cells adhere to the plastic surface of the culture flasks. These cells, when they are in the mid-logarithmic phase, were harvested by trypsinization as described below. One millilitre of the trypsin solution was added to each of the flasks and spread over the cell lawn by tilting the flask from side to side. This was followed by incubation at room temperature for 10–15 min. All the tumour cells released from the substratum were collected, washed three times with PBS, and resuspended in PBS.

Preparation of Microtitre Plates

For testing the immunoreactivity of the human MoAbs, aliquots of 50 μl cell suspension containing 5×10^5 cells per well were added to the troughs of a flat-bottom 96-well microtitre plate (Dynatech) and the plate was gently tapped to coat the bottom of the wells evenly with the cells. These plates were then incubated for 12 h at 37°C in a drying oven for non-specific attachment of the cells to the wells. After incubation, the plates were removed from the oven and 200 μl of FCS buffer was dispensed into each well in order to quench all the remaining non-specific binding sites of the wells. These plates were then either used immediately or sealed with plate-sealing devices for storage at 4°C.

Assay Procedure

The 200 μl of the FCS buffer in the wells of the prepared whole-cell ELISA plates were finger flicked out over a sink. Fifty-microlitre samples of partially purified VLN5C7 IgG MoAbs were added to triplicate wells, incubated for 60 min at room temperature and washed twice. Each wash consisted of adding 300 μl of gelatin buffer, incubating for 1 min, and forcefully flicking out. Each plate was then set at an angle of 45° for 1 min to allow the excess wash medium to pool on one side of the wells and then to be shaken off by flicking the plate. After two such washes 50 μl of HRP-conjugated secondary antibody were added to the appropriate wells and incubated for 45 min at room temperature. The wells were then washed three times as described before; 200 μl of the OPD substrate were then added to each well and incubated in the dark for 30 min at room temperature. Appropriate controls, one with irrelevant IgG and one without the secondary antibody–enzyme conjugates, were included in every plate. The enzyme reactions were stopped by adding 50 μl of 2.5 M H_2SO_4 to each well and the plate was read at 490 nm in a micro ELISA reader.

ENZYME IMMUNOFILTRATION ASSAY

EIFA, which blends the sensitivity of ELISA and the ease of washing, is highly suitable for the rapid detection of soluble, particulate, and cell bound antigens of biological materials (Cleveland *et al.*, 1979; Glassy and Surh, 1985). This assay procedure is similar to that of ELISA, but has variations. A typical EIFA is carried out in two main steps. In the first step, test antigens are immobilized in the wells of a microtitre plate and reacted with the antibody–enzyme conjugates. In the second step, free antibody–enzyme conjugates are separated from those reacted with the adsorbed antigens by suction under vacuum. The reaction is developed by adding the enzyme substrate to the wells, and the product formed is quantitated. Therefore, a method to immobilize antigens and a device to wash and develop the reaction, keeping the plate untouched, are the two important requirements of EIFA.

Antigen Immobilization

Antigens are attached either directly to the inner surface of the troughs or indirectly to the filters which conveniently fit into the wells of the microtitre plates (figure 6). Filters differing in surface area, flow rate and antigen-binding capacity are available in glass fibre, nitrocellulose and polycarbonate, depending on the requirements of the assay. The antigens are held in the wells by the non-specific interactions, irrespective of the method of immobilization.

Filtration Device

The filtration device plays an important role in the success of EIFA. A 96-well standard microtitre plate, modified with a small capillary-type hole in the bottom of each trough, equipped with an outlet to provide uniform suction to all the wells by vacuum, is used as the incubation and filtration device (see figure 6). The inner space of the wells serves as the incubation chamber. The surface tension forces of the liquid prevent reaction fluids from leaking until a vacuum is applied.

Reagents

See ELISA section (gelatin buffer, enzyme conjugates and OPD).

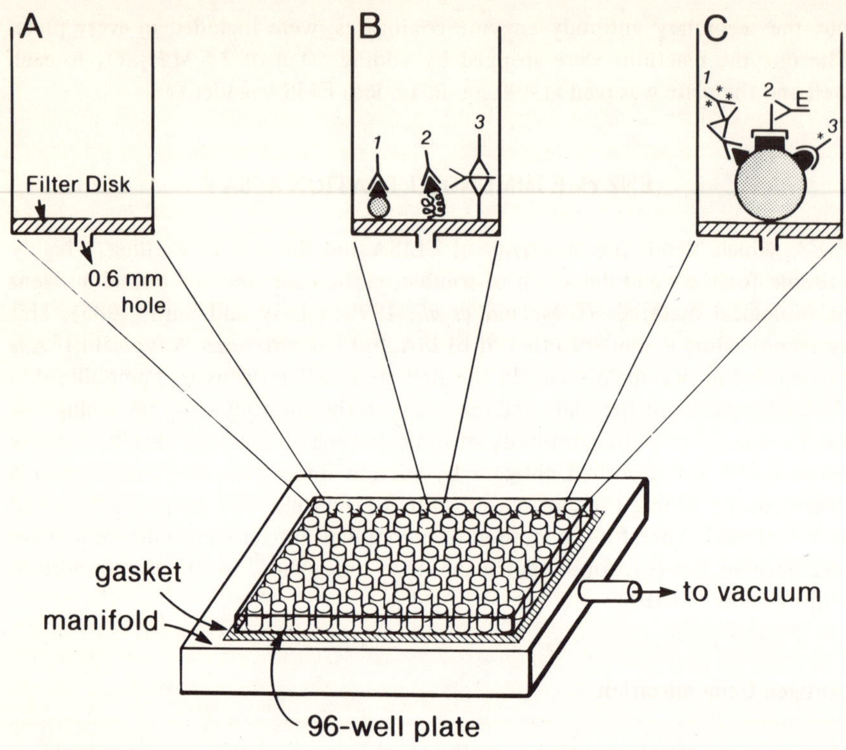

Figure 6 Enzyme immunofiltration manifold and plate. A specially designed 96-well plate (Cleveland *et al.*, 1979) sits on top of a vacuum manifold. (A) The filter disc in each well serves as the solid support for the incubation chamber and the liquid phase is evacuated through the 0.6 mm hole in the bottom. (B) Three types of antigens amenable to EIFA analysis include (1) cell bound or particulate antigens, (2) soluble antigens, such as a protein, and (3) antigens (including MoAbs themselves) captured by immobilizing antibody. (C) Options in immunoassay protocols with MoAbs reactive with a cell-bound antigen. The three types of assays used in conjunction with MoAbs are (1) amplification, such as an additional avidin-biotin or an anti-peroxidase step to boost greatly the signal-to-noise ratio, (2) the indirect type of EIFA which uses an Ig class specific affinity-purified antisera conjugated to an enzyme, such as HRP, and (3) the direct type, in which an enzyme or some other type of chromphore or fluorophore is directly conjugated to the test MoAb.

Procedure and Applications of EIFA

A basic requirement for the success of EIFA is reduction of the non-specific binding of the enzyme-antibody conjugates to either filters or wells of the microtitre plate. Therefore, addition of sufficient amounts of gelatin to the buffer used for the preparation and washing of the plate is essential. Since the reagents and purposes of EIFAs differ from one investigator to another, all experimental conditions such as concentration of reagents, time of coating, temperature, types of buffers and pH are to be standardized independently.

The procedure of EIFA as described below is a general one, but nevertheless applicable to determine the specificity, class and concentration of the MoAbs of any animal species (Glassy and Cleveland, 1986; Cleveland *et al.*, 1981). To each well of a microtitre plate, 50 μl of the test protein solution, for example A431 antigen extract, were applied onto the filter disk and dried under vacuum. The unbound proteins were removed from the filters by washing three times with the gelatin buffer. VLN5C7 IgG antibody was then added in 50 μl amounts to each well, and the plates were incubated for 30 min at room temperature. After washing the plates three times with the gelatin buffer, 50 μl of diluted HRP-conjugated goat anti-human IgG were added to each well and incubated for 30 min. The plate was washed three times to remove the unreacted enzyme-antibody conjugates. After sealing the bottom of the wells with a plate-sealing device to prevent leakage, 250 μl of the OPD solution was added to each well and the reaction was allowed to proceed in the dark. After 30 min of incubation, the reaction was terminated by the addition of 50 μl of 2.5 N H_2SO_4; 150 μl of the reaction product were then transferred from each well to the corresponding round-bottom troughs of a 96-well microtitre plate and the absorbance at 490 nm was recorded. A compilation of EIFA data demonstrating reactivity of a series of human MoAbs with human cell lines is shown in table 1. None of the human MoAbs was reactive with any kind of haemopoietic cell tested. The highest EIFA reactivity was with VLN3G2 and the A431 and T293 cell lines.

A variation of EIFA for the staining of the antigen positive target cells utilizes 3-amino-9-ethyl carbazole (AEC, Sigma) as the substrate of HRP (Glassy and Cleveland, 1986). Unlike OPD, the AEC product, which is red and insoluble, accumulates at the antigen–antibody reaction site on the cells. This type of product deposition on the cells helps antigen detection by means of the naked eye, hand lens or compound microscope.

The detection levels of EIFA can be increased further by using biotinylated-antibody and avidin–HRP conjugates. These reagents in particular decrease incubation time and background staining in the assay.

RESULTS

Harvesting of the VLN5C7 culture by centrifugation was performed after 4 days of growth, when cell viability and antibody secretion were optimal. This hybridoma supernatant was assayed with soluble ELISA and whole-cell ELISA in order to establish Ig concentration and to determine the immunoreactivity of the antibody molecules. Foetal calf serum proteins added to the growth medium showed no cross-reactivity with any of the immunological reagents employed in the assays.

Table 1 EIFA reactivity index with human MoAbs[a]

Cell types		IgM			IgG	
		8A1	CLNH5	MHG7	VLN3G2	VLN3F10
Myeloma:	SKO-007	–	–	–	–	–
	8226	–	–	–	–	–
Lymphoma:	Nalm-6	–	–	–	–	–
	8402	–	–	–	–	–
Leukaemia:	Molt-4	–	–	–	–	–
	CEM	–	–	–	–	–
Melanoma:	M21	–	N.T.	–	2	–
	SK-MEL-28	–	2	N.T.	1–2	–
Colon:	HT-29	–	–	–	1–2	–
	T-84	N.T.	2	2	3	–
Lung:	T293	–	3–4	2–3	5–6	4
	NCl-69	–	–	–	–	–
	Calu-1	–	2–3	–	3	–
	SK-MES-1	–	3	–	–	–
Stomach:	AGS	N.T.	–	–	5	–
	Kato-III	–	1–2	3	3	3
	MKN-74	–	–	–	4	4
	MKN-28	–	–	–	6	–
Prostate:	DU 145	–	–	–	3	–
	PC-3	–	–	2–3	4–5	2–3
	Ln-Cap	–	2–3	3	3	3
Cervix:	Hela	–	4	–	3	–
	CaSki	–	4	–	6	2
Bladder:	T24	–	N.T.	–	4–5	–
	Scaber	–	–	–	2–3	2–3
Kidney:	Caki-2	N.T.	–	–	2	–
Vulva:	A431	–	4	3	6–7	4–5
Fibroblasts:	350Q	–	–	–	1–2	–
	WI-38	–	–	–	–	–
Normal lymphocytes:	PBL	–	–	–	–	–

[a]Cells were used in the EIFA at 2.0×10^5/well. The reactivity index values were calculated from the following formula:

$$\text{reactivity index} = \frac{\text{OD}_{490} \text{ test MoAb} - \text{OD}_{490}, \text{ background}}{\text{OD}_{490}, \text{control MoAb} - \text{OD}_{490}, \text{background}}$$

The values in the table are the reactivity indices based on multiple experiments. The control MoAbs were either an irrelevant affinity-purified human IgG or an IgM. Negatives were unreactive. (N.T., not tested.)

Isolation and Estimation of VLN5C7 IgG

Human hybridoma supernatant was chromatographed on a G-200 gel column to isolate IgG antibodies from IgM and other proteins. Typically, two protein peaks were observed in the chromatographic run of VLN5C7 hybridoma (figure 2).

Proteins in fractions 43–65 of VLN5C7 hybrids reacted with goat anti-human IgG antibodies and also with A431 cell surface antigen(s). Also, higher molecular weight proteins in fractions 30–42 reacted with goat anti-human IgM antibodies but were not immunoreactive with the target cell antigens (data not shown). Both immunoreactivity and IgG antibody elution profile showed complete overlap in the G-200 fractions. Aggregates of IgG or monomers of IgM were not observed in any of the column fractions of VLN5C7.

The detection of tumour antigens by indirect immunofluorescence staining using Sephadex G-200 gel column fractionated VLN5C7 IgG MoAb is shown in figure 4.

Detection of Tumour Antigens by Immunofluorescence

MoAbs were noted to react with cell surface antigens of the A431 cell line, but not with the antigens of the control cell line (figures 2 and 4). Some tumour cells showed intense staining, while others exhibited a discontinuous and speckled nature of the membrane. Immunofluorescence was also associated with several small round vesicles dispersed in the cytoplasm; however, other cell organelles appeared negative. Cells treated with normal IgG showed no staining of either the cell membrane or the organelles.

DISCUSSION

Sephadex G-200 gel columns were used to separate IgG, IgM and other proteins present in VLN5C7 hybridoma supernatants. The void volume fractions of the gel column reacted only with the antibodies to μ chains, suggesting the presence of polymeric IgM, while lack of reactivity in other fractions implied the absence of any monomeric IgM or free μ heavy chains (figure 2). Similarly, reactivity of the column fractions with antibodies to human γ chains was always located in one region of the protein profile of the VLN5C7 hybridoma supernatant (figure 2). Lack of reactivity by proteins in the void volume with antibodies to γ chains indicates absence of aggregates of IgG and lack of hybrid molecules of IgG containing μ chains. Also, the IgG antibodies produced by this hybridoma were reactive with the A431 cell surface antigens. Overlapping peaks of protein concentration, immunoreactivity and corresponding elution volumes of standard IgG confirm the presence of native IgG molecules in these fractions. Although the monoclonal origin of these antibodies argues in favour of all the molecules being immunoreactive, the actual percentage of reactive antibodies was not determined.

The partially purified VLN5C7 IgG antibodies obtained by gel filtration were used to detect antigens on the A431 tumour cell line by immunofluorescence. The method of slide preparation described in figure 3 clearly offers several advantages over the conventional method of preparing slides, using the isolated antigen-positive target cells, one definite advantage being the rapid detection of antigens on the naturally anchored tumour cells. This method also prevents formation of cell clumps and damage to cell membranes or loss of antigen and, in particular, allows antibody to react with antigen without any induced alteration(s). The results of immunofluorescence staining of the A431 cells suggest that target antigen is located on the cell membrane. Association of immunofluorescence with the cytoplasmic vesicles could be due to internalization of portions of membrane with the antigen–antibody complexes.

Since the slides of antibody–fluorochrome conjugates cannot be stored indefinitely owing to quenching, other more permanent methods, such as immunoperoxidase staining, are being increasingly used. The coloured product formed by the action of the enzyme on the substrate is permanent and the specimens can be stored indefinitely.

ELISAs have great potential, not only in detecting antibodies and antigens but also in analysing large numbers of samples simultaneously and providing data rapidly. The results of these assays can be subjectively assessed by eye when a 'yes' or 'no' answer is required. This is because positive results are easily identified by the yellow product formed in the wells of the microtitre plate. However, other more sensitive methods of recording the results are available for accurate quantitation and comparison. In these methods, the product formed in the wells is read either in a spectrophotometer by transferring a portion of the product into microcuvettes or by measuring the absorbance of the product *in situ* in the microtitre plate by a micro ELISA reader. In general, the latter method of recording the results is found to be precise, time saving and not laborious. It is essential to include appropriate controls; for example in the soluble ELISA, one well with HRP-antibody conjugates plus OPD only, and another with OPD only. Because of difficulty in reproducing the exact assay conditions such as incubation time, temperature and reagents from one plate to another, titration of a standard protein in each microtitre plate is essential to ensure valid comparison. Improvements, by decreasing non-specific binding of the immuno-enzyme conjugates to the wells of the microtitre plates and by ensuring purity of the EIA reagents, can significantly increase analytical and diagnostic value of the ELISAs.

The results of an ELISA or any other IA are directly related to affinity and class of the antibody. A typical antibody required for an IA should have high affinity, belong to the IgG class and react with a unique immunodominant epitope of an antigen. A weakly reactive or low affinity antibody often gives inconsistent results because of its ready dissociation from the antigen and subsequent loss from the assay plate during incubation and washing procedures. Similarly, an antibody directed to a three-dimensional structural epitope of a protein antigen is least desired. Because most of the IA reactions, either specific or non-specific, induce some degree of conformational change in the antigen or antibody molecule, this in turn can create an alteration either in the epitope of the antigen or in the binding site of an antibody, resulting in loss of immune recognition. A high affinity antibody with some alteration in structure can still be useful in the IAs; however, an antibody with weak affinity may become totally inactive or poorly reactive with a high dissociation rate from the antigen. This could explain why purified, unlabelled VLN3G2 IgG antibody reacts with the antigen of the target cells but shows negligible reactivity with the same antigen after biotinylation (unpublished results).

The detection, as well as quantitation, of a cell-bound antigen by ELISA requires a different strategy from that for an antigen isolated from living cells or tissues. An ideal cell-bound antigen for IA should be an integral part of the membrane, well displayed on the surface, available in abundance for interaction with the antibody and not subjected to modulation by the cell. In our ELISAs, whole cells were immobilized as a source of antigen on the bottoms of wells of the microtitre plate. In such a method of immobilization, integrity of the antigen is generally protected because of the large number of other proteins present on the cells. In contrast, adsorption of isolated antigens requires special consideration, depending on the type of solid support and nature of the antigen. Since the interaction between surface of the microtitre plate and antigen is non-specific and charge dependent, the three-dimensional structure, including epitopes of the antigen, can be subjected to physical stress, which in turn can result in loss of recognition of the antigen by the antibody. Therefore, the pH of the buffer used for adsorption of the cells or antigens can play an important role in stabilizing structure and integrity of the epitopes of the antigen. However, this factor may not be important for the adsorption of small molecular weight antigens, because these haptens are first conjugated to a protein carrier such as albumin, and the complex is then adsorbed onto the well surfaces of the microtitre plate.

Based on design of the assay and the type of sample to be tested, a variety of enzymes, substrates and buffers are available in order to obtain satisfactory results. The ionic strength and pH of the buffer are to be optimized, taking all the experimental conditions into account. In our ELISAs, use of carbonate buffer for adsorbing antibodies onto the solid phase support, PBS with FCS for diluting the secondary reagents, and PBS containing gelatin for washing the plates, produced optimum results.

We have stored the plates coated with the antigen-positive target A431 cells at 4°C for up to 30 days and observed no loss of reactivity with human MoAbs. Once the plates are prepared, the whole-cell ELISA takes no more than 3 h to complete. This strategy of preparing and stacking the microtitre plates coated with the target cells in advance offers the investigator a rapid means of screening large numbers of hybridoma supernatants against the cell-bound target antigens. The whole-cell ELISA described in this paper easily detects the antigen in as few as 1×10^4 cells/well. Therefore, cell availability is not a limiting factor in screening hybridoma supernatants with this assay.

Recently, avidin–biotin linking systems (Guesdon *et al.*, 1979; Hsu *et al.*, 1981) have become important tools in amplifying the signal-to-background ratio in immunohistochemistry. Avidin, a 68 000 molecular weight glycoprotein of egg white, binds to 4 biotin molecules with exceptionally high affinity ($K_d = 10^{-15}$ M). Several biotin molecules in the form of hydroxysuccinimide derivatives can be coupled to an antibody molecule (Guesdon *et al.*, 1979). Using avidin as a bridge, the system is developed by adding biotinylated enzyme complexes and an insoluble substrate of the enzyme. The signal is greatly increased over the background staining because of the multiple binding sites of avidin.

Finally, a survey of the literature on IAs suggests that variations in design and purpose of these assays are limited only by the imagination of investigators. Applications of advanced computer and laser technologies to modify the IAs further will not only broaden the scope but also save precious time and the reagents of these assays.

ACKNOWLEDGEMENTS

We would like to thank Dorothy Kwiat for the preparation of this manuscript, and Charlie Surh and Robin Starr for expert technical assistance.

This work was partially supported by the National Institutes of Health (CA 32047, CA 37497), the Hagiwara Institute of Health, and the Arco Oil Foundation. MCG was the recipient of an NIH New Investigator Research Award.

REFERENCES

Anderson, G. W., Zimmerman, J. E., Callahan, F. M. (1960). Esters of N-hydroxysuccinimide in peptide synthesis. *J. Amer. Chem. Soc.*, **86**, 1839–1842

Avrameas, S. (1969). Coupling of enzymes to proteins with glutaraldehyde. Use of the conjugates for the detection of antigens and antibodies. *Immunochemistry*, **6**, 43–52

Berson, S. E., Yalow, R. S. (1957). Kinetics of reaction between insulin and insulin-binding antibody. *J. Clin. Invest.*, **36**, 873–878

Bloch, D. B., Smith, B. R., Ault, K. A. (1983). Cells on microspheres: a new technique for flow cytometric analysis of adherent cells. *Cytometry*, **3**, 449–452

Bretscher, M. S. (1984). Endocytosis: relation to capping and cell locomotion. *Science*, **224**, 681–686

Cleveland, P. H., Richman, D. D., Oxman, M. N., Wickham, M. G., Binder, P. S., Worthen, D. M. (1979). Immobilization of viral antigens on filter paper for a ^{125}I-staphylococcal protein A immunoassay: a rapid and sensitive technique for detection of herpes simplex virus antigens and antiviral antibodies. *J. Immunol. Meth.*, **29**, 369–386

Cleveland, P. H., Wickham, M. G., Goldbaum, M. H., Ryan, A. F., Worthen, D. M. (1981). Rapid and efficient immobilization of soluble and small particulate antigens for solid phase radioimmunoassays. *J. Immunoassay*, 2, 117–136

Coons, A. H., Creech, H. J., Jones, R. N. (1941). Immunological properties of an antibody containing a fluorescent group. *Proc. Soc. Exp. Biol.*, **47**, 200–202

Danliker, W. B., Hus, M. L., Vanderlaan, W. P. (1980). In Nakamura, R. M., Dito, W. R., Tucker III, E. S. (eds.) *Immunoassays: Clinical Laboratory Techniques for the 1980's*, Alan R. Liss, Inc., NY, 5–88

DeLuca, M. A. (1978). Bioluminescence and chemiluminescence. In DeLuca, M. A. (ed.) *Methods in Enzymology*, Vol. 57, Academic Press, NY

DiGuiseppi, J., Inman, R., Ishihara, A., Jacobson, K., Herman, B. (1985). Applications of digitized fluorescence microscopy to problems in cell biology. *BioFeature*, **3**, 394–403

Einstein, A. (1906). Zur theorie der brownschen bewegund. *Annalen der Physik*, **19**, 371–381

Gaffar, S. A., Surh, C. D., Glassy, M. C. (1986). Variations in the secretion of monoclonal antibodies by human–human hybridomas. *Hybridoma*, **5**, 93–105

Glassy, M. C. (1987). Immortalization of human lymphocytes from a tumor involved lymph node, *Cancer Res.*, **47**, 5181–5188

Glassy, M. C., Cleveland, P. H. (1986). Use of mouse and human monoclonal antibodies in enzyme immunofiltration. In DiSabato, G., Langone, J. J., Van Vunakis, H. (eds), *Methods in Enzymology*, Vol. 121, Academic Press, NY, pp. 525–541

Glassy, M. C., Gaffar, S. A. (1987). A simple procedure for the rapid immunofluoresence staining of human tumour antigens with human monoclonal antibodies. *J. Clin. Lab. Analysis*, **1**, 52–55

Glassy, M. C., Gaffar, S. A., Peters, R. E., Royston, I. (1985). In Reisfeld, R. A., Sell, S. (eds.) *Monoclonal Antibodies and Cancer Therapy*, Alan R. Liss, Inc., NY, 97–109

Glassy, M. C., Handley, H. H., Cleveland, P. H., Royston, I. (1983a). An enzyme immunofiltration assay useful for detecting human monoclonal antibody. *J. Immunol. Meth.*, **58**, 119–126

Glassy, M. C., Handley, H. H., Hagiwara, H., Royston, I. (1983b). UC 729-6, a human lymphoblastoid B cell line useful for generating antibody-secreting human–human hybridomas. *Proc. Natl. Acad. Sci. USA*, **80**, 6327–6331

Glassy, M. C., Surh, C. D. (1985). Immunodetection of cell bound antigens using both mouse and human monoclonal antibodies. *J. Immunol. Meth.*, **81**, 115–122

Guesdon, J. L., Ternynck, T., Avrameas, S. (1979). The use of avidin–biotin interaction in immunoenzymatic techniques. *J. Histochem. Cytochem.*, **27**, 771–776

Hamaguchi, Y., Yoshitake, S., Ishikawa, E., Endo, Y., Ohtaki, S. (1979). Improved procedure for the conjugation of rabbit IgG and Fab' antibodies with β-D-galactosidase from *Escherichia coli* using N,N,O-phenylenedimaleimide. *J. Biochem.*, **85**, 1289–1300

Hersh, L. S., Vann, W. P., Wilhelm, S. A. (1979). A luminol-assisted competitive-binding immunoassay of human immunoglobulin G. *Analyt. Biochem.*, **93**, 267–271

Hsu, S. M., Raine, L., Fanger, H. (1981). Use of avidin–biotin peroxidase complex (ABC) in immunoperoxidase techniques: a comparison between ABC and unlabeled antibody (PAP) procedures. *J. Histochem. Cytochem.*, **29**, 577–580

Kaptiza, H. G., McGregor, G., Jacobsen, K. (1985). Direct measurement of lateral transport in membranes using time-resolved spatial photometry. *Proc. Natl. Acad. Sci. USA*, **82**, 4122–4126

Kohen, F., Hollander, Z., Boguslaski, R. C. (1979). Non-radioisotopic homo-geneous steroid immunoassays. *J. Steroid Biochem.*, **11**, 161–167

Kohler, G., Milstein, C. (1975). Continuous cultures of fused cells secreting antibody of predefined specificity. *Nature*, **256**, 495–497

Maeda, H., Nakayama, M., Iwaoka, D., Sato, T. (1979). Assay of angiotensin I by fluorescence polarization method. In Moriya, H., Suzuki, T. (eds.) *Kinins II*, Part A, Plenum Press, NY, 203–211

McGregor, A. R., Crookall-Greening, J. O., Landon, J., Smith, D. S. (1978). Polarization fluoroimmunoassay of phenyltoin. *Clin. Chim. Acta*, **83**, 161–166

Nakane, P. K., Kawaoi, A. (1974). Peroxidase-labeled antibody: a new method of conjugation. *J. Histochem. Cytochem.*, **22**, 1084–1091

Nakane, P. K., Pierce, Jr., G. B. (1967). Preparation and application for the localization of antigens. *J. Histochem. Cytochem.*, **14**, 929–931

Plant, A. L., Benson, D. M., Smith, L. C. (1985). Cellular uptake and intra-cellular localization of benzo(a)pyrene by digital imaging microscopy. *J. Cell Biol.*, **100**, 1295–1308

Pratt, J. J., Woldring, M. G., Villerius, L. (1978). Chemiluminescence-linked immunoassay. *J. Immunol. Meth.*, **21**, 179–183

Reynolds, G. T. (1972). Image intensification applied to biological problems. *Q. Rev. Biophys.*, **5**, 295–347

Rubenstein, K. E., Schneider, R. S., Ullman, E. F. (1972). "Homogeneous" enzyme immunoassay. A new immunochemical technique. *Biochem. Biophys. Res. Comm.*, **47**, 846–851

Schroeder, H. R., Vogelhut, P. O., Carrico, R. J., Boguslaski, R. C., Buckler, R. T. (1976). Competitive protein binding assay for biotin monitored by chemi-luminescence. *Anal. Chem.*, **48**, 1933–1937

Simpson, J. S. A., Campbell, A. K., Ryall, M. E. T., Woodhead, J. S. (1979). A stable chemiluminescent-labeled antibody for immunological assays. *Nature*, **279**, 646–645

Smyth, D. G., Nagamatsu, A., Fruton, J. S. (1960). Some reactions of N-ethyl-maleimide. *J. Amer. Chem. Soc.*, **82**, 2414–2418

Soini, E., Hemmila, I. (1979). Fluoroimmunoassay: present status and key problems. *Clin. Chem.*, **25**, 353–361

Spencer, R. D. (1973). Applications of fluorescent polarization in clinical assays. In Kaplan, L. A., Pesce, A. J. (eds.) *Nonisotopic Alternatives to Radio-immunoassay. Principles and Applications*, Marcel Dekker, Inc., NY, 143–170

Spencer, R. D., Toledo, F. B., Williams, B. T., Yoss, N. L. (1973). Design, con-struction and two applications for an automated flowcell polarization fluoro-meter with digital read-out: enzyme–inhibitor (antitrypsin) assay and antigen-antibody (insulin–insulin antiserum) assay. *Clin. Chim. Acta*, **19**, 838–844

Voller, A., Bidwell, D. E. (1975). A simple method for detecting antibodies to Rubella. *Brit. J. Exp. Pathol.*, **56**, 338–339

Waart, M. V. D., Schuurs, A. H. W. M. (1976). Towards the development of a radioenzyme immunoassay. *Analyt. Chem.*, **279**, 142–150

Watson, R. A. A., Landon, J., Shaw, E. J., Smith, D. S. (1976). Polarization fluoroimmunoassay of gentamicin. *Clin. Chim. Acta*, **73**, 51–55

Weber, G. (1952). Polarization of the fluorescence of macromolecules. 1. Theory and experimental method. *Biochem. J.*, **51**, 145–167

Weiel, J., Hershey, J. W. (1981). Fluorescent polarization studies of the inter-actions of *Escherichia coli* protein synthesis initiation factor 3 with 30S ribosomal subunits. *Biochemistry*, **20**, 5859–5865

Yoshitake, S., Hamaguchi, Y., Ishikawa, E. (1979). Efficient conjugation of rabbit Fab' with β-D-galactosidase from *Escherichia coli. Scand. J. Immunol.*, **10**, 81–86

7. Adaptation of Enzyme Labelled Immunoassay (ELISA) for Measurement of Biosynthesis of Human and Rat Complement Components

L. MORRISON, A. HAMILTON, R. ANTHONY, D. LAPPIN

AND K. WHALEY

INTRODUCTION

A number of cell types are now known to produce complement proteins, although the sites of synthesis of late-acting components, such as C7 and C9, still remain unclear (Colten, 1976). Identification of these sites has been achieved by using both *in vivo* and *in vitro* systems, the former involving study of changes in the allotypes of certain complement proteins such as C3, C6, C8 and factor B following human orthotopic liver transplantation. *In vitro* techniques which have been more widely employed consist of the maintenance of specific cell types or cell lines in culture in order to study their products. Complement proteins are detected, if active, either by functional assay or by the incorporation of radio-labelled amino-acids into the protein, which can then be identified by specific antibody precipitation or by radioimmunoassay.

In most of our previous studies on complement biosynthesis (Lappin and Whaley, 1980; Lappin and Whaley, 1982), we have used functional haemolytic assays for measurement of complement components. This particular type of assay, although exquisitely sensitive and capable of measuring nanogram quantities of material, is not capable of measuring absolute quantities of individual components, as the haemolytic efficiency of individual components varies considerably. For instance, one molecule of C1 will produce one haemolytic site (Colten *et al.*, 1967), whereas as many as 300 C3 molecules are required to achieve the same result (Colten and Alper, 1972). Furthermore, this technique does not detect components which are functionally inactive. Thus the presence of inactive precursor molecules and degraded components would be overlooked. Haemolytic assays also tend to have the additional problem of inter-assay variation.

In an attempt to overcome some of these problems, we have used an adaptation of the non-competitive double-antibody sandwich enzyme-labelled immunoassay (ELISA) for detection and measurement of the biosynthesis of a wide variety of complement components and other proteins. This technique was developed for the purpose of antigen detection by Beards and Bryden (1981) from the original ELISA technique developed independently by two groups of

147

workers (Engvall and Perlmann, 1971; Van Weeman and Shuuo, 1971). Table 1 gives a brief description of the basic ELISA method that we have employed throughout our studies. The availability of high affinity antisera specific for individual complement components has made the establishment of these assays relatively simple. ELISA has the advantage of great sensitivity, combined with the ability to detect functionally active precursor and degraded molecules. In addition, complement biosynthesis may be fully quantified in terms of molecules produced per cell per hour by using this versatile technique; moreover, inter-assay variation is found to be minimal. Precise quantification of individual complement components by means of the ELISA technique, in conjunction with the determination of their functional activities by haemolytic assay, has allowed us to compare the specific activities of individual complement components synthesised by different cell types with that of the corresponding component present in the plasma or serum. We have also used the ELISA technique extensively in studies of modulation of complement biosynthesis by various agents.

MATERIALS AND METHODS

Choice of Solid Phase

We have used Linbro Titertek polystyrene EIA microtitration plates obtained from Flow Laboratories, Irvine, Scotland, for all ELISAs. These are prepared non-sterile and consist of 96 flat-bottom wells (0.35 ml capacity).

Choice of Antisera

In order to develop ELISAs with maximum sensitivity, high affinity antisera are required. We have screened antisera from a wide variety of commercial and non-commercial sources. For most of our assay systems we have used the IgG fraction of goat anti-human complement component antisera obtained from Atlantic Antibodies (American Hospital Supplies, Didcot, Oxfordshire, England). For most other ELISAs we have used the IgG fraction of rabbit anti-human complement component antisera raised in our own laboratory, with the exception of anti-C2 which was a gift from Dr. Michael Kerr (Ninewells Hospital, Dundee, Scotland).

For each individual ELISA, the IgG fraction of the antisera was used for both initial adsorption onto the solid phase to act as 'trapping' antibody and also as the antibody from which the horseradish peroxidase (HRP) conjugate was prepared and used as the enzyme probe at a later stage in the assay.

We have used the IgG fraction of the antiserum in order to eliminate non-specific reactivity.

Table 1 Basic ELISA method

Step	Reagent	Volume per well	Diluent	Concentration range	Incubation time and temperature storage conditions
Coating	IgG# fraction of antiserum	100 μl	0.05 M carbonate–bicarbonate	1–10 μg/ml	Overnight at 4°C humidity
Wash × 5	PBS + 0.05% Tween 20				
Blocking	PBS + 0.1% BSA	250 μl	–	–	1 h R.T. humidity
Wash × 5	As above				
Standards + sera to be assayed	Normal sera pool or purified component	100 μl	PBS–Tween	Standard = 1000 → 3 ng/ml	At least 2 h R.T. humidity
Wash × 5	PBS + 0.05% Tween 20				
Enzyme-conjugated IgG# of antiserum (as for coating)	HRP + IgG# of antiserum (used)	100 μl	PBS–Tween	–	1 h R.T. humidity
Aspiration + wash × 10	PBS + 0.05% Tween 20	–	–	–	–
Substrate	o-phenylene diamine (OPD) + H_2O_2	100 μl	Phosphate–citrate buffer, pH 5.6	34 mg OPD + 20 μl H_2O_2–100 ml buffer	$\frac{1}{2}$ h R.T. humidity + darkness
Stop reaction	4 N H_2SO_4	25 μl	–	–	–

Choice of Standards

A standard serum pool was prepared from 40 normal human volunteers. The level of the particular complement component to be assayed was previously determined by either nephelometry or radial immunodiffusion (Whaley, 1985).

Purified rat complement components or other serum proteins were used as standards for ELISAs wherever possible. However, for most rat ELISAs (as also for human assays), a pool of 20 normal rat sera was used as a standard. The concentrations of the individual complement components were determined by radial immunodiffusion (Dr. Mohammed Daha, Leiden, Netherlands).

Preparation of Conjugate

Choice of Enzyme

HRP was selected as the enzyme to be used for the preparation of all conjugates, as it has been shown (Avrameas and Uriel, 1966; Nakane and Pierce, 1967; Nakane, 1975) to be a good choice of enzyme for conjugation. Like alkaline phosphatase, HRP possesses high activity, but is less expensive.

Conjugation Method

We have used both of the two-step glutaraldehyde (Avrameas and Ternynak, 1971; Nakane and Kawaoi, 1974) methods for coupling HRP to antibodies. Although both methods produce reasonable conjugates, in our hands the periodate method consistently produces higher titre conjugates.

In the preparation of our HRP-Ab conjugates, we have found it unnecessary to separate the Ab-bound fraction from the free enzyme, as the presence of free enzyme does not cause interference in the double-Ab sandwich ELISA. The fact that we use most of our conjugates at a working titre similar to that of commercial conjugates indicates that the percentage of antibody conjugated to HRP by the periodate method is probably quite high. In any case, the high titre at which we use most of our conjugates has meant that we have never found it necessary to separate enzyme-bound from free antibody.

Preservation and Storage of ELISA Reagents

Thimerosal (Sigma) at a concentration of 0.01% (w/v) was used as a preservative in all ELISA reagents.

Conjugates were aliquoted and stored at 4°C, whereas antisera and standards were stored in aliquots at −20°C. Under these storage conditions the majority of conjugates were found to have a lifespan of $1-1\frac{1}{2}$ years at 4°C.

ELISA Standardisation Procedure

The optimum concentrations of reagents are determined, initially, by three-dimensional checkerboard titration. Usually, a wide range of concentrations of antibody, covering three logarithmic dilutions ranging from 0.1 to 10 μg/ml, is used to trap standard antigen, which also spans three logarithmic dilutions of $10-10^3$ ng/ml, with PBS + 0.05% TWEEN, as diluent, for the control. The appropriate conjugate is then used at three wide-ranging concentrations in order to detect the presence of standard antigen.

The optimum concentrations of coating antibody and conjugate are subsequently determined from this initial checkerboard at a point where the highest concentration of standard gives an optical density reading of between 1 and 1.2, where the lowest concentration of the standard gives an optical density reading of between 0.1 and 0.2, and where the PBS-TWEEN control is negative at 492 nm on a standard micro ELISA reader.

These optimum concentrations of coating antibody and conjugate are then used in a subsequent ELISA, in which the standard is diluted out in a series of approximately 12 doubling dilutions from the original top concentration of standard to determine the lower limit of detection of the assay. Again, PBS-TWEEN alone is used as the control. The OD_{492} of each of the standard serial dilutions is then plotted in a semi-logarithmic plot against concentration of the standard to construct the standard curve. The linear portion of the curve is used to determine the range of standard concentrations employed in subsequent assays.

The optimum incubation conditions for each stage of the ELISA were determined using a range of different incubation times and temperatures. The time, temperature, and storage conditions for each individual step listed in the basic ELISA method (table 1) were found to be optimal for each of the ELISAs developed.

Concentrations of Reagents Used

For most of the ELISAs developed, the IgG fractions of the coating antisera were used at concentrations of either 5 or 10 μg/ml. Standard antigen was generally used within a range of 1–1000 ng/ml. The appropriate dilution for test samples was determined by titration. HRP–Ab conjugates were used at titres of between 1/200 and 1/10T in PBS + 0.05% TWEEN. The limit of detection of the majority of ELISAs lay within the range of 1–5 ng/ml.

Adaptation of Human ELISA for Detection of Rat Complement Components

High affinity antisera to rat complement components and the corresponding HRP–Ab conjugates are not yet widely available on a commercial basis. In order to overcome this problem, we have tested the majority of our goat anti-human

Table 2a ELISAs for human complement components and other human proteins

Protein	Source of antisera	Concentration of coating antibody (μg/ml)	Standard and concentration range	Special adaptations	Dilution of HRP conjugate
C1q	Atlantic Antibodies; IgG fraction goat and human	5	NHS pool $\approx$ 250 μg/ml; 1/200 $\rightarrow$ 1/102400		1/10T
C1r	Atlantic Antibodies; IgG fraction goat and human	10	NHS pool $\approx$ 100 μg/ml; 1/100 $\rightarrow$ 1/51200		1/200
C1s	Atlantic Antibodies; IgG fraction goat and human	10	NHS pool $\approx$ 80 μg/ml; 1/80 $\rightarrow$ 1/40860		1/200
C1–inhibitor	Atlantic Antibodies; IgG fraction goat and human	5	NHS pool = 220 μg/ml (nephelometry); 1/500 $\rightarrow$ 1/256T		1/2T
C2	Laboratory-produced (M. Kerr, Ninewells, Dundee); rabbit and human	10	NHS pool $\approx$ 20 μg/ml; 1/50 $\rightarrow$ 1/256T		1/500
C3	Atlantic Antibodies; IgG fraction goat and human	5	NHS pool = 1085 μg/ml (nephelometry); 1/T $\rightarrow$ 1/1024T		1/5T
C4	Atlantic Antibodies; IgG fraction goat and human	5	NHS pool = 472 μg/ml (nephelometry); 1/250 $\rightarrow$ 1/32T		1/5T
C5	Atlantic Antibodies; IgG fraction goat and human	5	NHS pool $\approx$ 75 μg/ml; 175 $\rightarrow$ 1/38400	Block with PBS + 0.2% BSA	1/T
C8	Atlantic Antibodies: IgG fraction goat and human	5	NHS pool $\approx$ 80 μg/ml 1/5T $\rightarrow$ 1/256T		1/T
Factor B	Atlantic Antibodies; IgG fraction goat and human	5	NHS pool = 270 μg/ml (nephelometry); 1/200 $\rightarrow$ 1/204T		1/5T
Factor P (properdin)	Atlantic Antibodies; IgG fraction goat and human	5	NHS pool $\approx$ 30 μg/ml; 1/50 $\rightarrow$ 1/25T		1/2T
Factor H (β1H)	Atlantic Antibodies; IgG fraction goat and human	5	NHS pool $\approx$ 300 μg/ml; 1/500 $\rightarrow$ 1/512T		1/10T
Albumin	Atlantic Antibodies; IgG fraction goat and human	5	HSA (Sigma) 1 mg/ml; 1/T $\rightarrow$ 1/1024T		1/5T
Lysozyme	Dako; rabbit and human whole antiserum	10	Sigma purified lysozyme (from human milk) 1 mg/ml		1/2T
CRP	Atlantic Antibodies; IgG fraction goat and human	5	Boehringer CRP standard (high) 60 μg/ml; 1/500 $\rightarrow$ 1/356T		1/10T

Table 2b   ELISAs for rat complement components and other rat proteins

Protein	Source of antisera	Concentration of coating antibody (μg/ml)	Standard and concentration range	Special adaptations	Dilution of HRP conjugate
Serum albumin	Cappel Worthington; goat and rat IgG fraction	5	Purified RSA (Sigma) 1 mg/ml; $1/T \rightarrow 1/4M$		$1/7T$
C3	Cappel Worthington; goat and rat IgG fraction	5	NRS pool $1/T \rightarrow 1/200T$		$1/5T$
C4	ATAB; goat and human C4 IgG fraction	10	NRS pool ≈ 200 μg/ml; $1/20 \rightarrow 1/20T$		$1/T$
C5	ATAB; goat and human C5 IgG fraction	10	NRS pool ≈ 75 μg/ml; $1/10 \rightarrow 1/5T$		$1/200$
P	ATAB; goat and human P IgG fraction	10	NRS pool ≈ 30 μg/ml; $1/5 \rightarrow 1.5120$		$1/50$
β1H	ATAB; goat and human β1H IgG fraction	10	NRS pool ≈ 300 μg/ml; $1/10 \rightarrow 1/5T$		$1/500$

NRS, normal rat serum.

complement component antisera from Atlantic Antibodies for cross-reactivity against rat complement components, and we have found that some of these antisera are indeed suitable for the development of a sufficiently sensitive ELISA for rat complement components. Usually, for these assays, all reagents are used at a much greater concentration than for the corresponding human ELISAs, i.e. trapping antibody at a concentration of 10 μg/ml, HRP–Ab conjugate at a titre of between 1/50 and 1/T, and a range of concentrations of the standard of between 5 ng/ml and approximately 30 μg/ml. The specificity of these cross-reactions was proved by SDS–PAGE analysis of immunoprecipitates of ^{35}S-labelled rat and human complement components from macrophage and hepatocyte culture supernatants.

For all double-antibody sandwich ELISAs developed to date see tables 2a and 2b.

Cell Culture Techniques

Human peripheral blood monocytes and human synovial fluid macrophages were isolated and maintained in culture as described previously (Hamilton and Whaley, 1985).

Rat hepatocytes were isolated from rat liver and maintained in culture according to the technique described (Berry and Friend, 1969).

RESULTS

Biosynthesis of Rat Complement Components

Hepatocytes isolated from the perfused livers of Charles River rats were cultured *in vitro* and ELISAs were used to measure production of albumin, C3 and C4 by these cells. In a preliminary study (Anthony *et al.*, 1985) ELISA was used for the assay of albumin levels in supernatants of cultured rat hepatocytes. Complement component biosynthesis by these cells was measured by haemolytic assay. Measurable amounts of albumin, a constitutive protein, and also C4, C2, C3 and factor B were demonstrated in the culture supernatants. The patterns of cumulative synthesis of all four complement components and albumin were similar. However, in those cultures from which only small portions of medium were removed, the amount of all five proteins synthesised was considerably less after 24 h of culture. This observation may indicate negative feedback control of biosynthesis of these proteins. This difference was least marked with albumin and most obvious with C3 and C4. Within 9 h, the hepatocytes synthesised 7.5 μg of albumin/10^6 cells and, in cumulative experiments, 12.5 μg of albumin/10^6 cells. Assuming 1 g of liver wet weight contains 1.7×10^8 hepato-cytes (Weibler *et al.*, 1969), the cultures synthesised 142 μg of albumin/h per gram of liver in the continuous system, and 236 μg of albumin/h per gram in the cumulative method of sampling. Addition of cyclohexamide decreased the production of albumin by 73%. Within 6 h of replacement of cyclohexamide-containing medium with fresh culture medium, synthesis of albumin was restored.

In further, unpublished, studies on the biosynthesis of complement compo-nents and albumin by cultured rat hepatocytes, the ELISA was used to assay C3 and C4 production in addition to albumin. With respect to albumin biosynthesis, the following observations were made.

(i) During the acute phase, induced by intraperitoneal injection of rats with 3 g of casein, albumin synthesis was reduced from a normal control level of 163 μg to 58 μg/10^6 cells per 24 h.

(ii) Rates of synthesis of albumin were found to be similar for both male and female rats.

(iii) The rate of synthesis of albumin increased with age, e.g. female rats of 3 months produced approximately 35 μg albumin/10^6 cells per 24 h and 9 month old female rats produced approximately 100 μg/10^6 cells per 24 h.

With respect to C3 and C4 biosynthesis, the following observations were made.

(i) Unlike the effect on albumin synthesis, C3 levels were increased from 2.0 μg/10^6 cells per 24 h in hepatocytes from control rats to 3.75 μg/10^6 cells per 24 h in hepatocytes from acute phase rats, and C4 synthesis was also increased from 3.5 to 5.6 μg/10^6 cells per 24 h under similar conditions.

(ii) For both C3 and C4, synthesis rates were found to be higher in females than in males.

(iii) C3 and C4 synthesis rates were found to increase with age, that for C3 in 3 month old rats being 1.4 μg/10^6 cells per 24 h and in 9 months old rats being 2.45 μg/10^6 cells per 24 h. Synthesis of C4 in 3 month old rats was 0.6 μg/10^6 cells per 24 h, and in 9 month old rats it was 2.8 μg/10^6 cells per 24 h.

The effect of recombinant γ-interferon and interleukin I on the biosynthesis of C3 and C4 by cultured rat hepatocytes was also examined. It was found that a dose of 1 μg interferon/ml culture medium increased C3 synthesis by 70% but had no effect on C4 synthesis. Interleukin I (1 unit/ml) of culture medium was shown to increase C3 synthesis by 25% but decreased C4 synthesis by 30%.

In a further, unpublished, study the ELISA technique was used to study the effect of addition of culture supernatants from both resident and elicited rat peritoneal macrophages on the biosynthesis of C3 by cultured rat hepatocytes. Preliminary results have shown that the addition of supernatants from cultures of elicited rat peritoneal macrophages significantly reduced the biosynthesis of C3 by cultured rat hepatocytes over a period of 48 h. Further, direct co-culture of elicited rat macrophages with rat hepatocytes had a relatively greater inhib-itory effect on C3 biosynthesis.

Table 3a   Synthesis rates for complement components by monocytes and macrophages[a]

	Monocytes			Macrophages		
	ng/μg DNA per 24 h[b]	mol $\times 10^{-3}$/cell per hour[c]	Lysozyme (%)	ng/μg DNA per 24 h	mol $\times 10^{-3}$/cell per hour[d]	Lysozyme (%)
Lysozyme	278 ± 47[e]	4700 ± 80	–	254 ± 6	4300 ± 100	–
C2	1.3 ± 0.1	3.2 ± 0.2	0.068	3.4 ± 0.2	8.6 ± 0.5	0.18
C3	2.4 ± 0.5	3.2 ± 0.6	0.068	8.9 ± 0.4	11.8 ± 0.6	0.25
B	0.4 ± 0.1	1.1 ± 0.2	0.23	2.2 ± 0.1	5.5 ± 0.2	0.12
C1–inhibitor	0.6 ± 0.1	1.5 ± 0.2	0.032	3.7 ± 0.3	9.3 ± 0.8	0.20

[a] From Lappin *et al.* (1986), courtesy of the Editor.
[b] Average rate of accumulation per 24 h based on increase in levels between days 3 and 5.
[c] Molecular weights of lysozyme (14 800), C2 (100 000), C3 (190 000), B (95 000) and C1–inhibitor (105 000) were assumed.
[d] Secretion rate (molecules/cell per hour) of component as percentage of secretion rate of lysozyme.
[e] Mean ± SEM of three separate experiments.

Biosynthesis of Human Complement Components

We have also used ELISAs to study the biosynthesis of various complement components by cultured human monocytes and macrophages, and we have made the following observations (table 3a).

(i) With respect to rates of synthesis of lysozyme and complement components by monocytes and synovial macrophages as determined by ELISA, the following were found.

Lysozyme: the synthesis rate for lysozyme between days 3 and 5 in monocytes (4700×10^3 molecules/cell per hour) did not differ significantly from the synthesis rate in macrophages (4300×10^3 molecules/cell per hour) over the same period.

Complement: in contrast to lysozyme, the synthesis rates for the complement components (factor B, C1–inhibitor, C3 and C2) were higher in macrophages than in monocyte cultures. The percentage increase was more marked for factor B (400%) and C1–inhibitor (540%) than for C3 (260%) and C2 (170%).

By virtue of the sensitivity of the ELISA assay it was possible to detect C3 in monocyte cultures as early as day 1, at very low levels. In contrast to monocyte cultures, C3, C2, factor B and C1–inhibitor could all be detected by ELISA

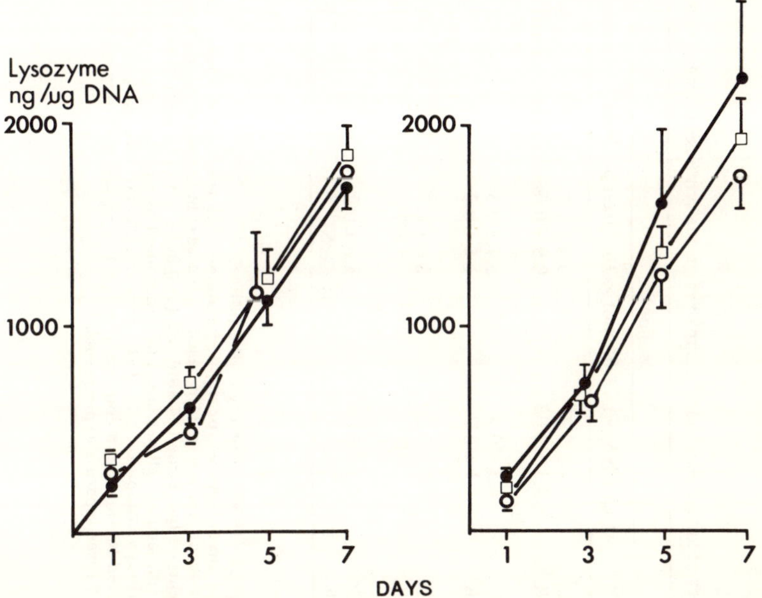

Figure 1   Synthesis of lysozyme by synovial fluid macrophages (left) and monocytes (right) in the presence of untreated (●——●) or serum-treated (○——○) BSA–anti-BSA immune complexes and control cultures (□——□). Each point represents the mean (± SEM) of three cultures. (From Lappin *et al.* (1986), courtesy of the Editor.)

Table 3b   Effect of antigen–antibody complexes on the synthesis rates for complement components by monocytes and macrophages[a,b]

		Monocyte			Macrophage		
		ng/μg DNA per 24 h[c]	mol $\times$ 10^{-3}/cell per hour[d]	Lysozyme (%)	ng/μg DNA per 24 h	mol $\times$ 10^{-3}/cell per hour[e]	Lysozyme (%)
C2	IC[f]	3.8 ± 0.7[h]	9.5 ± 1.7	0.18	7.7 ± 0.8	19.3 ± 2.1	0.49
	SIC[g]	0.4 ± 0.02	0.9 ± 0.05	0.02	1.4 ± 0.15	3.4 ± 0.1	0.08
C3	IC	4.3 ± 0.4	5.7 ± 0.5	0.11	14.7 ± 3.0	19.4 ± 3.9	0.50
	SIC	1.1 ± 0.2	1.5 ± 0.2	0.004	3.6 ± 1.4	4.7 ± 1.9	0.12
B	IC	0.8 ± 0.20	2.0 ± 0.5	0.04	5.6 ± 0.02	14.1 ± 0.5	0.36
	SIC	ND	ND	ND	1.4 ± 0.08	3.5 ± 0.2	0.09
C1–inhibitor	IC	1.23 ± 0.04	3.0 ± 0.2	0.06	6.6 ± 0.6	16.5 ± 1.5	0.43
	SIC	ND	ND	ND	2.2 ± 0.3	5.5 ± 0.7	0.13

ND = not determined.

[a] From Lappin *et al.* (1986), courtesy of the Editor.
[b] The untreated control cultures for these experiments are the same as those shown in table 1.
[c] Average rate of accumulation in 24 h based on increase in levels between days 3 and 5.
[d] Molecular weights of lysozyme (14 800), C2 (100 000), C3 (190 000), B (95 000) and C1–inhibitor (105 000) were assumed.
[e] Secretion rate (molecules/cell per hour) of component as a percentage of the secretion rate of lysozyme.
[f] IC–antigen–antibody complexes added at a concentration of 600 ng IgG antibody/ml culture medium.
[g] SIC–serum-treated IC added at a concentration of 150 ng IgG antibody/ml of culture medium.
[h] Mean ± SEM of three separate experiments.

in macrophage culture supernatants on the first day of culture. It probably would have been impossible to detect such low levels at so early a stage of culture by functional assay.

(ii) The effect of various agents on the synthesis rates of lysozyme and complement components, produced by human monocytes and synovial macrophages, was examined, and the following observations were made.

(a) Neither serum-treated (bearing C3b and reacting with C3b receptors) nor untreated (reacting with Fc receptors) immune complexes altered the rate of synthesis of lysozyme by monocytes or macrophages (figure 1).

(b) Untreated immune complexes were found to stimulate the synthesis of all four complement components.

(c) In contrast, serum-treated immune complexes suppressed the production of these components by both monocytes and macrophages (table 3b).

(d) γ-interferon did not affect lysozyme production by either monocytes or macrophages but was found to enhance synthesis of C1–inhibitor, factor B and C2 by both monocytes and macrophages.

(e) In contrast to this, γ-interferon was found to inhibit C3 production. γ-interferon was thus shown to have a selective effect on the biosynthesis of these complement components by monocytes and macrophages.

It would seem possible, therefore, to use the ELISA technique to examine and compare biosynthesis of complement components not only by different types of human cells but also by different cell types derived from various species of animal.

Determination of Specific Activity of Complement Components and Other Serum Proteins

Accurate quantification of total protein by ELISA, in conjunction with determination of the corresponding functional activity by appropriate assay, e.g. haemolytic assay, has permitted determination of the specific activity of individual complement components and other proteins. It has, therefore, been possible to compare the specific functional activities of lysozymal and complement components synthesised by cultured cells with those of their serum counterparts.

(i) Detection of the functional activity of lysozyme by bacterial lysis, in conjunction with accurate quantification of the total amount of lysozyme present by ELISA, has permitted determination of the specific activity of lysozyme derived from both human monocytes and synovial macrophages. This was found to be 120 000 units/mg lysozyme, which is in agreement with other similar data reported (Gordon *et al.*, 1974).

(ii) Although the functional activity of C2 in monocyte culture supernatants correlated with the quantity of C2 protein as measured by ELISA (figure 2), it was found that the specific activity of monocyte C2 was approximately five-fold greater than functionally purified C2. One possible explanation for this was that the C2 formed a more stable complex with EAC14, as occurs when C2 is oxi-

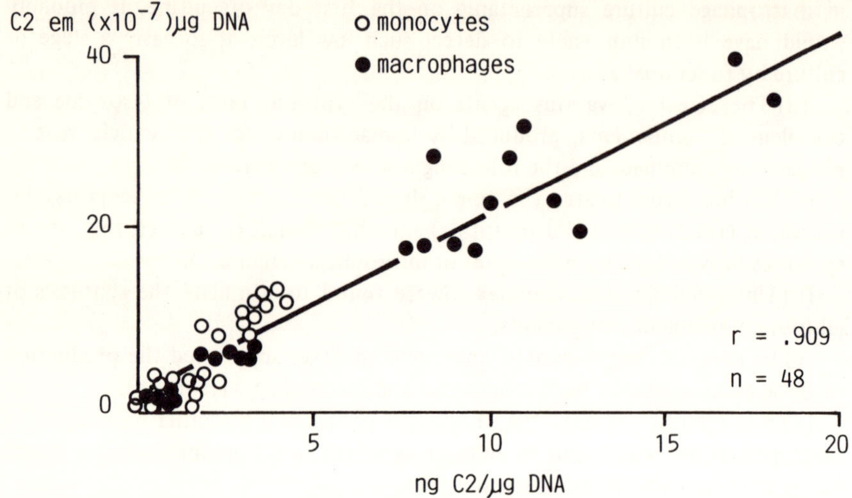

Figure 2   Correlation of functional activity of C2 in monocyte and macrophage culture supernatants with the quantity of C2 protein as measured by ELISA.

dised. To test this hypothesis, we prepared EAC142 with both monocyte C2 and purified C2, and measured the rate of decay from the cells. The results showed (figure 3) that EAC142 prepared with monocyte C2 ($C2_M$) had a significantly longer half-life (13.5 min) than EAC142s prepared with purified C2 ($C2_S$) (4.5 min). This interesting observation may indicate that C2 produced locally by monocytes at the site of inflammation may promote more efficient activation of the classical pathway by way of formation of a more stable C42 classical pathway C3 convertase than when complement activation occurs in serum. Similar studies on the specific activity of C1–inhibitor and C3 have indicated that monocyte C1–inhibitor has a similar functional activity to that of its serum counterpart. In contrast, monocyte C3 has a much lower specific activity than serum C3. The significance of these observations is unclear. However, monocyte C3 possesses an internal thiol ester but does not appear to form an effective C3 convertase with B and D (Hamilton and Whaley, unpublished observations).

The specific activity of other complement components, produced by various other cell types, could also be determined in a similar manner by accurate quantification by ELISA in conjunction with determination of functional activity.

Assay of Complement Components in Human Serum

We have used the double-antibody sandwich ELISA for assay of the various complement components in human serum. The ease with which these assays can be carried out and the degree of sensitivity obtained have rendered them particularly suitable for the rapid screening of patients' sera for deficiency of individual

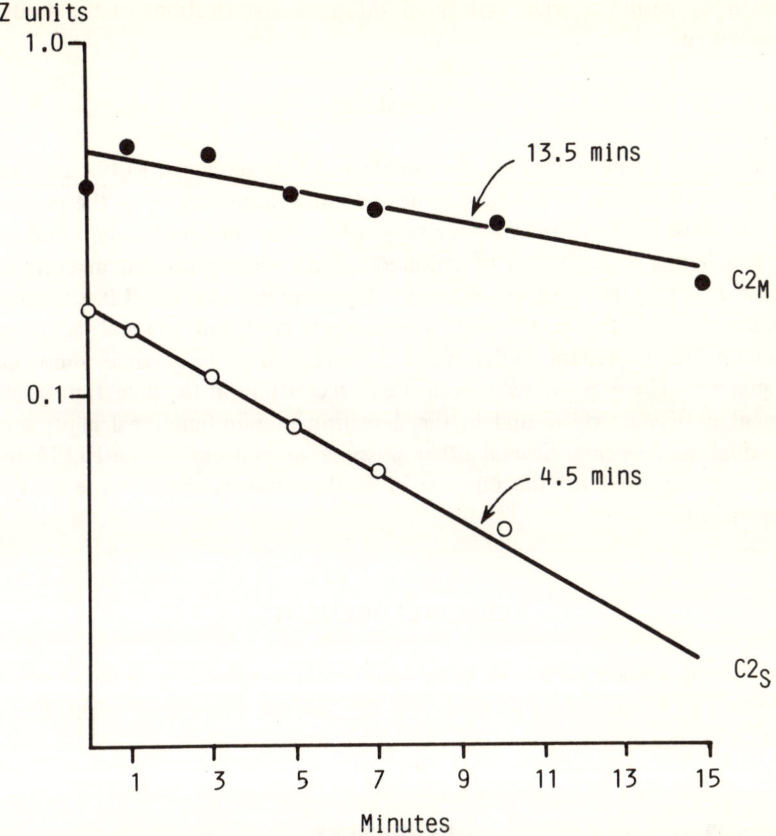

Figure 3   EAC142 prepared with monocyte C2 (C2$_M$) has a significantly longer half-life (13.5 min) than EAC1425 prepared with purified C2 (C2$_S$) (4.5 min). (From Lappin *et al.* (1986), courtesy of the Editor.)

complement components. In addition, measurement of the functional activity, relative to the total quantity of an individual complement component as measured by ELISA, may elucidate further the specific nature of some complement component deficiencies and may lend itself to the quantitation of C4A and C4B gene production in whole serum.

As most of the ELISAs which we have developed are capable of detecting, with accuracy, very small quantities of protein, i.e. 2–4 ng/ml, it should be possible, in future, to use these assays for the examination of other body fluids such as CSF, urine and also pleural and peritoneal exudates for the presence of complement components and other proteins. Moreover, it should also prove possible to adapt the basic ELISA technique to permit detection of complement activation products, e.g. Clr Cls C1-inhibitor complexes and C5b-9 membrane attack complexes. The basic ELISA technique is, therefore, highly versatile and may be adapted to permit a wide variety of different investigations in the study of complement.

SUMMARY

In summary, we have adapted the double-antibody sandwich ELISA technique and, in combination with HRP-conjugated antisera, produced by the periodate method, have used it to assay a wide range of complement components and other proteins in the supernatants of cultured human monocytes and macrophages, and rat hepatocytes. We have also used this adaptation of the ELISA technique to quantify individual complement components in human sera and, in conjunction with functional data, to determine the specific activity of some complement components. These assays have been used successfully in the detection of complement deficiency states and in the detection of non-functional allotypes of individual components. Several other possible adaptations of the ELISA technique are suggested for the purpose of further investigations in the study of complement.

ACKNOWLEDGEMENTS

Some of the research reported in this paper was supported by grants from the Arthritis and Rheumatism Council and the Scottish Home and Health Department.

REFERENCES

Anthony, R., Morrison, L., MacSween, R. N. M., Whaley, K. (1985). Biosynthesis of complement components by cultured rat hepatocytes. *Biochem. J.*, **232**, 93–98

Avrameas, S., Ternynak, T. (1971). Peroxidase labelled antibody and Fab conjugates with enhanced intracellular penetration. *Immunocytochemistry*, **8**, 1175–1179

Avrameas, S., Uriel, J. (1966). Method de marquage d' antigenes et d'anticorps avec des enzymes et sans application en immunodiffusion. *C.R. Acad. Sci.*, *Ser. D*, **262**, 2543–2545

Beards, G. M., Bryden, A. S. (1981). Evaluation of a new enzyme-linked immunosorbent assay test for rotavirus antigen in faeces. *J. Clin. Path.*, **34**, 1388–1391

Berry, U. N., Friend, D. S. (1969). High-yield preparation of isolated rat liver parenchymal cells. *J. Cell Biology*, **43**, 506–520

Colten, H. R. (1976). Biosynthesis of complement. *Adv. Immunol.*, **22**, 67–118

Colten, H. R., Alper, C. A. (1972). Haemolytic efficiencies of genetic variants of human C3. *J. Immunol.*, **108**, 1184–1187

Colten, H. R., Borsos, T., Rapp, H. J. (1967). Efficiency of the first component of complement in the hemolytic reaction. *Science*, **158**, 1590–1592

Engvall, E., Perlmann, P. (1971). Enzyme-linked immunosorbent assay (ELISA). *Immunochemistry*, **8**, 871–874

Gordon, S., Todd, J., Cihn, Z. A. (1974). *In vitro* synthesis and secretion of lysosyme by mononuclear phagocytes. *J. Exp. Med.*, **139**, 1228–1248

Hamilton, A. D., Whaley, K. (1985). In Whaley, K. (ed.), *Methods in Complement for Clinical Immunologists*, Churchill Livingstone, Edinburgh, 238–265

Lappin, D., Whaley, K. (1980). Effects of histamine on monocyte complement production. I. Inhibition of C2 production mediated by its action of H_2 receptors. *Clin. Exp. Immunol.*, **41**, 497–504

Lappin, D., Whaley, K. (1982). Prostaglandins and prostaglandin synthetase inhibitors regulate the synthesis of complement components by human monocytes. *Clin. Exp. Immunol.*, **49**, 623–630

Lappin, D., Hamilton, A. O., Morrison, L., Aret, M., Whaley, K. (1986). Synthesis of complement components (C3, C2, B and C1-inhibitor) and lysozyme by human monocytes and macrophages. *J. Clin. Lab. Immunol.*, **20**, 101–105

Nakane, P. K. (1975). Recent progress in the peroxidase-labelled antibody method. *Ann. N.Y. Acad. Sci.*, **254**, 203–211

Nakane, P. K., Kawaoi, A. (1974). Peroxidase labelled antibody. A new method of conjugation. *J. Histochem. Cytochem.*, **22**, 1084–1091

Nakane, P. K., Pierce, G. B. (1967). Enzyme-labelled antibodies: preparation and application for the localization of antigens. *J. Histochem. Cytochem.*, **14**, 929–931

Van Weeman, B. K., Shuuo, A. H. W. M. (1971). Immunoassay using antigen-enzyme conjugates. *FEBS Letters*, **15**, 232–235

Weibler, E. R., Staubli, W., Gnagi, H. R., Hess, F. A. (1969). Correlated morphometric and biochemical studies on the liver cell. I. Morphometric model stereologic methods and normal morphometric data for rat liver. *J. Cell. Biol.*, **42**, 68–91

Whaley, K. (1985). In Whaley, K. (ed.), *Methods in Complement for Clinical Immunologists*, Churchill Livingstone, Edinburgh, 77–139

8. Immunofluorescent Methods for the Assay of Cytoskeleton Antibodies in Human Sera

D. ZAULI, C. CRESPI, F. B. BIANCHI, M. MUSIANI
AND P. TAZZARI

Antibodies reacting with the three major components of the cytoskeleton have been found in human sera from a variety of diseases using immunofluorescence (IFL) techniques (Toh *et al.*, 1979; Pedersen *et al.*, 1982; Kurki *et al.*, 1983a, Dellagi *et al.*, 1984; Zauli *et al.*, 1985a, Zauli *et al.*, 1985b; Kurki *et al.*, 1983b). Although the significance and role of such autoantibodies are still far from clear, it is suggested that they are not simply serological markers of other more important immune events but that they might, on the contrary, play some primary role by interfering with components expressed on the cell membrane which share common antigenic determinants with intracellular cytoskeleton structures (Dales *et al.*, 1983). This mechanism might be of particular importance if one considers that these cytoskeleton constituents are also present in cells of the immune system, as we have recently shown (Zauli *et al.*, 1985c). It is, therefore, important to develop reliable and reproducible methods for the detection of such autoantibodies in human sera.

This Chapter will review some of the IFL methods employed to date for this purpose and will also provide some of our personal findings. Before going into methodological details, it is essential to give a brief introduction to the main characteristics of the structures which make up the cytoplasmic cytoskeleton in order to have a better understanding of some of the problems encountered in the development of such methods.

THE CYTOSKELETON COMPONENTS

The complex of cellular filamentous structures not extractable by detergents and buffers of different ionic strengths represents the 'cytoplasmic cytoskeleton'. The cytoskeleton plays a fundamental role in maintaining and regulating cellular integrity, shape and motility of most (and probably all) eukaryotic cells. It consists of three major filamentous components of different sizes, which mutually interact both structurally and functionally: microfilaments (MF), intermediate filaments (IMF) and microtubules (MT).

As regards the biochemical and antigenic composition of these structures, it is well established that the main protein of MF is actin although, in non-muscle cells, several actin-associated proteins have been identified (Stossel, 1984). The actin filament structures revealed by electron microscopy are of a cellular type (parallel bundles, stress fibres, annular ring etc.), depending on the type and functional status of the cell. This microfilament network can be disrupted by drugs (cytochalasin), which do not interfere with the other cytoskeletal constituents (Weber *et al.*, 1976; Norberg *et al.*, 1975).

Despite morphological and structural similarities, at least five different types of IMF have been identified on the basis of biochemical and immunological properties (Lazarides, 1980). Cytokeratin filaments are found in epithelial cells (Sun and Green, 1978). At least 19 different keratins have been characterized, with molecular weights ranging from 40 000 to 70 000 (Sun *et al.*, 1983). Vimentin filaments are present in all mesenchymal cells (Franke *et al.*, 1979), whereas desmin filaments are characteristic of muscle cells (Lazarides and Balzer, 1978). Neurofilaments, which contain three main polypeptides, are present in neuronal cells (Liem *et al.*, 1978) and glial filaments, composed of the glial fibrillary acidic protein, in glial cells, especially astrocytes (Bignami *et al.*, 1980). By using monoclonal antibodies, however, it has been found that the different types of IMF may share common antigenic determinants (Pruss *et al.*, 1981). Furthermore, in cultured cells, two types of IMF can be expressed simultaneously by individual cells (Virtanen *et al.*, 1981).

The main protein of cytoplasmic MT is tubulin, but there are several MT-associated proteins (Valee, 1980). MT can be disrupted by various drugs (colchicine, vinca alkaloids, griseofulvin) which also alter the organization of IMF with the formation of thick perinuclear bundles of filaments. In addition, vinblastine is able to induce the formation of tubulin paracrystals (De Robertis and De Robertis, 1980; Bryan, 1972), easily identifiable at the optical microscopy level. Thus, vinblastine-treated cells represent a useful substrate for the IFL demonstration of antibodies reacting with each of the three components of the cytoskeleton (Kurki and Virtanen, 1984).

It should also be emphasized that alterations of the cytoskeletal structures are linked with well-defined morphological phenomena associated with a variety of diseases. Well-known examples are damage to pericanalicular actin filaments and cholestasis, pathologic cytokeratins and Mallory bodies, microtubular dysfunction and the 'immotile cilia syndrome' (Denk and Krepler, 1982). Such pathological tissues might also represent suitable substrates for the demonstration of cytoskeleton antibodies, as has been done for anti-Mallory body antibody in cases of alcoholic liver disease.

IFL METHODS FOR THE ASSAY OF CYTOSKELETON ANTIBODIES

The technique currently used for the demonstration of these antibodies in human sera is the indirect IFL on various cell substrates. Such a technique, however, obviously does not identify the nature of the autoantigens involved. To date, however, other more sophisticated and more specific techniques (ELISA, RIA) have only occasionally been used for clinical purposes (Bretherton *et al.*, 1983). This is probably due to the difficulties encountered during the purification procedures of the various autoantigens.

In IFL, the most widely employed cell type is represented by cultured fibroblasts (Toh *et al.*, 1979; Pedersen *et al.*, 1982; Dellagi *et al.*, 1984; Zauli *et al.*, 1985a; Zauli *et al.*, 1985b; Kurki *et al.*, 1983b) of different origin (rat, mouse, human) previously exposed to the action of microtubule-disrupting agents (mainly vinblastine and colchicine). As already mentioned, vinblastine treatment allows the IFL identification of three antibody patterns on the same cell by inducing the formation of tubulin paracrystals and of thick filamentous coils of vimentin IMF and by leaving the microfilament network intact. This may be clinically relevant, as in some disease sera the various patterns may be variably associated. Therefore, cells are usually incubated in medium containing the drug at a concentration of 10 μg/ml for 4 h at 37°C before fixation.

Fixation is a crucial step for the success of this IFL method. Different fixation procedures have been employed (acetone, methanol, formaldehyde) and, sometimes, treatment with detergents has been suggested, before fixation, to enhance the penetration of the antibodies (Kurki and Virtanen, 1984). It seems, however, that acetone at -20°C for 10 min is the most frequently used fixation procedure. As reported later, when other cell types have been employed instead of fibroblasts, acetone fixation at 4°C for 2–5 min has proved best for achieving well-preserved morphology and antigenicity (Zauli *et al.*, 1985c).

Other cell types, such as cultured epithelial cells, lymphoblastoid and myeloid leukemic cell lines, have occasionally been used by some workers as substrate for the assay of cytoskeleton antibodies (Linder *et al.*, 1979). It should, however, be emphasized that primary cultures may contain several types of cells with different cytoskeleton composition (IMF in particular) and that established cell lines may express two types of IMF simultaneously (Virtanen *et al.*, 1981). We have, in fact, recently shown that IMF of K562 leukaemic cells (myeloid) can be stained by both anti-vimentin and anti-keratin monoclonal antibodies (Zauli *et al.*, 1986). Therefore, when testing human sera for anti-IMF antibodies on this substrate, the specificity of the antibodies (anti-vimentin or anti-keratin) cannot be established.

For these reasons, and as the availability of cell cultures may be a problem for some laboratories, we have recently developed an IFL method for the detection of cytoskeleton antibodies using vinblastine-treated, freshly isolated, normal peripheral blood mononuclear cells (Zauli *et al.*, 1985c). Other cell types have been subsequently evaluated in order to identify the ideal substrate for each of the three different antibody specificities.

METHODS USED

When cultured fibroblasts were used, the method of Kurki *et al.* (1983b) was adopted.

We have shown that density gradient separated normal peripheral blood mononuclear cells express the three major components of the cytoskeleton, which are readily distinguishable when cells are treated with vinblastine (Zauli *et al.*, 1985c). A dose–response curve was made and we found that a 20 μg/ml vinblastine concentration was ideal to induce morphological alterations of the cytoskeleton components. After incubating cells with the drug for 4 h at 37°C, they were quickly washed (the effect of the drug is reversible) and cytocentrifuged. Various fixation procedures were tested and we prefer acetone for 2–3 min at 4°C. Slides were then stored at −20°C for a long period of time without any loss of morphological or antigenic integrity.

Before using these cells for clinical purposes, i.e. as substrate for the detection of autoantibodies in human sera, we have shown that both polyclonal and monoclonal antibodies to the main subunit proteins of the cytoskeleton structures (actin, vimentin and tubulin) adorn actin–MF (figure 1), vimentin–IMF (figure 2) and tubulin paracrystals (figure 3) respectively.

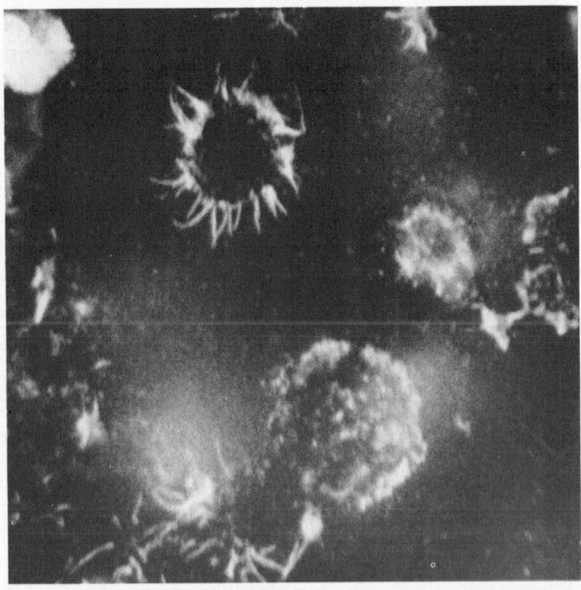

Figure 1 Immunofluorescence pattern of anti-actin microfilament antibodies using mononuclear cells. Magnification: 50×.

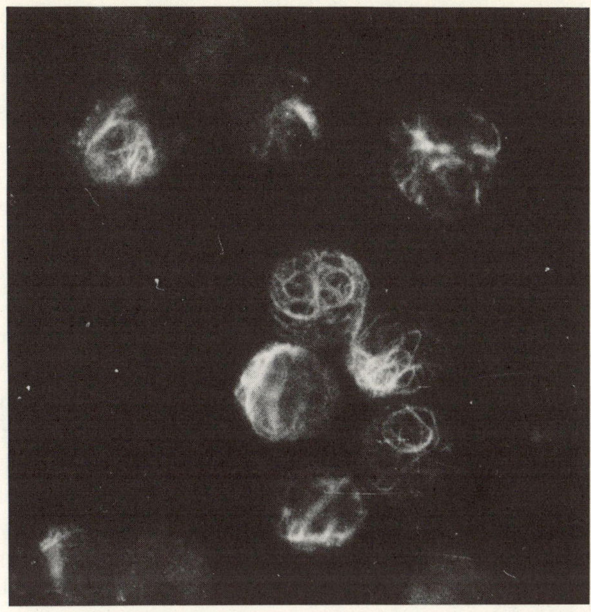

Figure 2   Immunofluorescence pattern of anti-vimentin intermediate filament antibodies using vinblastine-treated mononuclear cells. Magnification: 50×.

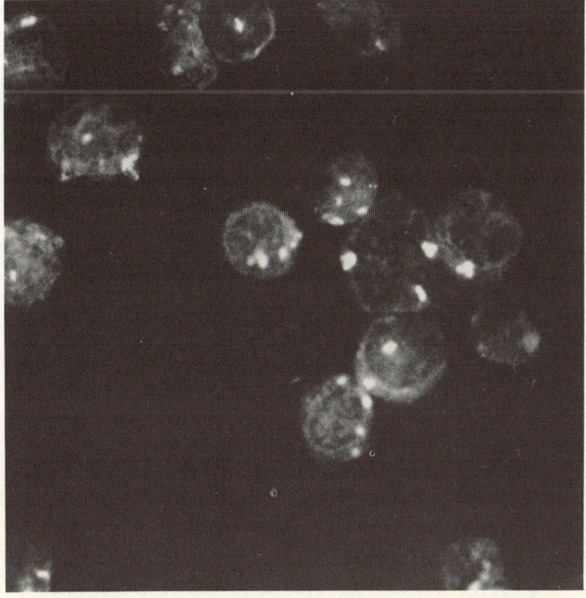

Figure 3   Immunofluorescence pattern of anti-tubulin antibodies using vinblastine-treated mononuclear cells. Magnification: 50×.

For the identification of MF-containing microvilli, cells should be suspended in 0.034 M sodium citrate (Fagraeus *et al.*, 1974). Furthermore, platelets (always contaminating cell preparations) are also stained by anti-actin antibodies. It is, in fact, well established that platelets are extremely rich in actin (Rosenberg *et al.*, 1981). The specificity of the reaction was also confirmed by treating cells with cytochalasin B, which disrupts actin–MF into actin-containing granular or asterisk-like material, similarly to what has been found with other cell types (Weber *et al.*, 1976; Norberg *et al.*, 1975). Moreover, direct IFL with rhodamine-labelled phalloidin (a kind gift from T. Wieland, Heidelberg) showed staining of MF identical to that of anti-actin antibodies.

In an attempt to identify the ideal substrate for each of the three different types of antibodies, we have studied other cell types. The following commercially available cell lines have been evaluated: the K562 leukaemic cell line, EBV-infected Raji and P3HR1 lymphoblastoid cells and the T lymphocyte leukaemic HPB-MLT cell line. Native 'hairy' leukaemic cells were also studied. In all these different cell types, organization of the cytoskeleton has been studied before and after vinblastine treatment, using both monoclonal and polyclonal antibodies to the various cytoskeleton constituents, as described for mononuclear cells. The results obtained using all these cell types will be discussed later.

OCCURRENCE OF CYTOSKELETON ANTIBODIES IN HUMAN SERA

Anti-MF antibodies have been found essentially in the sera of patients with autoimmune (smooth muscle antibody positive) chronic active hepatitis (CAH)

Table 1   Prevalance (%) of anti-microfilament antibodies using various cell substrates

	Fibroblasts	Mononuclear cells	Raji cells
Autoimmune CLD	38[a], 55[b], 67[c]	90[a]	86[a]
HBV–CLD	8[a]	0[a]	NT
HDV–CLD	NT	5[a]	NT
ALD	13[a], 25[c]	14[d]	NT
IBD	6[e]	NT	NT
Neuroblastoma	35[f]	NT	NT
Controls	3[c], 2[e]	0[a]	0[a]

CLD = chronic liver disease; HBV = hepatitis B virus; HDV = hepatitis delta virus; ALD = alcoholic liver disease; IBD = inflammatory bowel disease; NT = not tested.
[a] Present work.
[b] Pedersen *et al.* (1982).
[c] Kurki *et al.* (1983b).
[d] Crespi *et al.* (1986).
[e] Zauli *et al.* (1985a).
[f] Zauli *et al.* (1985b).

and primary biliary cirrhosis (PBC) (Pedersen *et al.*, 1982; Kurki *et al.*, 1983b). They are only occasionally present in other types of chronic liver disease and other diseases and in healthy subjects. The results of the anti-MF assay obtained by various authors and our personal findings are summarized in table 1.

We have tested the sera from autoimmune liver disease on three different cell types: fibroblasts, mononuclear cells and Raji cells, which proved to contain enormous amounts of actin (figures 4 and 5). When we compared the results obtained, we found that the highest prevalence and best agreement were reached with mononuclear and Raji cells. We conclude, therefore, that, in our hands at least, fibroblasts are not the substrate of choice for the demonstration of anti-MF antibodies in sera from autoimmune liver disease. The clinical relevance of this conclusion emerges from the consideration that anti-actin positive CAH cases are universally recognized as the true autoimmune cases, potentially susceptible to immunomodifying treatment. Furthermore, we have recently found that 'hairy' cells display an extremely rich network of actin filaments (figure 6) and might, therefore, be a suitable substrate for the demonstration of anti-MF antibodies in human sera. The immunoglobulin class of anti-MF antibodies is mainly IgG in autoimmune chronic liver disease but may also be IgA in alcoholic cirrhosis (43%) (Crespi *et al.*, 1986) and IgM in virus-induced chronic liver disease (100%) (personal findings).

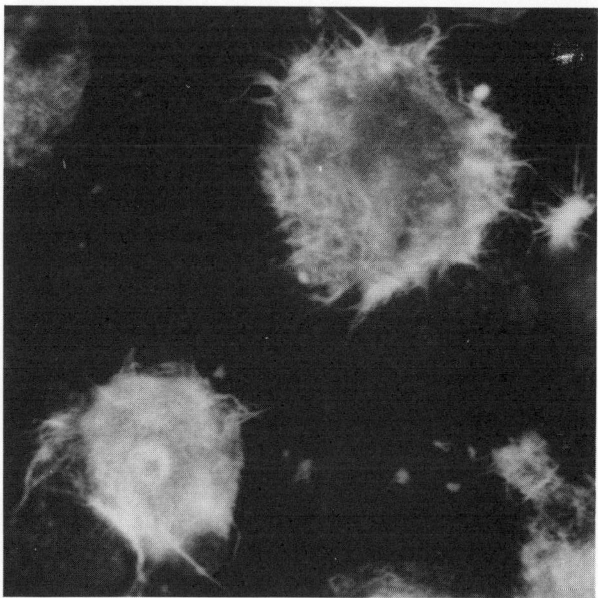

Figure 4   Immunofluorescence appearance of Raji cells using anti-actin antibodies. Magnification: 50×.

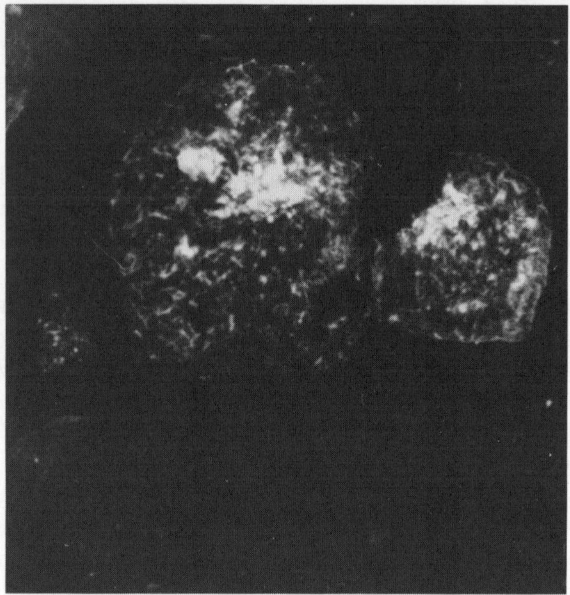

Figure 5   Immunofluorescence appearance of Raji cells using anti-actin antibodies after treatment with cytochalasin B. Actin microfilaments are disrupted. Magnification: 50×.

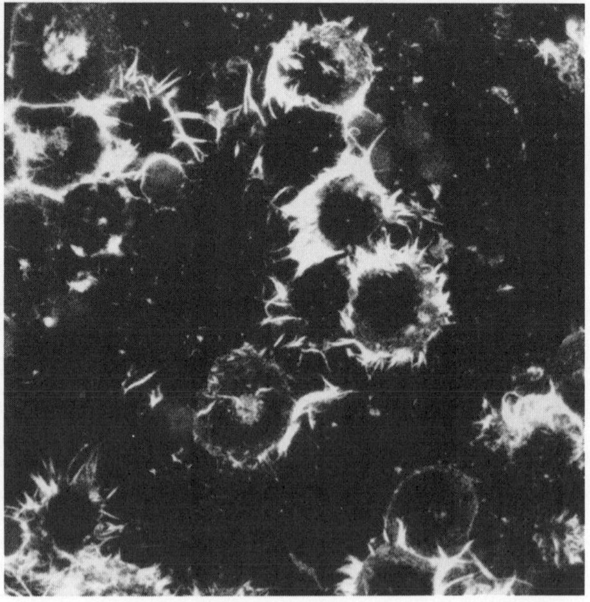

Figure 6   Immunofluorescence appearance of native leukaemic 'hairy' cells using anti-actin antibodies. Magnification: 50x.

Anti-IMF antibodies have been reported in a wide variety of human diseases as well as in healthy controls (Toh *et al.*, 1979; Pedersen *et al.*, 1982; Dellagi *et al.*, 1984; Kurki *et al.*, 1983b). The prevalence of anti-vimentin IMF in human sera is shown in table 2. It is clear from this table that mononuclear cells are less sensitive, but seem to be more specific, than fibroblasts for the assay of anti-IMF antibodies. In fact, no anti-IMF reactivity was found in the sera of healthy controls. These antibodies are more frequently IgM although, in alcoholic and inflammatory bowel disease (IBD) cases, we have also found reactivity in the IgA class (Zauli *et al.*, 1985a). IgM anti-IMF antibodies have been reported in 80% of the sera from infectious mononucleosis using K562 cells (Linder *et al.*, 1979). However, for the reasons mentioned above, the specificity of these antibodies remains to be elucidated. We are currently studying the IMF system of normal lymphocyte subsets, of native leukaemic cells and of various leukaemic cell lines. Preliminary results seem to indicate that T lymphocytes (both normal and leukaemic) are particularly rich in vimentin IMF. Further investigation will show how suitable these cells may be for the IFL assay of anti-IMF autoantibodies.

Anti-MT antibodies were initially reported in infectious mononucleosis (Mead *et al.*, 1980) and, more recently, in alcoholic liver disease (Kurki *et al.*, 1983b). Using vinblastine-treated fibroblasts, we have found antibodies reacting with tubulin paracrystals in 58% of the sera from children affected by neuroblastoma (Zauli *et al.*, 1985b). More recently, using mononuclear cells, we have obtained a high frequency of anti-tubulin antibodies both in alcoholic and in hepatitis

Table 2 Prevalence (%) of anti-vimentin intermediate filament antibodies using various cell substrates

	Fibroblasts	Mononuclear cells
Autoimmune CLD	15[a], 88[b]	11[c]
PBC	93[b]	25[c]
ALD	26[c], 50[b]	37[c]
HBV–CLD	34[a]	39[c]
HDV–CLD	NT	71[c]
Viral infections	65[d]	NT
IBD	37[e]	NT
Neuroblastoma	46[f]	NT
Controls	29[e]	0[c]

CLD = chronic liver disease; PBC = primary biliary cirrhosis; ALD = alcoholic liver disease; HBV = hepatitis B virus; HDV = hepatitis delta virus; IBD = inflammatory bowel disease; NT = not tested.
[a] Pedersen *et al.* (1982).
[b] Kurki *et al.* (1983b).
[c] Present work.
[d] Toh *et al.* (1979).
[e] Zauli *et al.* (1985a).
[f] Zauli *et al.* (1985b).

delta virus-induced chronic liver disease, as shown in table 3. Interestingly, in alcoholic cases, 53% of the anti-MT antibodies are also IgA, whereas in all the other conditions they are IgG.

While studying the cytoskeletal organization of various cell lines, we have observed that vinblastine-treated K562, Raji and P3HR1 cell lines express a consistent number of large tubulin paracrystals (figure 6). These cell lines might, therefore, represent an excellent substrate for the study of anti-tubulin antibodies.

As regards the titres of cytoskeleton antibodies, they have been reported to be low. In chronic liver disease they only occasionally exceed 1:60 (Kurki *et al.*, 1983b). However, in acute hepatitis A, titres up to 1:512 have been described (Pedersen *et al.*, 1981). Preliminary results obtained in our laboratory seem to indicate that, in graft-*versus*-host disease of bone-marrow transplant patients, titres of anti-IMF antibodies may be very high (up to 1:1024).

Table 3   Prevalence (%) of anti-microtubule antibodies using various cell substrates

	Fibroblasts	Mononuclear cells
ALD	50[a]	47[b]
HBV–CLD	NT	9[c]
HDV–CLD	NT	44[c]
IBD	19[d]	NT
Neuroblastoma	58[e]	NT
Controls	3[d], 9[a]	0[c]

ALD = alcoholic liver disease; HBV = hepatitis B virus; HDV = hepatitis delta virus; CLD = chronic liver disease; IBD = inflammatory bowel disease; NT = not tested.
[a] Kurki *et al.* (1983b).
[b] Crespi *et al.* (1986).
[c] Present work.
[d] Zauli *et al.* (1985a).
[e] Zauli *et al.* (1985b).

CONCLUSIONS

This chapter has reviewed the results obtained by various authors, and by ourselves, in the study of cytoskeleton antibodies using the indirect IFL technique in different cell substrates.

The conclusions we have reached are that, although cultured fibroblasts have been the most frequently used cell substrate to date, other cell types have more recently been shown to be not only as suitable as, but also superior to, fibroblasts for several reasons. After studying various cell types, we believe that normal mononuclear cells are an ideal substrate for the following reasons: ready availability of these cells in almost any laboratory, low cost of the method, no cell cultures required and no culture-induced alterations of the original cytoskeleton composition. However, if other cell types are available in some laboratories (i.e. Raji cells for the detection of circulating immune complexes), they might be usefully employed in the assay of some anti-cytoskeleton specificity.

REFERENCES

Bignami, A., Dahl, D., Rueger, D. C. (1980). Glial fibrillary acidic protein (GFA) in normal neural cells and in pathological conditions. *Adv. Cell. Neurobiol.*, 7, 285–310

Bretherton, L., Brown, C., Pedersen, J. S., Toh, B. H., Clarke, F. M., Mackay, I. R., Gust, I. D. (1983). ELISA assay for IgG autoantibody to G-actin: comparison of chronic active hepatitis and acute viral hepatitis. *Clin. Exp. Immunol.*, 51, 611–616

Bryan, J. J. (1972). Vinblastine and microtubules. *J. Mol. Biol.*, 66, 157–163

Crespi, C., Zauli, D., Miserocchi, F., Bianchi, F. B., Pisi, E. (1986). IgA anti-cytoskeleton antibodies in alcoholic liver disease (ALD). *Ital. J. Gastro-enterol.*, 18, 55–56

Dales, S., Fujinami, R. S., Oldstone, M. B. A. (1983). Serologic relatedness between Thy-1.2 and actin revealed by monoclonal antibody. *J. Immunol.*, 131, 1332–1338

De Robertis, E. D. P., De Robertis, E. M. F. (1980). The cytoskeleton and cell motility: microtubules and microfilaments. In *Cell and molecular biology*, Saunders, Philadelphia, 179–205

Dellagi, K., Brouet, J.-C., Seligman, M. (1984). Antivimentin autoantibodies in angioimmunoblastic lymphoadenopathy. *N. Engl. J. Med.*, 310, 215–218

Denk, H., Krepler, R. (1982). The cytoskeleton in pathologic conditions. *Path. Res. Pract.*, 175, 180–195

Fagraeus, A., Lidman, K., Biberfeld, G. (1974). Reaction of human smooth muscle antibodies with human blood lymphocytes and lymphoid cell lines. *Nature*, 252, 246–247

Franke, W. W., Schmid, E., Winter, S., Osborn, M., Weber, K. (1979). Widespread occurrence of intermediate sized filaments of the vimentin type in cultured cells from diverse vertebrates. *Exp. Cell. Res.*, 123, 25–46

Kurki, P., Helve, T., Virtanen, I. (1983a). Antibodies to cytoplasmic intermediate filaments in rheumatic diseases. *J. Rheumatol.*, 10, 558–562

Kurki, P., Miettinen, A., Salaspuro, M., Virtanen, I., Stenman, S. (1983b). Cytoskeleton antibodies in chronic active hepatitis, primary biliary cirrhosis and alcoholic liver disease. *Hepatology*, 3, 297–302

Kurki, P., Virtanen, I. (1984). The detection of human antibodies against cyto-skeletal components. *J. Immunol. Methods*, 67, 209–223

Lazarides, E. (1980). Intermediate filaments as mechanical integrators of cellular space. *Nature*, 283, 249–256

Lazarides, E., Balzer, D. R. (1978). Specificity of desmin to avian and mammalian muscle cells. *Cell*, 14, 429–438

Liem, R. K. H., Yen, S.-H., Salomon, G. D., Shelanski, M. L. (1978). Intermediate filaments in nervous tissue. *J. Cell. Biol.*, 79, 637–645

Linder, E., Kurki, P., Andersson, L. C. (1979). Autoantibody to intermediate filaments in infectious mononucleosis. *Clin. Immunol. Immunopathol.*, 14, 411–417

Mead, G. M., Cowin, P., Whitehouse, J. M. A. (1980). Anti-tubulin antibody in healthy adults and patients with infectious mononucleosis and its relationship to smooth muscle antibody (SMA). *Clin. Exp. Immunol.*, **39**, 328–336

Norberg, R., Lidman, K., Fagraeus, A. (1975). Effects of cytochalasin B on fibroblasts, lymphoid cells and platelets revealed by human anti-actin antibodies. *Cell*, **6**, 507–512

Pedersen, J. S., Toh, B.-H., Locarnini, S. A., Gust, B. D., Shyamala, G. N. S. (1981). Autoantibody to intermediate filaments in viral hepatitis. *Clin. Immunol. Immunopathol.*, **21**, 154–161

Pedersen, J. S., Toh, B.-H., Mackay, I. R., Tait, B. D., Gust, I. D., Kastelan, A., Hadzic, N. (1982). Segregation of autoantibody to cytoskeletal filaments with two types of chronic active hepatitis. *Clin. Exp. Immunol.*, **48**, 527–532

Pruss, R. M., Mirsky, R., Raff, M. G., Thorpe, R., Dowding, A. J., Anderton, B. H. (1981). All classes of intermediate filaments share a common antigenic determinant defined by a monoclonal antibody. *Cell*, **27**, 419–428

Rosenberg, S., Stracher, A., Lucas, R. C. (1981). Isolation and characterization of actin and actin-binding protein from human platelets. *J. Cell. Biol.*, **91**, 201–211

Stossel, T. P. (1984). Contribution of actin to the structure of the cytoplasmic matrix. *J. Cell. Biol.*, **99**, 15s–21s

Sun, T.-T., Green, H. (1978). Immunofluorescent staining of keratin fibres in cultured cells. *Cell*, **14**, 469–476

Sun, T.-T., Eichner, R., Nelson, W. G., Scheffer, C. G., Weiss, R. A., Jarvinen, M., Woodcock-Mitchell, J. (1983). Keratin classes: molecular markers for different types of epithelial differentiation. *J. Invest. Dermatol.*, **81**, 109–115

Toh, B.-H., Yildiz, A., Sotelo, J., Osung, O., Holborow, E. J., Kanakoudi, F., Small, J. V. (1979). Viral infections and IgM autoantibodies to cytoplasmic intermediate filaments. *Clin. Exp. Immunol.*, **37**, 76–82

Valee, R. (1980). Structure and phosphorylation of microtubule-associated protein. 2. *Proc. Natl. Acad. Sci.*, **77**, 3206–3210

Virtanen, I., Lehto, V. P., Lehtonen, E., Vartio, T., Stenman, S., Kurki, P., Wager, O., Small, J. V., Dahl, D., Badley, R. A. (1981). Expression of intermediate filaments in cultured cells. *J. Cell. Sci.*, **50**, 45–63

Weber, K., Rathke, P. C., Osborn, M., Franke, W. W. (1976). Distribution of actin and tubulin in cells and in glycerinated cell models after treatment with cytochalasin B (CB). *Exp. Cell. Res.*, **102**, 285–297

Zauli, D., Crespi, C., Dall'Amore, P., Bianchi, F. B., Pisi, E. (1985a). Antibodies to the cytoskeleton components and other autoantibodies in inflammatory bowel disease. *Digestion*, **32**, 140–144

Zauli, D., Crespi, C., Mancini, A. F., Zerbini, M., Bianchi, F. B., Pisi, E. (1985b). Relationship between smooth muscle and cytoskeleton antibodies in neuroblastoma. *Tumori*, **71**, 425–430

Zauli, D., Crespi, C., Bianchi, F. B., Pisi, E. (1985c). Immunofluorescent detection of anti-cytoskeleton antibodies using vinblastine-treated mononuclear cells. *J. Immunol. Methods*, **82**, 77–82

Zauli, D., Gobbi, M., Crespi, C., Tazzari, P. L., Miserocchi, F., Magnani, M., Testoni, N. (1986). Vimentin and keratin intermediate filaments expression by K562 leukemic cell line. *Leuk. Res.*, **10**, 29–33

9. The Use of Western Blot Procedures in the Analysis of Herpes Simplex Virus Proteins

J. KÜHN, G. DUNKLER, K. MUNK AND R. BRAUN

During the past few years a multitude of different experimental approaches have been developed to assess the interaction between proteins, of which the use of cross-linking agents and immune electrophoresis are the most widespread. With the introduction of blotting techniques by electrophoretic transfer of proteins to filter membranes (Towbin *et al.*, 1979), however, the possibility of assessing protein–protein interactions at molecular level has been extended, especially in the analysis of antibody reactivity and specificity. By the transfer of an exact image of electrophoretically separated proteins to a filter membrane, the Western blot technique offers a series of advantages in comparison with other techniques, the most obvious being the ease and practicability of the procedure and the interpretation of results. It is thus that Western blot techniques have also been widely applied to the routine diagnosis of viral infections (e.g. as confirmatory tests in the diagnosis of HIV).

Moreover, besides their ability to detect antibody-reactive proteins, Western blot procedures may also be used in the detection of protein functions other than antibody antigen interactions (e.g. in the analysis of the ability of proteins to bind nucleic acids).

However, all the above-mentioned experiments require careful selection of specific blotting, incubation, and binding conditions, to avoid possible pitfalls and nonspecific results in the respective protein binding assays. It is the intention of this article to give an overview of the various Western blot procedures, examples of which will be shown for proteins of herpes simplex virus type 1.

GENERAL REMARKS ON A WESTERN BLOTTING STRATEGY

The individual goal of a Western blotting experiment (e.g. assessment of protein-protein or assessment of protein–nonprotein ligand interaction) requires the careful selection of a blotting strategy which should consider the following points: (1) transfer of proteins from the separating gels to membranes; (2) binding of proteins to the surface of membranes; (3) blocking of free binding sites to reduce background; (4) binding of ligands to membrane bound proteins; (5) further incubation steps with second ligands (sandwich-type assays); (6) detection of bound ligands.

Transfer of Polypeptides

Polypeptide transfer from gels to filter membranes may be achieved either by diffusion or by side-directed solvent flow (Aubertin *et al.*, 1983; Reinhart and Malamud, 1982; Smith and Summers, 1980; Peferoen *et al.*, 1982) similarly to the method first described for transfer of DNA to nitrocellulose (NC) membranes (Southern, 1975). Electro-elution, however, appears to be the most widely used principle in Western blotting (Towbin *et al.*, 1979; Burnett, 1981; Gershoni and Palade, 1983; Towbin and Gordon, 1984; Tsang *et al.*, 1983). Originally, electro-elution was performed in a gel destainer. Today, however, a number of electro-blotting chambers are commercially available.

Polypeptides separated by SDS–PAGE leave the gel as anions, and the filter membrane has to be positioned at the side of the gel directed towards the anode of the electrophoretic transfer chamber. If electro-elution is performed from gels run without SDS, or if transfer buffers with other compositions are used as described below, the membrane has to be positioned according to the resulting electric charge of the proteins to be transferred. During electrotransfer of proteins, electrolytes are eluted from the gel together with the proteins, which results in a decreasing resistance of the transfer unit and a consequent increase of current. Therefore, when power supplies keeping a constant current up to 1 A or even more are used, the Joule heating of the blot chamber must be taken into consideration. Generally, low ionic strength of transfer buffers allows higher voltage and, therefore, less time-consuming blotting procedures. The efficiency of electro-elution from the gel at constant voltage is dependent on the molecular weight of the protein and — to a lesser degree — on the composition of the gel, i.e. percentage of polyacrylamide, amount of crosslinking, and differences between the various crosslinking agents. Poor transfer of small proteins may be due to their precipitation in the gel or due to the fact that these proteins are at their IEP and thus without charge.

Transfer buffers for electro-elution are normally of relatively low ionic strength (25 mM Tris, 192 mM glycine, 20 vol% methanol, pH 8.3 (Towbin *et al.*, 1979)) and may contain methanol. In the presence of 20 vol% methanol, proteins adsorb better to NC and swelling of the gel (and resulting broadening of the bands) in low ionic strength buffers can be avoided. In contrast to these advantages, methanol reduces the efficiency of protein transfer from SDS–PAGE, which results in prolonged incubation times (Burnett, 1981).

Thus, the efficiency of protein elution from gels has to be carefully determined, e.g. by silver staining of the remaining proteins in the gel. In case of insufficient transfer of proteins, the blotting time should be extended or other transfer buffers should be used.

Binding of Proteins to Membranes

Immobilisation of the proteins on membranes can be achieved by adsorption to NC (Towbin *et al.*, 1979; Aubertin *et al.*, 1983; Peferoen *et al.*, 1982; Burnett, 1981; Gershoni and Palade, 1983; De Blas and Cherwinski, 1983; Erickson *et al.*, 1982; Glass *et al.*, 1981; Lin and Kasamatsu, 1983; Ramirez *et al.*, 1983) or nylon membranes (Zetabind (ZB) (Gershoni and Palade, 1982, 1983)) or by covalent linkage to chemically activated papers, e.g. diazobenzyloxymethyl (DBM)-paper (Smith and Summers, 1980; Renart *et al.*, 1979; Schaltmann and Pongs, 1980; Symington *et al.*, 1981) or diazophenylthioether (DPT)-paper (Olmsted, 1981; Reiser and Wardale, 1981). For most purposes NC membranes appear to be superior to other materials in terms of availability, costs, binding capacity, and reduction of background binding of ligands.

The interaction of NC with proteins is only poorly understood. It is likely, however, that hydrophobic effects play an important role in protein immobilisation. The pore size of the NC membranes used may also have an influence on their binding capacity. In this context, the migration of small proteins through NC membranes has been reported (Burnett, 1981; Lin and Kasamatsu, 1983). The use of less porous material (0.2 μm instead of 0.45 μm) was recommended to increase the binding capacity.

ZB (Gershoni and Palade, 1982, 1983) is a nylon membrane with numerous positively charged groups on the surface. Because of its positive charge, this type of membrane offers very high binding capacity, especially when proteins are transferred from SDS–PAGE (negative charge of the polypeptides). ZB, however, also needs extensive blocking procedures to reduce the background binding of second-step ligands sufficiently.

In order to obtain stable binding of transferred proteins, DBM-, DPT- or CNBr-activated papers may also be used, which offer the advantage of covalent linkage of the polypeptides to the paper matrix. However, these papers have to be activated before use and this might present a possible hazard for laboratory personnel handling toxic activation substances. Furthermore, when using this material, a slight loss in resolution from gel to blot, due to the intrinsic coarseness of these papers, has been reported (Burnett, 1981).

In most experiments it is desirable to visualise the total membrane-bound protein pattern, besides the protein bands detected by immunostaining. Whereas the work with radioactively labelled proteins causes hazards in handling, the staining and destaining of blotted proteins with dyes such as amido black, fast green, Ponceau red S (10% in water) or India ink stain (Hancock and Tsang, 1983) has proved to be a useful tool to compare immunoreactive protein bands with the total protein profile of the blot. Recently, fluorescent labelling of proteins with 2-methoxy-2,4-diphenyl-3(2H)-furanone (MDPF) before SDS–PAGE was found to be a sensitive method for monitoring polypeptides during gel electrophoresis and Western blotting (Falk and Elliott, 1985). Staining of proteins on the blot, however, may interfere with the subsequent immuno-detection and cause a loss of sensitivity.

Blocking of Free Binding Sites

Filter areas not covered with transferred protein bands may nonspecifically adsorb second-step ligands, as added in the subsequent incubation steps, and this would result in high background staining. In order to reduce such a back-ground binding of second-step ligands, the blots must be blocked prior to addition of ligands. When using chemically activated paper, the remaining untreated binding sites must be inactivated after protein blotting by adding reactive groups in excess. A variety of different substances have been used to block the adsorb-ing membranes such as whole animal sera (i.e. 10% horse serum, foetal calf serum) (Peferoen *et al.*, 1982; Burnett, 1981; Towbin and Gordon, 1984), BSA, gelatine or haemoglobin (Towbin *et al.*, 1979; Gershoni and Palade, 1982, 1983). The use of ovalbumin and mild detergents has also been recommended (De Blas and Cherwinski, 1983; Spinola and Cannon, 1985).

Another major aspect of the preincubation of blots with protein and deter-gent solutions is the removal of SDS and the renaturation of antigenic sites. Although complete renaturation of proteins by such procedures is not possible, there is still some effect on the renaturation of antigenic domains and a high percentage of the SDS may be removed by such procedures.

However, blocking agents in turn may cause variation in the immunologic detection of proteins transferred to NC membranes. By comparing bovine serum albumin with commercial nonfat dry milk and Tween 20 as blocking and renatur-ing agents in the immunologic detection of bacterial proteins transferred to nitrocellulose, quantitative and qualitative differences in specifically detected antigens were found (Spinola and Cannon, 1985). Thus, different blocking agents should be tested when evaluating a blotting strategy in order to achieve optimal results.

Another reason for artificial and nonspecific results may be the use of protein-contaminated solutions, reagents and equipment in SDS–PAGE. It was shown that such contaminating proteins were mainly skin proteins, especially keratins (Ochs, 1983). Therefore, handling of the gel electrophoresis buffers, equipment etc. without the wearing of gloves should be avoided.

Binding of Ligands to Membrane-bound Proteins

In a widely spread modification of Western blot procedure, proteins transferred to NC membranes are detected by further incubation of blots with specific monoclonal or polyclonal antibodies which are directly labelled either with an enzyme or with radioactivity or which are detected by further incubation with a second antibody. In this step also incubation conditions have to be carefully selected to avoid nonspecific false positive or false negative results. Although antigen–antibody reactions, in general, proceed faster at 37°C than at 4°C, the reaction appears to be more specific at 4°C and thus incubation of ligands with blots at low temperature is generally recommended. It has been shown, however, that with certain proteins antigen–antibody reactions are more specific and have higher affinity constants at 37°C than at 4°C and vice versa. In addition, the use of blocking substances in binding buffers is also recommended, in order to reduce nonspecific binding of antibodies to membrane-fixed proteins to a minimum. This may also include the use of proteinase inhibitors such as phenylmethyl-sulfonylfluoride (PMSF) to avoid degradation of antigens and antibodies.

It has been the experience of this laboratory that even extensive blocking of membranes with nonfat dry milk, BSA, Tween 20 and other substances does not always sufficiently reduce background binding when human sera are used to detect virus-specific proteins in infected cell lysates. It is recommended that, for such experiments, lysates of mock infected cells be added to antibody binding buffers, in order to remove competitively such nonspecific reactions. Furthermore, a variety of cells and viruses have been shown to possess receptors for the Fc part and other domains of antibodies which might result in nonspecific binding. Such interactions may be avoided by using purified $F(ab')_2$ fragments as first and second antibodies, or using rheumatoid factor to detect binding of the first ligand. The use of protein A or the recently introduced protein G (Akerström *et al.*, 1985) as a second ligand cannot be recommended, owing to their restricted reactivity with certain IgG subclasses and also to their reactivity with unbound antibodies in general. It should be noted that whole animal sera cannot be used as blocking agents if protein A or protein G (Akerström *et al.*, 1985) is involved in the immunodetection steps.

Further Incubation Steps with Second Ligands

If labelled ligands for detection of membrane-bound proteins are not available, or the antigen specificity of first-step ligands has to be assessed, further incubation of blots with a second-step ligand, binding to the first ligand protein or antibody, must be performed. This generally has the advantage of enhancing sensitivity of the procedure by multiplying the effect of antibody–antibody reaction. The choice of a second-step ligand depends on the nature of the first-step ligand used and is dependent on the rationale of the experiment. Most frequently, horseradish-peroxidase-labelled antibodies are used. In order to enhance further the sensitivity of the procedure, however, biotin-labelled second antibodies may also be used which, in a further incubation step, may be detected by their reactivity with a peroxidase-labelled streptavidin complex.

Furthermore, the appropriate selection of second-step antibodies may also be helpful in the detection of binding of specific immunoglobulin classes (e.g. IgG or IgM) to membrane-bound proteins. In such experiments, however, competition of different immunoglobulin classes for antigenic binding sites may occur, requiring the preparative separation of these antibody classes before their application in Western blots. An example of this is given in figure 2, in which the binding of human IgM antibodies to HSV proteins is shown before and after removal of serum IgG.

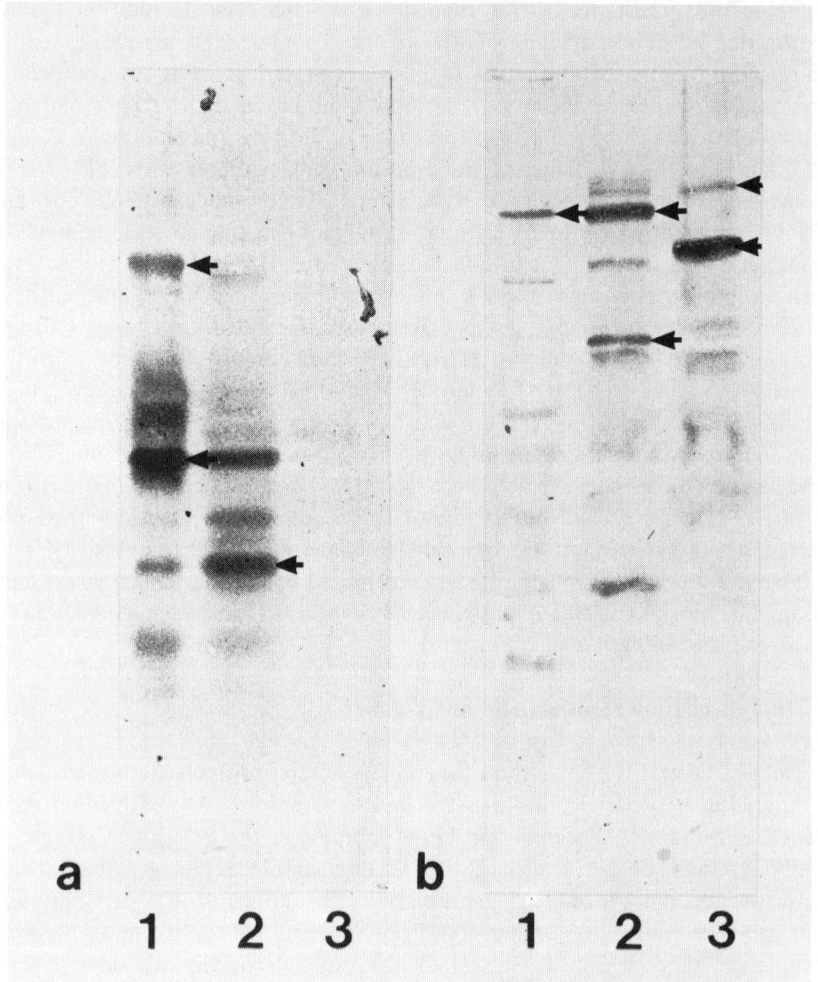

Figure 1   Humoral immune response in acute primary HSV infection. Figure 1a shows a typical IgG immune response against HSV-1 late proteins (lane 1), early proteins (lane 2) and immediate–early proteins (lane 3). Characteristic proteins recognised by the antibodies are marked by arrow heads (from high to low molecular weight). Lane 1 gB, gD; lane 2 50 kD capsid protein. Figure 1b shows a typical IgM immune response against HSV-1 specified late proteins (lane 1), early proteins (lane 2) and immediate–early proteins (lane 3). Proteins typically recognised are marked by arrow heads (from high to low molecular weight). Lane 1, VP5; lane 2, ICP8 and a nonstructural protein with an approximate molecular weight of 75 kD; lane 3, ICP4 and ICP0.

Detection of Bound Ligands

Immunodetection of membrane-bound proteins and other ligands is generally performed similarly to other (already established) solid-phase immunoassays. In order to save monoclonal antibodies or precious sera, antibodies with high avidity should be preferentially applied in high dilutions for long incubation periods. Low avidity antibodies, by contrast, should be used in low dilutions and for shorter incubation periods. Although a steadily increasing number of reagents, i.e. nearly all reagents developed for immunohistochemistry, have been adopted for immunoblotting (Brada and Roth, 1984; Burnett, 1981; Hierholzer *et al.*, 1984; Knecht and Dimond, 1984; Ramirez *et al.*, 1983), peroxidase-labelled antibodies seem to be the most used and convenient label (Gershoni and Palade, 1983; Towbin and Gordon, 1984; Ashley and Corey, 1984). It is noteworthy that diaminobenzidine $(DAB)-H_2O_2$ as substrate for peroxidase possesses a carcinogenic risk and should therefore be replaced by 4-chloronaphthol-H_2O_2.

General Remarks

In means of detection of macromolecular interaction, the fact that many proteins fixed to membranes retain their ability not only to react with antibodies but also to bind to specific receptor or effector molecules is promising. For example, protein–hormone interactions between a 150 kD membrane protein of human epidermoid cancer cells and epidermal growth factor (EGF) could be demonstrated by reacting transferred cell membrane proteins with EGF and subsequently labelling with radioactive antibodies directed against EGF (Fernandez-Pol, 1982). In a similar way, a large number of protein–ligand interactions have already been studied (Gershoni and Palade, 1983), including demonstration of specific interaction between proteins and DNA or RNA (Bowen *et al.*, 1980). Even specific binding of whole cells to blotted adhesion factors was shown (Hayman *et al.*, 1982). In order to retain specific reactivity of blotted proteins, denaturation during gel electrophoresis and blotting should be minimised (Cohen *et al.*, 1984). Afterwards, blotted proteins should be carefully renatured. The preservation of disulphide bridges in proteins by non-reducing gel conditions may be of relevance (Gershoni and Palade, 1983).

ANALYSIS OF THE HUMORAL IMMUNE RESPONSE TO HSV

During the last decades, the humoral immune response to HSV-1 and HSV-2 infection has been extensively studied and serological methods monitoring this humoral immune response have been widely used in the laboratory diagnosis of acute HSV infections. Acute primary infection with HSV can easily be detected by standard serological methods or by modern solid-phase immunoassays, when seroconversion, a significant rise in antibody titres or virus-specific IgM anti-bodies (eventually IgA) are demonstrated. However, in episodes of recurrent HSV infection, serological methods are often unsatisfactory for the detection of an acute recrudescence. Many patients will not show a signficiant increase in antibody titres or the appearance of virus-specific IgM antibodies.

Recent interest has been focused on the immune response to single HSV-encoded polypeptides during different clinical manifestations of HSV infection, e.g. (i) on the appearance of antibodies against single HSV polypeptides follow-ing primary type 1 and type 2 infections, (ii) on the demonstration of differences in pattern of antibody reactivity between primary and secondary infection, and (iii) on the demonstration of type-common and type-specific epitopes on single HSV polypeptides.

Because conventional serological methods generally use crude extracts of HSV-infected cells or HSV virions, antibody response against HSV can be measured only quantitatively. Evaluation of antibodies specific for single poly-peptides would require large scale purification of HSV peptides prior to their use in these serological tests and thus appears to be inconvenient. To overcome these problems, analysis of humoral immune response has been performed by immuno-blotting (WBA) (Eberle and Mou, 1983; Eberle *et al.*, 1985; Bernstein *et al.*, 1984; Norrild *et al.*, 1981; Bernstein *et al.*, 1985a, 1985b; Lehtinen *et al.*, 1986) and radioimmunoprecipitation followed by polyacrylamide gel electrophoresis (RIPA–PAGE) for analysis of specifically precipitated viral polypeptides (Ashley and Corey, 1984; Eberle and Courtney, 1981; Ashley *et al.*, 1985).

In RIPA–PAGE, viral proteins are reacted in a native state with virus-specific antibodies; an analysis of insoluble polypeptides, however, cannot be performed. Thus, only the immune response to a limited number of soluble viral proteins, such as glycoproteins, can be investigated. Western blotting, by contrast, allows investigation of the immune response to virtually all polypeptides specified by HSV, but alteration of antigenic determinants due to protein denaturation during gel electrophoresis and protein blotting must be taken into consideration.

During replication of HSV, the production of approximately 80 virus-specific polypeptides is induced, of which up to 25 proteins are structural proteins. In WBA, antibodies directed against up to 31 HSV-1 specified polypeptides and up to 27 HSV-2 specified polypeptides of infected cells may be recognised. Analysis of the humoral immune response to HSV-1 polypeptides in patients with recurrent HSV infections (Eberle and Mou, 1983) showed high antibody titres against the major glycoproteins gB, gC and gD and a number of uncharacterised proteins with low molecular weight. In addition, nonglycosylated structural proteins were also recognised by the human antibodies. No consistent differences between patients experiencing frequent recurrent HSV infections and those with infre-quent recurrent lesions could be demonstrated.

However, in primary genital HSV-2 infections, marked differences between acute phase sera and reconvalescent sera were reported (Eberle *et al.*, 1984). The first detectable and strongest antibody response in acute phase sera was not directed against viral glycoproteins but rather to an internal capsid protein of HSV-2 with an approximate molecular weight of 66 kD. Reconvalescent sera resembled those of patients with recurrent genital HSV-2 infection; antibodies detectable in WBA were directed primarily against the viral glycoproteins gD and gG and several other non-glycosylated structural proteins. In primary HSV-1 infections located at various anatomical sites, similar results have been reported (Eberle *et al.*, 1985). In early sera from previously seronegative patients, only low levels of antibodies directed against the major viral glycoproteins gB, gC and gD were found as compared with patients with recurrent HSV infections. However, acute phase antibodies were strongly reactive with several low molecular weight antigens (MW 34–49 kD), probably components of the viral nucleocapsid.

Analysis of the humoral immune response by RIPA–PAGE yields different results from WBA. In primary first-episode genital herpes infection, an early seroconversion of HSV-1 infected patients to VP 5, gB and gC was shown (Ashley *et al.*, 1985), followed by an antibody response to gD and an 88 kD protein; finally, antibodies against gE and a 66 kD protein appeared. In HSV-2 infected patients, antibodies against p148 (VP 5), gB and an 88 kD protein appeared within one week, after onset of the symptoms. Seroconversion to gD, gC and gE and a 66 kD protein was demonstrated later. These authors also pointed out that early seroconversion to the HSV-2 polypeptides gD, g80 and p66 was associated with a longer time interval to the first recrudescence in HSV-2 infected patients.

Several workers have studied the influence of therapy with the antiviral drug acyclovir on the humoral immune response (Bernstein *et al.*, 1984; Ashley and Corey, 1984). In agreement with a reduced expression of viral polypeptides after acyclovir treatment, a lower immune response to HSV-specified polypeptides has been reported in patients with primary infections treated with acyclovir as compared with an untreated control group. Predominantly lower antibody titres against gD and gE were found in patients treated with acyclovir. This correlates well with the acyclovir-induced block of DNA replication and a subsequent delay of late, i.e. structural, polypeptide synthesis in HSV.

In order to show the qualitative and quantitative differences in IgM and IgG immune response not only to viral structural proteins, i.e. late proteins (L), but also to immediate–early (IE) and early (E) peptides, we analysed 100 sera from patients with acute primary infection and from patients with acute recrudescent infection in WBA. Exemplary immunoblots are shown in figures 1–3.

IgM antibody response: although individual variation in IgM antibody responses occurred, IgM antibodies strongly recognised IE proteins, namely ICP4 and ICP0, in primary infections. In recrudescent infections, however, the antibody response to ICP4 was clearly reduced. The IgM immune response to E and L proteins appeared to be similar in primary and secondary infections.

IgG antibody response: in contrast to the IgM response, IE proteins were recognised at a low rate in primary infections, whereas in secondary infections antibodies directed against IE proteins could be detected frequently. A variety of E proteins were recognised in both primary and secondary infections, e.g. poly-

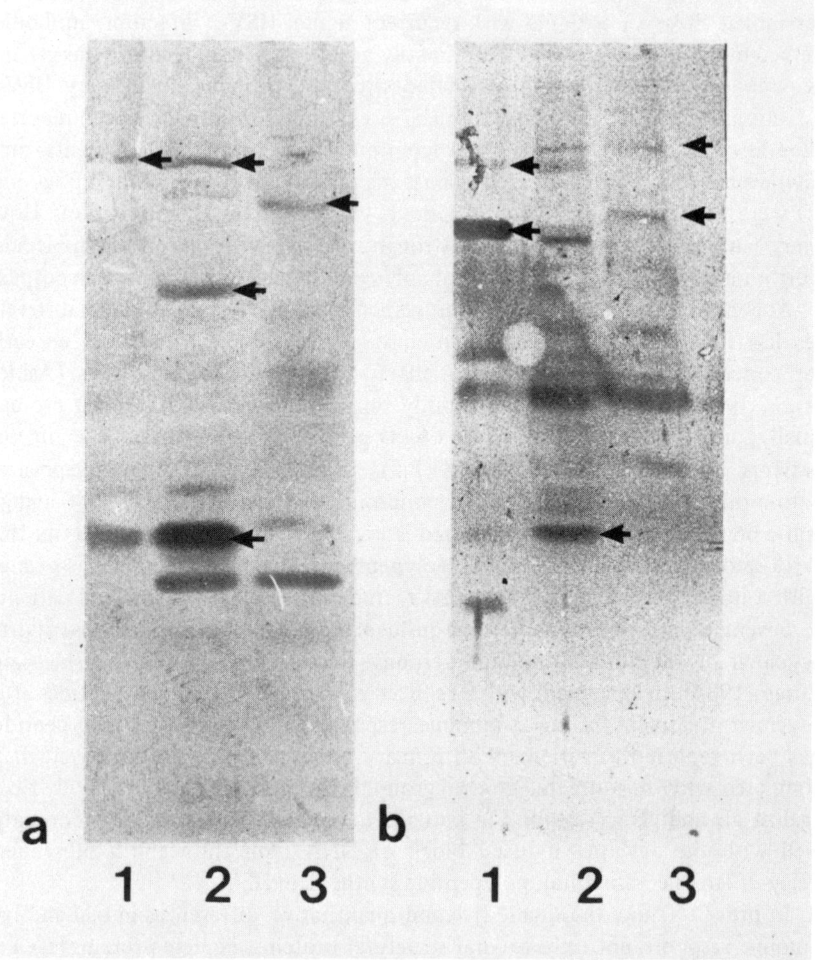

Figure 2   Effect of IgG–IgM competition on the demonstration of a protein-specific IgM antibody response. (a) Protein-specific binding of IgM antibodies (patient with acute primary infection) without preadsorption of IgG antibodies. HSV-1 polypeptides characteristically recognised by IgM antibodies are indicated by arrow heads (with decreasing molecular weight). Lane 1 (late proteins), VP5; lane 2 (early proteins), ICP10, a nonstructural 75 kD protein and a 50 kD capsid protein; lane 3 (immediate–early proteins), ICP0. (b) Preadsorption of IgG antibodies prior to analysis of IgM antibody response. The following proteins are marked by arrow heads: lane 1 (late proteins), VP5, gB; lane 2 (early proteins), 50 kD capsid protein; lane 3 (immediate–early proteins), ICP4, ICP0. Note the appearance of IgM antibodies strongly reactive for gB after preadsorption of IgG antibodies.

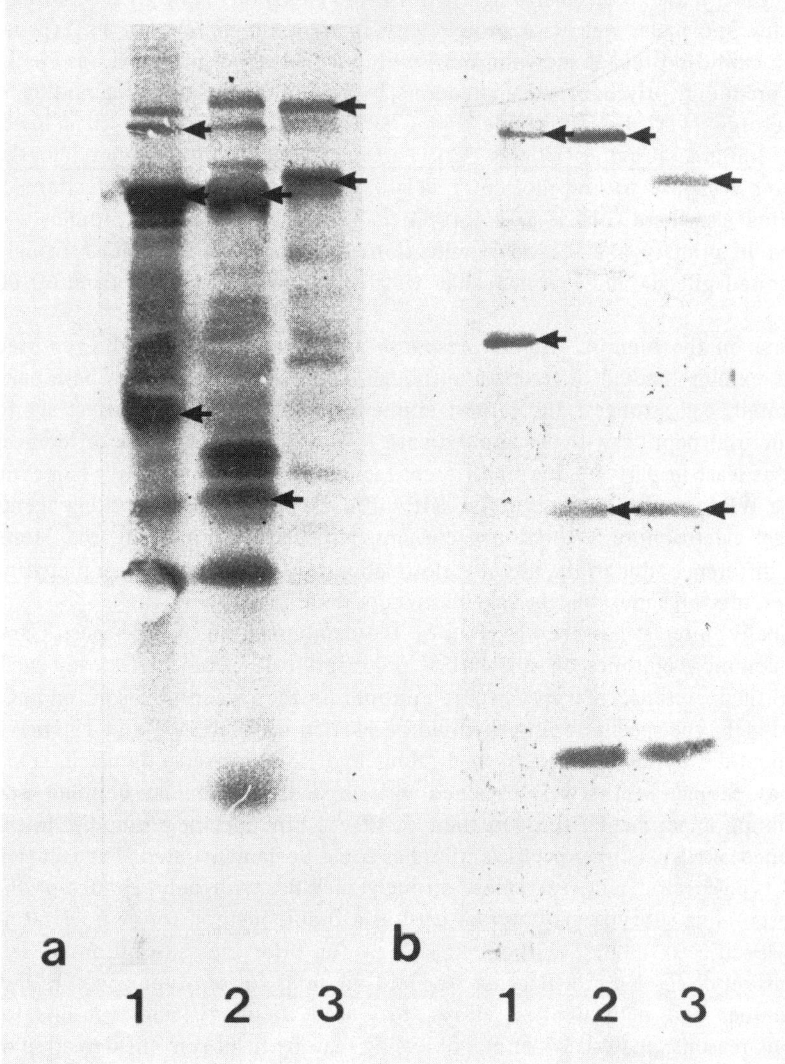

Figure 3   Typical immune response in an acute secondary HSV infection. (a) shows the IgG immune response against HSV-1 late (lane 1), early (lane 2) and immediate–early (lane 3) proteins. The following specifically recognised polypeptides are indicated by arrow heads: VP5, gBand gD in lane 1; gB and a 50 kD capsid protein; lane 3 (immediate–early proteins), ICP0. (b) Preadsorption of weight). (b) depicts a characteristic IgM immune response against HSV proteins. Protein-specific binding of IgM antibodies is indicated by arrow heads. Lane 1 (late proteins), VP5; lane 2 (early proteins), ICP10 and a 50 kD capsid protein; lane 3 (immediate–early proteins), ICP0 and a 50 kD capsid protein. The appearance of a viral structural protein among viral immediate–early proteins is possibly due to an insufficient block in synthesis of viral early and late proteins.

peptides with high molecular weight from 160–110 kD including gB and proteins with low molecular weight. A protein with an approximate MW of 50 kD (probably a capsid protein as shown in WBA with purified capsid proteins) was identified, predominantly in primary infections, by IgG antibodies (specific binding to this protein was also detectable under 'late' conditions; however, at a lower rate). Immune response to this 50 kD protein might well correspond to the immune response to low molecular weight polypeptides early in infection, as reported elsewhere (Eberle *et al.*, 1984, 1985). Recognition of L proteins was similar in primary and secondary infections; in most cases antibodies strongly recognised gB, gD and low molecular weight polypeptides ranging from 60–90 kD.

Data on the humoral immune response against HSV polypeptides reported so far exhibit marked differences, although some common findings have been presented, e.g. strongest and earliest immune response in primary infections to a structural peptide with an approximate MW of 40–50 kD. These differences may, at least in part, be due to different techniques, most obviously when comparing WBA results with results in RIPA–PAGE, but different blocking agents and gel electrophoresis conditions etc. may also play an important role. Moreover, differences due to the use of various laboratory viral strains when preparing antigen mixtures must also be taken into consideration.

Finally, interest has been focused on the demonstration of type-specific and type-common epitopes on single HSV polypeptides. Besides the already well-established presence of type-specific epitopes on the glycoproteins gC and gG, additional type-specific epitopes could be located on 11 HSV-1 and 13 HSV-2 polypeptides by using crossadsorbed rabbit hyperimmune sera (Bernstein *et al.*, 1985a). Similar results were obtained with crossadsorbed human immune sera. In mixing experiments, the detection of HSV-2 type-specific antibodies in the presence of HSV-1 type-specific antibodies could be demonstrated. The fact that HSV type-specific sera react more strongly in WBA with polypeptides of the corresponding subtype may also be used as a simple method for demonstrating type-specific antibodies without the need for prior crossadsorption of sera (Bernstein *et al.*, 1985b). Because standard methods for serotyping, e.g. ELISA techniques and neutralisation assays, may lead to unsatisfactory results for various reasons, analysis by immunoblotting may be helpful in the detection of type-specific antibodies.

RECOVERY OF ANTIBODIES SPECIFIC FOR VIRAL PROTEINS

Western blot procedures not only have proved to be useful tools in the analysis of protein–protein interactions but also may be used for the preparation of monospecific, although not monoclonal, antibodies against a specific protein (Olmsted, 1981). This is easily achieved by application of the Western blot procedure to two different lanes of a blot, which are run in parallel. One of these lanes is incubated with the first antibody only, but not with the second peroxidase-labelled antibody; the other lane is reacted with the first and second antibodies. The appropriate band is cut out from the protein lane, minced and incubated for 15 min on ice with 0.1 M Tris–glycine (pH 2.8). Subsequently, the mixture is brought to a neutral pH by the addition of a requisite amount of 0.1 N NaOH and the NC particles are centrifuged. The supernatant containing the corresponding antibody is dialysed against TBS and may be used for further applications. If the relative antibody content of the supernatant is too low, a precipitation step may become necessary. Protein-specific antibodies selected by this procedure have retained their original specificity and may be used in further experiments to identify specific viral proteins (figure 4).

Furthermore, it is possible to remove preparatively proteins bound directly to the NC membrane. For this purpose, the minced NC band is incubated for 1 h at 37°C with 6 M guanidine–isothiocyanate containing 0.1 M 2-mercapto-ethanol and 0.5% sarcosyl. Subsequently, the NC particles are centrifuged and the supernatant is dialysed against buffer or the protein is precipitated by the addition of 20% TCA.

ANALYSIS OF INTERACTIONS BETWEEN VIRAL PROTEINS AND DNA

Western blot procedures may not only be used to determine interactions between proteins but may also be used in the analysis of interactions between proteins and nucleic acids (Gilmour *et al.*, 1981; Hoch, 1982; Jack *et al.*, 1981). A typical example of such an assay was originally developed by Bowen *et al.* (1980), who showed specific interaction of the lac repressor with the lac operator. In such experiments, however, it is very important to achieve renaturation of proteins after SDS–PAGE as quantitatively as possible. Since SDS is a major factor in the denaturation of proteins, and is hardly ever completely removed by any renaturation processes, it might be advantageous to run gels for the assessment of protein–DNA interactions under 'native' conditions, i.e. omitting SDS. Our own experiments with this method, however, yielded poor results in terms of resolution of protein bands and, therefore, this method is not to be generally recommended. In contrast, we did achieve clear-cut results by transferring SDS–PAGE-separated proteins to NC membranes, with subsequent extensive renaturation including treatment of membranes with 0.1% Triton X-100. Thus, we were able to analyse DNA binding properties of HSV immediate early proteins, as given in figure 5. For this purpose, the blotted proteins were first incubated with herring sperm DNA to block non-specific DNA binding. Subsequently, in a series of experiments, different ^{32}P-labelled viral and nonviral DNA sequences of interest were added. Figure 5 shows binding of the promotor region of the HSV early gene thymidine kinase (TK) to ICP0, a viral immediate–early gene product.

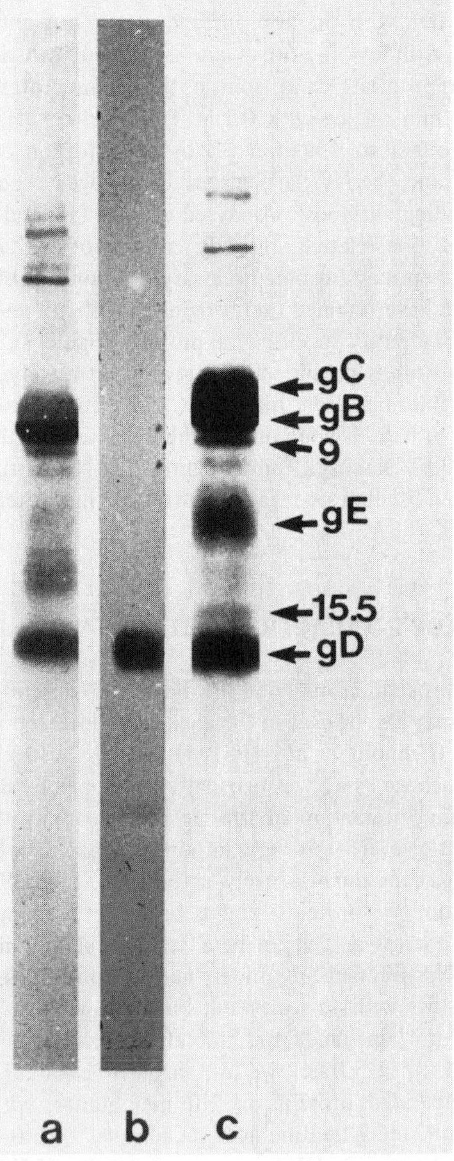

Figure 4   Reisolation of monospecific antibodies from Western blots. Lane (a) proteins specifically recognised by a rabbit hyperimmune serum raised against HSV-1 structural proteins. Lane (b) rabbit antibodies exhibiting monospecific binding properties against gD after their recovery from the blot. Antibodies were isolated from a lane identical to (a) but containing only the first rabbit antibody. After recovery from the blot antibodies were again allowed to react with blotted HSV polypeptides. Lane (c) autoradiography of blotted HSV structural proteins.

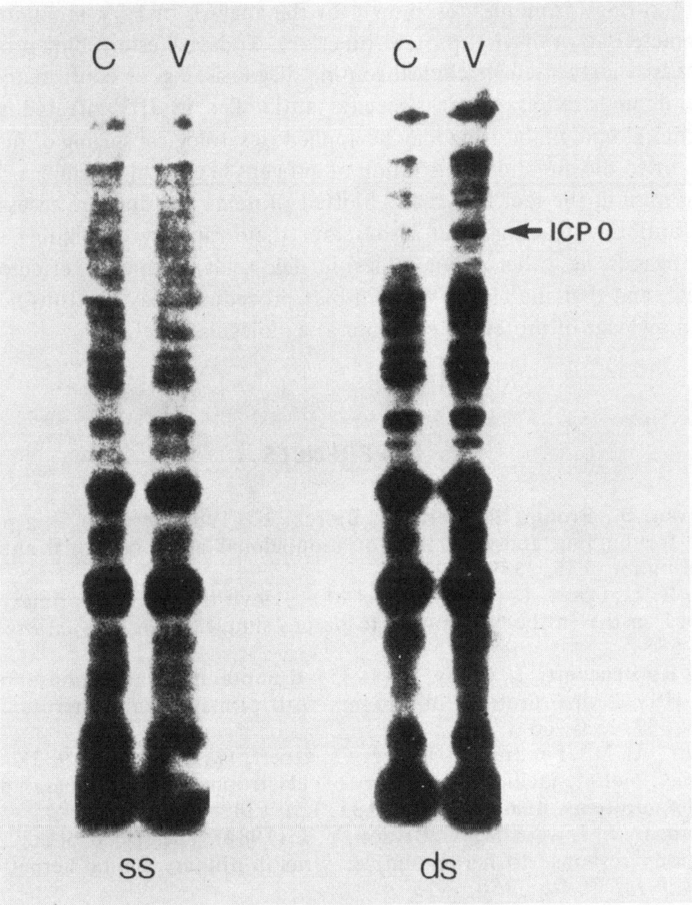

Figure 5   DNA binding properties of blotted HSV immediate–early proteins. Proteins of HSV-infected cells (V) containing viral immediate–early proteins and of mock-infected cells (C) were incubated with a ^{32}P-labelled DNA sequence, including the promotor region of the thymidine kinase (TK) gene, a viral early gene. In this experiment single-stranded DNA (ss) and double-stranded DNA (ds) was used. Arrow indicates the DNA binding of the viral immediate–early protein ICP0.

CONCLUSIONS

Successfully combining the high resolution power of protein gel electrophoresis and the sensitivity and specificity of modern solid-phase immunoassays, Western blot procedures proved to be extremely helpful for our understanding of macro-molecular interactions. It has been the intention of this chapter to present some protein blotting techniques, as shown for the analysis of HSV immunobiology and characterisation of viral protein functions. Today, Western blot procedures are already widely used in clinical routine diagnosis, e.g. as confirmatory tests for the demonstration of virus-specific antibodies in HIV-infected persons. Furthermore, immunoblotting may be applied to serological staging of infectious diseases or to the direct demonstration of antigens in clinical specimens. There is great promise in the fact that many blotted proteins not only are accessible for antigen-antibody reactions but also retain their capacity of binding to their specific ligands, i.e. other polypeptides, nucleic acids, hormones, effector molecules, etc. and that the use of Western blot procedures may be fruitful for our future knowledge of protein interactions at a molecular level.

REFERENCES

Akerström, B., Brodin, T., Reis, K., Björck, L. (1985). Protein G: a powerful tool for binding and detection of monoclonal and polyclonal antibodies. *J. Immunol.*, **135**, 2589–2592

Ashley, R. L., Corey, L. (1984). Effect of acyclovir treatment of primary genital herpes on the antibody response to herpes simplex virus. *J. Clin. Invest.*, **73**, 681–688

Ashley, R., Benedetti, J., Corey, L. (1985). Humoral immune response to HSV-1 and HSV-2 viral proteins in patients with primary genital herpes. *J. Med. Virol.*, **17**, 153–166

Aubertin, A. M., Tondre, L., Lopez, C., Obert, G., Kirn, A. (1983). Sodium dodecyl sulfate-mediated transfer of electrophoretically separated DNA-binding proteins. *Anal. Biochem.*, **131**, 127–134

Bernstein, D. I., Lovett, M. A., Bryson, Y. J. (1984). The effects of acyclovir on antibody response to herpes simplex virus in primary genital herpetic infections. *J. Infect. Dis.*, **150**, 7–13

Bernstein, D. I., Bryson, Y. J., Lovett, M. A. (1985a). Antibody response to type-common and type-unique epitopes of herpes simplex virus polypeptides. *J. Med. Virol.*, **15**, 251–263

Bernstein, D. I., Garratty, E., Lovett, M. A., Bryson, Y. J. (1985b). Comparison of Western blot analysis to microneutralization for the detection of type-specific herpes simplex virus antibodies. *J. Med. Virol.*, **15**, 223–230

Bowen, B., Steinberg, J., Laemmli, U. K., Weintraub, H. (1980). The detection of DNA-binding proteins by protein blotting. *Nucleic Acids Res.*, **8**, 1–20

Brada, D., Roth, J. (1984). "Gold Blot" – detection of polyclonal and monoclonal antibodies bound to antigens on nitrocellulose by protein A–gold complexes. *Anal. Biochem.*, **142**, 79–83

Burnett, W. N. (1981). "Western blotting": electrophoretic transfer of proteins from sodium dodecyl sulfate–polyacrylamide gels to unmodified nitrocellulose and radiographic detection with antibody and radioiodinated protein A. *Anal. Biochem.*, **112**, 195–203

Cohen, B. B., Moxley, M., Crichton, D., Deane, D. L., Steel, C. M. (1984). A mild procedure for separating polypeptide chains prior to immunoprecipitation and Western blotting analysis. *J. Immunol. Methods*, **75**, 99–105

De Blas, A. L., Cherwinski, H. M. (1983). Detection of antigens on nitrocellulose paper immunoblots with monoclonal antibodies. *Anal. Biochem.*, **133**, 214–219

Eberle, R., Courtney, R. J. (1981). Assay of type-specific and type-common antibodies to herpes simplex virus types 1 and 2 in human sera. *Infect. Immun.*, **31**, 1062–1070

Eberle, R., Mou, S.-W. (1983). Relative titers of antibodies to individual polypeptide antigens on herpes simplex virus type 1 in human sera. *J. Infect. Dis.*, **148**, 436–444

Eberle, M., Mou, S.-W., Zaia, J. A. (1984). Polypeptide specificity of the early antibody response following primary and recurrent genital herpes simplex virus type 2 infections. *J. Gen. Virol.*, **65**, 1839–1843

Eberle, R., Mou, S.-W., Zaia, J. A. (1985). The immune response to herpes simplex virus: comparison of the specificity and relative titers of serum antibodies directed against viral polypeptides following primary herpes simplex virus type 1 infections. *J. Med. Virol.*, **16**, 147–162

Erickson, P. F., Minier, L. M., Lasher, R. S. (1982). Quantitative electrophoretic transfer of polypeptides from SDS polyacrylamide gels to nitrocellulose sheets: a method for their re-use in immunoautoradiographic detection of antigens. *J. Immunol. Methods*, **51**, 241–249

Falk, B. W., Elliott, C. (1985). Fluorescent monitoring of proteins during sodium dodecyl sulfate–polyacrylamide gel electrophoresis and Western blotting. *Anal. Biochem.*, **144**, 537–541

Fernandez-Pol, J. A. (1982). *FEBS Lett.*, **143**, 86–92

Gershoni, J. M., Palade, G. E. (1982). Electrophoretic transfer of proteins from sodium dodecyl sulfate–polyacrylamide gels to a positively charged membrane filter. *Anal. Biochem.*, **124**, 396–405

Gershoni, J. M., Palade, G. E. (1983). Protein blotting: principles and applications. *Anal. Biochem.*, **131**, 1–15

Gilmour, R. S., Lang, A., Gu, J. R., Johnston, C., Paul, J. (1981). DNA binding proteins in chromatin structure and function. *Cell Biol. Int. Rep.*, **5**, 45–53

Glass, W. F., Briggs, R. C., Hinlica, L. S. (1981). Identification of tissue-specific nuclear antigens transferred to nitrocellulose from polyacrylamide gels. *Science*, **211**, 70–71

Hancock, K., Tsang, V. C. W. (1983). India ink staining of proteins on nitrocellulose paper. *Anal. Biochem.*, **133**, 157–162

Hayman, E. G., Engvall, E., A'Hearn, E., Barnes, D., Pierschbacher, M., Ruoslahti, E. (1982). Cell attachment on replicas of SDS polyacrylamide gels reveals two adhesive plasma proteins. *J. Cell Biol.*, **95**, 20–23

Hierholzer, J. C., Coombs, R. A., Anderson, L. J. (1984). Spectrophotometric quantitation of peroxidase-stained protein bands following gel electrophoresis and the Western blot transfer technique with respiratory syncytial virus. *J. Virol. Methods*, **8**, 265–268

Hoch, S. O. (1982). DNA-binding domains of fibronectin probed using Western blots. *Biochem. Biophys. Res. Comm.*, **106**, 1353–1358

Jack, R. S., Gehring, W. J., Brack, C. (1981). Protein component from Drosophila larval nuclei showing sequence specificity for a short region near a major heat-shock protein gene. *Cell*, **24**, 321–331

Knecht, D. A., Dimond, R. L. (1984). Visualization of antigenic proteins on Western blots. *Anal. Biochem.*, **136**, 180–184

Lehtinen, M., Koivisto, V., Lehtinen, T., Paavonen, J., Leinikki, P. (1986). Immunoblotting and enzyme-linked immunosorbent assay analysis of serological responses in patients infected with herpes simplex virus types 1 and 2. *Intervirology*, **24**, 18–25

Lin, W., Kasamatsu, H. (1983). On the electrotransfer of polypeptides from gels to nitrocellulose membranes. *Anal. Biochem.*, **128**, 302–311

Norrild, B., Pedersen, B., Roizman, B. (1981). Immunological reactivity of herpes simplex virus 1 and 2 polypeptides electrophoretically separated and transferred to diazobenzyloxymethyl paper. *Infect. Immun.*, **31**, 660–667

Ochs, D. (1983). Protein contaminants of sodium dodecyl sulfate–polyacrylamide gels. *Anal. Biochem.*, **135**, 470–474

Olmsted, J. B., (1981). Affinity purification of antibodies from diazotized paper blots of heterogeneous protein samples. *J. Biol. Chem.*, **256**, 11955–11957

Peferoen, M., Huybrechts, R., De Loof, A. (1982). Vacuum-blotting: a new simple and efficient transfer of proteins from sodium dodecyl sulfate–polyacrylamide gels to nitrocellulose. *FEBS Lett.*, **145**, 369–372

Ramirez, P., Bonilla, J. A., Moreno, E., León, P. (1983). Electrophoretic transfer of viral proteins to nitrocellulose sheets and detection with peroxidase-bound lectins and protein A. *J. Immunol. Methods*, **62**, 15–22

Reinhart, P. M., Malamud, D. (1982). Protein transfer from isoelectric focusing gels: the native blot. *Anal. Biochem.*, **123**, 229–235

Reiser, J., Wardale, J. (1981). Immunological detection of specific proteins in total cell extracts by fractionation in gels and transfer to diazophenythioether paper. *Eur. J. Biochem.*, **114**, 569–575

Renart, J., Reiser, J., Stark, G. R. (1979). Transfer of proteins from gels to diazobenzyloxymethyl–paper and detection with antisera: a method for studying antibody specificity and antigen structure. *Proc. Natl. Acad. Sci. USA*, **76**, 3116–3120

Schaltmann, K., Pongs, O. (1980). A simple procedure for blotting of proteins to study antibody specificity and antigen structure. *Hoppe-Seyler's Z. Physiol. Chem.*, **361**, 207–210

Smith, G. E., Summers, M. D. (1980). The bidirectional transfer of DNA and RNA to nitrocellulose or diazobenzyloxymethyl–paper. *Anal. Biochem.*, **109**, 123–129

Southern, E. M. (1975). Detection of specific sequences among DNA fragments separated by gel electrophoresis. *J. Mol. Biol.*, **98**, 503–517

Spinola, S. M., Cannon, J. G. (1985). Different blocking agents cause variation in the immunologic detection of proteins transferred to nitrocellulose membranes. *J. Immunol. Methods*, **81**, 161–165

Symington, J., Green, M., Brackmann, K. (1981). Immunoautoradiographic detection of proteins after electrophoretic transfer from gels to diazo–paper: analysis of adenovirus encoded proteins. *Proc. Natl. Acad. Sci. USA*, **78**, 177–181

Towbin, H., Gordon, J. (1984). Immunoblotting and dot immunobinding – current status and outlook. *J. Immunol. Methods*, **72**, 313–340

Towbin, H., Staehelin, T., Gordon, J. (1979). Electrophoretic transfer of proteins from polyacrylamide gels to nitrocellulose sheets: procedure and some applications. *Proc. Natl. Acad. Sci. USA*, **76**, 4350–4354

Tsang, V. C. W., Peralta, J. M., Simons, A. R. (1983). Enzyme-linked immuno-electrotransfer blot techniques (EITB) for studying the specificities of antigens and antibodies separated by gel electrophoresis. *Methods Enzymol.*, **92**, 377–392

10.   Non-isotopic Studies of the TSH Receptor

N. R. FARID AND G. FAHRAEUS-VAN REE

INTRODUCTION

Thyrotropin (TSH) is a heterodimeric glycoprotein with an α subunit common to FSH, LH and hCG and a unique β subunit: dissociated subunits are without biological activity (Pierce and Parsons, 1981). TSH interacts with specific binding sites on the basal aspect of the thyroid cell membrane; ^{125}I-TSH binding sites have also been described on polymorphonuclear leucocytes and cells in both testicular and fat tissues (Farid *et al.*, 1983). Hormone binding is associated with a number of changes in the plasma membrane, including activation of adenylate cyclase, synthesis of prostaglandins, activation of protein kinase C and inward movement of calcium ions. The possible involvement of the phosphatidyl inositol cycle is unclear. Whether or not TSH is a growth factor for the thyrocyte in its own right may depend on the species studied. Some authors have shown that the epidermal growth factor, as well as insulin and insulin-like growth factors, can act as growth stimulants and that TSH inhibits this effect (Gartner *et al.*, 1985; Errick *et al.*, 1985). However, other workers have indicated that TSH is a thyroid cell mitogen (Lewinski *et al.*, 1983; Valente *et al.*, 1983). Physiological polarity appears to be of prime importance in the retention of physiological sensitivity to TSH and to growth factors (Gartner *et al.*, 1985); single-cell suspensions of thyroid cells allowed to make follicles invariably have an inside-out follicle orientation; this may account for some of, but not all, the discrepancies in the literature.

In addition to the TSH, epidermal growth factor and insulin receptors, thyrocytes have receptors for acetylcholine, catecholamines, prostaglandin (Dumont and Vassart, 1979) and vasoactive inhibitory peptide. These receptors may interact and influence receptor number affinity as well as post-receptor mediated events.

TSH RECEPTOR ANTIBODIES

Graves's Disease was one of the first anti-receptor antibody diseases to be recognized (Farid *et al.*, 1983). It is now known that a family of antibodies exists which apparently interact with different epitopes of the TSH receptor. Some of these antibodies inhibit ^{125}I-bTSH binding to thyroid plasma membranes without stimulating adenylate cyclase; others stimulate adenylate cyclase without inhibiting ^{125}I-bTSH binding. Some antibodies apparently augment ^{125}I-bTSH binding to the membrane, while others inhibit TSH-mediated adenylate cyclase activity (Kohn *et al.*, 1985). It is unclear at this juncture whether the thyroid antibodies associated with thyroid cell growth are directed against the receptor.

THE STRUCTURE OF THE TSH RECEPTOR

The association of a common disease with antibodies against the TSH receptor led to a search for its structure. We have suggested that the TSH receptor is a symmetrical heterotetrameric glycoprotein of $Mr \approx 200\,000$. As shown in figure 1 the two $Mr \approx 35\,000$ light (ϵ) chains are held together by disulphide bonds, each of which interacts non-covalently with a δ subunit of $Mr \approx 66\,000$. The locus of TSH binding is between the two ϵ subunits, and its integrity as well as that of the receptor as a whole are dependent on the reduced form of these bonds. The δ subunits appear to act as stabilizers or affinity regulators (Islam and Farid, 1985; Farid *et al.*, 1985). Both chains appear to be exposed to the external aspects of the cell (Islam and Farid, 1985; Farid *et al.*, 1985). Thyroid cells have a number of previously unrecognized proteolytic activities, the inactivation of which yields a chain of $Mr \approx 95\,000$; the ϵ and δ subunits thus appear as a result of proteolytic digestion in the course of receptor isolation.

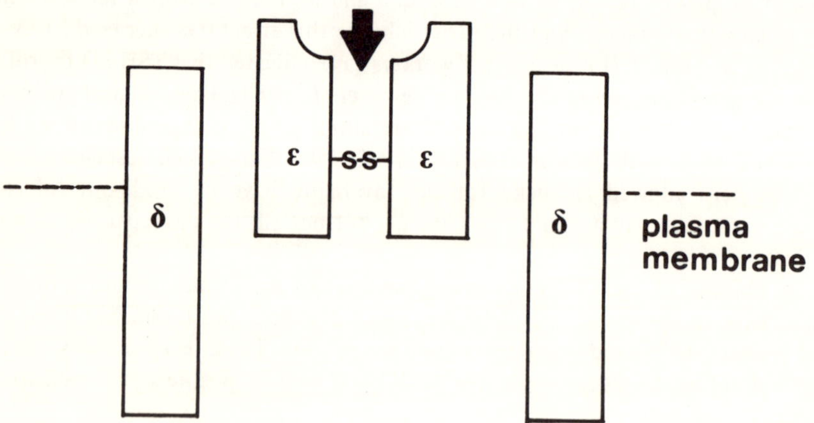

Figure 1   The TSH receptor is a heterotetrameric glycoprotein of $Mr \approx 200\,000$. The arrow indicates the locus of TSH binding. In view of the designation of the two TSH subunits α and β, and electing to continue the use of the Greek alphabet, we designated the receptor heavy chain δ and light chain ϵ.

Many TSH receptor structures have been proposed, based on photoaffinity cross-linking (Kajita *et al.*, 1985), target size analysis (Nielsen *et al.*, 1984) and immunoprecipitation (Heyma and Harrison, 1984; Kohn *et al.*, 1983) as well as gel filtration (see Farid *et al.* (1983) for review and Koizumi *et al.* (1982) and Iida *et al.* (1983)). Photoaffinity cross-linking yielded a porcine receptor composed of $Mr \approx 45\,000$ and $Mr \approx 25\,000$ covalently linked subunits (Kajita *et al.*, 1985). Deducing subunit structure and its organization into the receptor solely on the basis of photoaffinity cross-linking is fraught with problems, e.g. ^{125}I-bTSH may be cross-linked to membrane components other than the receptor, binding to the TSH receptor may protect disulphide bonds between subunits from reduction and may induce receptor proteolysis, the change of electrophoretic mobility after cross-linking with ^{125}I-bTSH does not allow calculation of receptor subunit size by subtraction of the M.W. of TSH or its subunits (Farid *et al.*, 1983; Bako *et al.*, 1985; Islam *et al.*, 1983a). Target site analysis has suggested a TSH binding unit of $Mr \approx 70\,000$ (Nielsen *et al.*, 1984), although the data could accommodate a structure of up to $Mr \approx 100\,000$. Receptor subunits of $Mr \approx 38\,000$ and $66\,000$ have been described (Koizumi *et al.*, 1982) and an ^{125}I-bTSH receptor has been eluted with a profile compatible with M.W. $180\,000$ (Iida *et al.*, 1983). Bands of $Mr \approx 100\,000$–$110\,000$, $80\,000$–$90\,000$ and $60\,000$–$70\,000$ were precipitated by Graves's IgG (Heyma and Harrison, 1984), whereas a receptor-specific monoclonal precipitated $Mr \approx 50\,000$–$55\,000$ species as well as $Mr \approx 18\,000$–$23\,000$ species (Kohn *et al.*, 1983). Graves's IgG in the former study (Kajita *et al.*, 1985) had high microsomal antibody titre and also precipitated thyroid microsomal antigens (see below). Several studies (Farid *et al.*, 1983; Nielsen *et al.*, 1984; Heyma and Harrison, 1984; Koizumi *et al.*, 1982) are in agreement with our conclusions that an $Mr \approx 65\,000$–$70\,000$ peptide constitutes at least fragments of the TSH receptor, and one study (Heyma and Harrison, 1984) confirms our findings that an $Mr \approx 35\,000$ peptide has similar properties.

INTERACTION OF THYROID PLASMA MEMBRANE PROTEINS WITH NATURALLY OCCURRING AUTOANTIBODIES

A number of approaches, including protein blotting techniques, were used to examine the nature of the interaction of antibodies found in the sera of patients with Graves's disease (Islam *et al.*, 1983a) and Hashimoto's thyroiditis (Islam *et al.*, 1987) with antigens in thyroid plasma membranes. We have previously shown that TSH interacted on protein blots with a band of $Mr \approx 197\,000$ and that this interaction only took place when thyroid plasma membranes were resolved under non-reducing conditions. The interaction was not inhibited by a 5000-fold greater amount of insulin and only to a small degree by human chorionic gonadotropin (Islam *et al.*, 1983a).

Graves's IgG interacted (at 1 mg/ml) with the same $Mr \approx 200\,000$ band to which TSH was bound. Interaction of Graves's IgG with the receptor peptide was blocked by pre-incubation with TSH, suggesting that they bind to the same receptor domain, as does TSH itself (figure 2). Using purified human thyroid membranes in an immunoblotting dot assay (figure 3) (Gyula Bako *et al.*, manuscript in preparation), IgG from at least 95% of 120 patients with active Graves's disease was found to be positive in this assay; pre-incubation of dotted membranes with TSH blocked the interaction. Most patients in remission after treatment with anti-thyroid drugs were negative. The results correlated very well with ^{125}I-bTSH displacement and cyclic AMP stimulation assays.

No binding of TSH or anti-receptor antibody was observed when the membranes were resolved on reducing SDS–polyacrylamide gel before blotting, con-

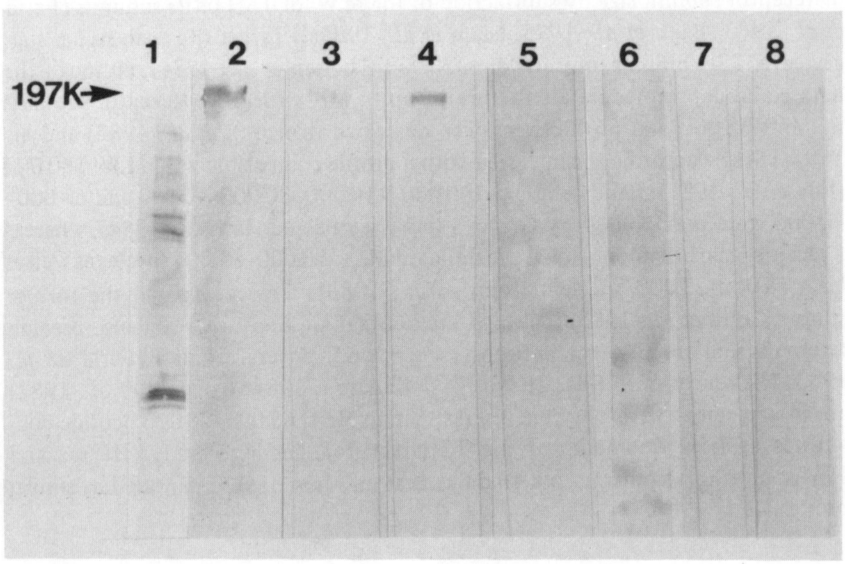

Figure 2   Binding of bTSH and Graves's IgG to the TSH holoreceptor. Individual lanes were incubated with TSH for 4 h followed by anti-TSH or IgG for 14 h at 4°C, the strips then being thoroughly washed and developed with peroxidase-conjugated species-specific anti-IgG and chromogen. Lane 1 shows the bands protein blotted from non-reduced gels and stained with Coomassie blue. bTSH (1 U/ml) (lane 2) and Graves's IgG (1 mg/ml), whether tested with porcine (lane 3) or human (lane 4) thyroid membrane, interacted with a single $Mr \approx 197\,000$ holoreceptor band. Preincubation of transferred material with native bTSH (1 U/ml) caused a decrease in the binding of the $Mr \approx 197\,000$ band (lane 5). IgG from patients with autoimmune thyroiditis with an anti-microsomal antibody titre of $1/256\,000$ in the sample, in lane 6, showed no binding to the receptor band, as did most healthy controls (lane 8). Lane 7 shows the reaction of IgG from a technician who was involved in TSH receptor purification: she remains euthyroid 18 months after this study. It is important to note that in this study IgG was tested at a concentration of 1 mg/ml.

firming the importance of the $-S-S-$ bridges for TSH receptor function (Islam and Farid, 1985; Farid *et al.*, 1985).

Unexpectedly, when the concentration of IgG was increased to 2 mg/ml from patients with Hashimoto's thyroiditis and was tested (see the legend to figure 4), interaction with a variable number of bands (including the Mr ≈ 200 000 holo-receptor polypeptide) was observed. This interaction was not blocked by TSH, implying that Hashimoto's IgG interacted with an epitope on the TSH receptor separate from that to which TSH and Graves's IgG bind (Islam *et al.*, 1987).

We developed the studies of Hashimoto's IgG to investigate the nature of the 'microsomal autoantigen', and selected sera with high anti-microsomal antibody titre (≥ 1/1600) but negative for thyroglobulin antibody activity. We investigated the pattern of interaction with protein blots of purified plasma and light microsomal membranes. The pattern of interaction of Hashimoto's IgG was similar for both plasma and microsomal membrane preparations, strongly supporting the sharing of antigenic determinants by these two cellular components (Islam *et al.*, 1987), and in keeping with the now well-established dynamic interrelationship between them (Khoury *et al.*, 1981; Khoury *et al.*, 1984). The

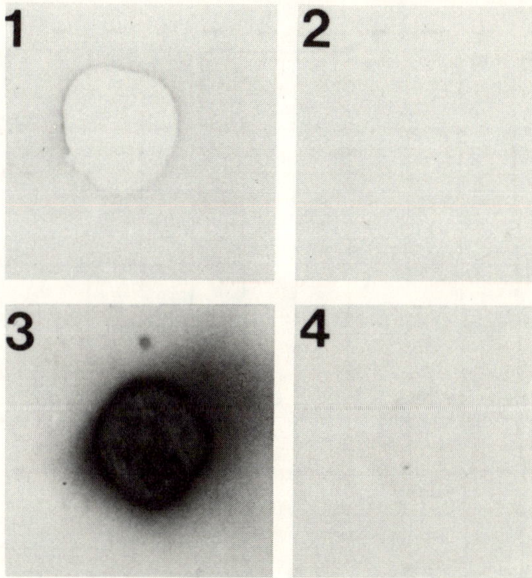

Figure 3 Binding of putative anti-TSH receptor antibodies with thyroid plasma membrane dotted onto NC paper. Bound IgG was detected with peroxidase-conjugated species-specific anti-IgG and developed with 4-chloro-1-naphthol and hydrogen peroxide. A strong positive reaction is seen with anti-TSH anti-idiotype IgG (300 μg) (3). A weaker reaction is seen with the same concentration of Graves's IgG (4). Both of these interactions were blocked by prior incubation with TSH (not shown). Rabbit IgG (1) (the control for anti-idiotype) and normal human IgG (2) (the control for Graves's IgG) were negative. This figure stresses the relative potency of anti-idiotype (by a factor of 20–50) compared with Graves's IgG.

results of the studies with the light microsome were not due to cross-contamination with thyroid plasma membrane. Mr ≈ 200 000 receptor peptide was present both in plasma and microsomal membrane, resolved by SDS–PAGE in the absence but not in the presence of reductant (figures 4–6).

A large number of bands, in addition to that of the TSH receptor, visualized with Hashimoto's IgG, were common to both plasma and microsomal membrane patterns. Some bands became more distinct when membranes were resolved under reducing rather than non-reducing conditions. A number of unique antigens were of particular note. One was estimated at Mr ≈ 210 000, the second at Mr ≈ 22 000 and the third at Mr ≈ 103 000. In the presence of reductant, the mobilities of the first two types of antigens changed to Mr ≈ 180 000 and Mr ≈ 12 500 respectively (figures 4–6). A high titre of IgG antibody Mr ≈ 210 000 was seen in patient 1, although immune reactions were discernable for most of the patients with Hashimoto's thyroiditis. Autoantibodies to Mr ≈ 22 000 peptides were detected in only 1 of over 20 patients studied to date. Mr ≈ 103 000 was detected most distinctly in patient 4, but was also seen in patients 1 and 3. Intensity of the bands was not affected by TSH. This band was even more

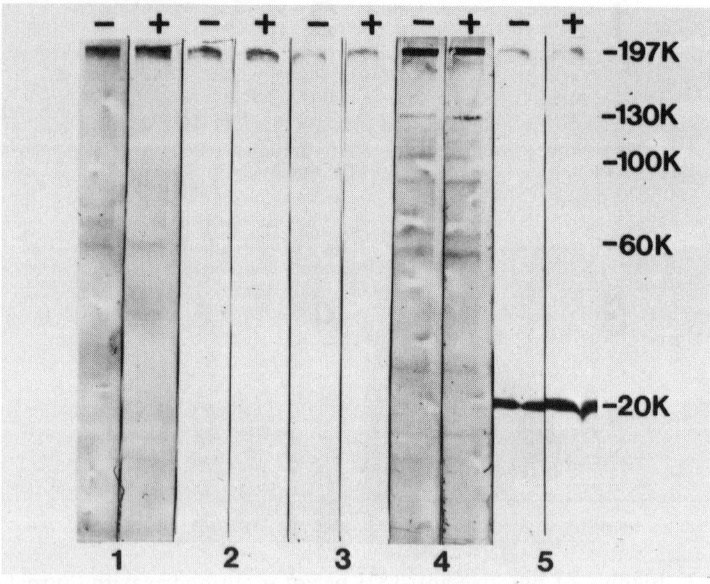

Figure 4   The interaction of Hashimoto's IgG with thyroid plasma membrane peptides. These were resolved by SDS–PAGE in the absence of reductant and transferred to NC paper. Binding of Hashimoto's IgG was tested in the presence (+) and absence (−) of native TSH. Samples from patients 3 and 5 stimulated AC and those from patients 1 and 2 inhibited TSH-stimulated AC whereas IgG from patient 4 had no effect on AC activity. Note that sample 4 has a distinct band, heavier than TSH receptor shown as 197K, and that sample 5 has a unique 20 000 polypeptide.

marked in the light microsomal fraction of these patients; it corresponds to thyroid peroxidase, recently described by several investigators (Nagakawa *et al.*, 1985; Czarnocka *et al.*, 1985).

The Mr ≈ 210 000 peptide was further investigated. Immunization of BALB/c mice with thyroid plasma membranes, and subsequent hybridization of their splenocytes with SP/20 myeloma cells, resulted in a number of hybrid clones producing monoclonal antibodies against the Mr ≈ 210 000 polypeptide (Islam

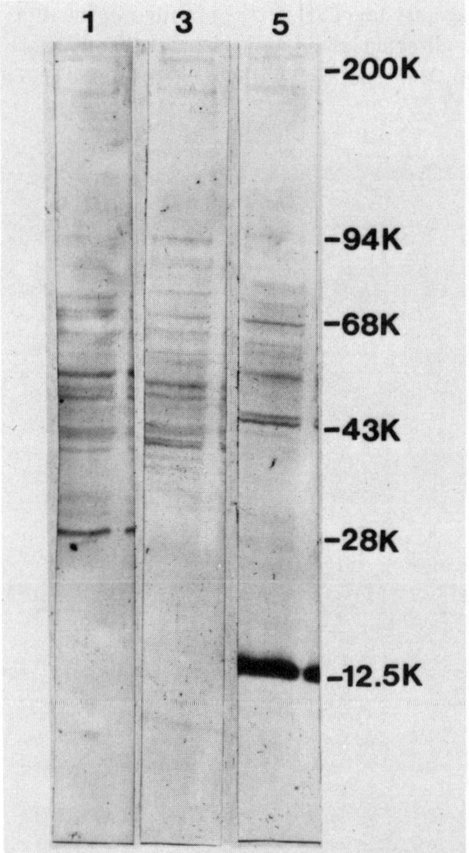

Figure 5   Pattern of interaction of selected Hashimoto's IgG with plasma membrane protein resolved under reducing conditions and transferred to NC paper. The numerals above the lanes correspond to the samples numbered in figure 15. A faint band may be seen at Mr ≈ 180 000 in all three lanes, suggesting that all these sera have low concentrations of antibodies against Mr ≈ 210 000, which migrates faster under reducing conditions. The 'unique' patterns of antibody interaction described in the text are relative rather than absolute. The 197 000 band is no longer visible and a distinct Mr ≈ 28 500 band appears in lane 1. The fine band Mr ≈ 66 000 in the three lanes probably represents a TSH receptor subunit.

et al., 1987). This peptide was shown to be related to thyroglobulin in that it could be visualized with rabbit polyclonal antibodies against thyroglobulin (figure 7) and its interaction with specific monoclonals was abolished when these were absorbed with thyroglobulin (not shown).

It is clear from these studies that patients with Hashimoto's thyroiditis appear to have auto-antibodies against a variety of thyroid cell components, including the TSH receptor, thyroid microsomal antigens, thyroglobulin and its breakdown products, even though they may be negative in standard clinical assays. Autoantibodies against the TSH receptor found in the sera of these patients are, however, clearly directed at domains separate from those to which TSH and Graves's IgG bind. Many patients with Graves's disease also have anti-microsomal

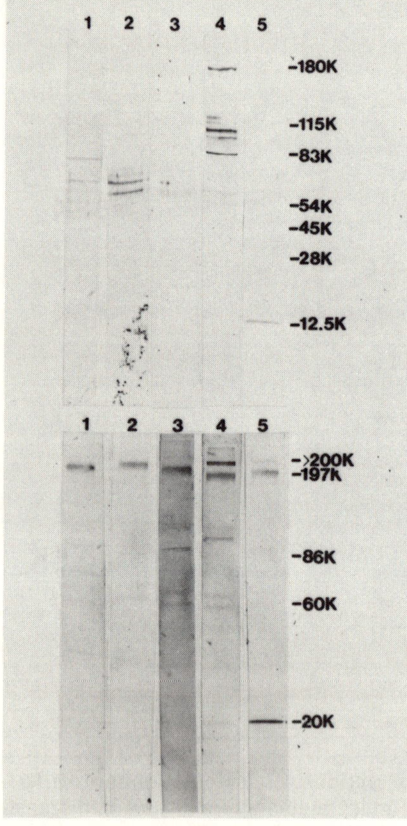

Figure 6   Binding of light microsome proteins resolved in the presence (upper panel) and absence (lower panel) of reductant. Note should be made of the substantial reduction in the mobility of several bands on the addition of reductant. Numerals above the lanes refer to sample numbers. Further investigation indicated that pp 210 (lower panel, lane 4) and Mr ≈ 180 000 (upper panel, lane 4) are degradation derivatives of thyroglobulin.

antibodies, and their sera may, therefore, be expected to show activity, not only against the TSH binding site but also against other TSH receptor domains. Depending on the relative predominance of one or the other of the antibodies, the sera of these patients may behave differently in *in vitro* assay for thyroid

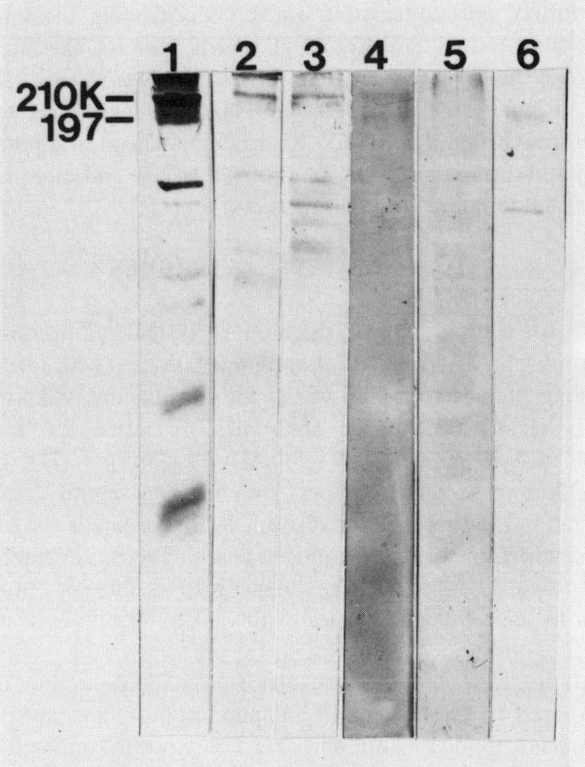

Figure 7   Interaction of Hashimoto's IgG, Graves's IgG and anti-thyroglobulin antibody with commercial thyroglobulin and plasma membranes, resolved under non-reducing conditions: lane 1, interaction of thyroglobulin with anti-thyroglobulin; lane 2, interaction of sucrose-gradient-purified thyroid plasma membranes with anti-thyroglobulin; lane 3, binding of Hashimoto's IgG to protein-blotted thyroglobulin; lane 4, binding of Hashimoto's IgG to protein blots of thyroid plasma membranes; lane 5, interaction of Graves's IgG with thyroglobulin; lane 6, interaction of Graves's IgG with thyroid plasma membrane. The rabbit polyclonal antibody interacts with a variety of thyroglobulin-related polypeptides including those of $Mr \approx 210\,000$ and $180\,000$. Hashimoto's IgGs, which were negative by haemagglutination assay, are strongly positive to these two polypeptide bands when allowed to interact with either thyroglobulin or plasma membranes. The reaction with Graves's IgG results in faint bands with thyroglobulin which can barely be seen but a distinct band with the TSH receptor. The band of $Mr \approx 165\,000$ in lane 6 is unrelated to thyroglobulin and is often obtained with normal rabbit IgG.

stimulating IgG compared with the sera of patients where the predominance of antibodies is against the TSH binding site. The anti-microsomal antibody studies were heterogeneous in that some induced adenylate cyclase, some inhibited TSH-driven cyclase activation and others had no effect on cyclase activity; the degree to which each class interacts with a separate receptor epitope is unclear.

Clearly, future work directed towards understanding the immunology of autoimmune disorders of the thyroid gland will have to take into account the fine structure of the TSH receptor. This is becoming feasible now that an increasing number of monoclonal antibodies are available which interact with specific receptor epitopes (Kohn *et al.*, 1985). Such immunochemical approaches, applied to other thyroid-specific antigens, may provide a new and more revealing basis for classifying autoimmune thyroid disease.

ANTI-IDIOTYPIC ANTIBODIES

When confronted with an antigen, the immune system synthesizes specific antibodies. Additionally, a second set of antibodies is raised with specificity for the antigen binding site (paratope) as well as the surrounding backbone structures. Determinants against which such antibodies are raised are 'idiotopes', and collections of such determinants are referred to as 'idiotypes'. The second class of antibodies is known as 'anti-idiotypes'; they fall into several classes (Farid and Lo, 1985; Farid, 1985). The most relevant in this review is the subclass which encodes an 'internal image' of the antigen (Farid, 1985). The interaction of this anti-idiotype class is inhibited by the antigen with its idiotype but also simulates many of the biological characteristics of the antigen itself (Farid and Lo, 1985; Farid, 1985).

Anti-idiotypic antibodies have regulatory functions in that they are able either to suppress or to augment an immune response; not unexpectedly, idiotypic determinants found on antibodies are also expressed on the B cell receptor. The paradox of T regulatory cells' influencing the synthesis of both idiotypes and anti-idiotypes to a fine specificity, with the knowledge that the T cell receptor appears to be constructed as a result of rearrangement of a set of genes other than immunoglobulins, has been resolved recently. Seemingly, T regulatory cells with receptors specific for idiotypic determinants on B cell receptor or circulating antibodies are generated (Farid and Lo, 1985); these are functionally anti-idiotypic in nature. A matter of interest is the fact that the idiotypic repertoire in the mouse is reached within the first few weeks of life. Inability to establish the appropriate repertoire may lead to occurrence of autoimmune responses in adult animals (Martinez *et al.*, 1985).

The first indication that the anti-idiotypic antibody approach could be used to examine the receptors for hormones was a demonstration that anti-insulin anti-idiotypic antibodies had insulin-like effects (Sege and Peterson, 1978).

In order to investigate the possibility that an anti-ligand anti-idiotype may interact with a ligand receptor, we have raised two classes of anti-idiotypes over the past few years: anti-TSH anti-idiotypes and anti-TSH subunit antibodies, with which we have studied the TSH receptor, interaction of the TSH with its receptor as well as biosynthesis and turnover of the receptor.

Anti-TSH Anti-idiotypic Antibody

In brief, anti-TSH anti-idiotypes were raised by immunizing Sprague-Dawley rats with human TSH, and subsequently immunizing rabbits with affinity-purified TSH specific IgG. The IgG fraction of rabbit immune sera was absorbed with pooled rat IgG to obtain idiotype-specific antibodies. The binding of radio-labelled anti-idiotype with anti-TSH was dose-dependently inhibited by TSH but not by human chorionic gonadotropin, suggesting that the antibody preparation contained internal image anti-idiotypes. These anti-idiotypes bound to the TSH receptor, with affinity in the order of 7×10^{-9} M (*vs.* 1.3×10^{-10} M for bTSH). They had higher affinity for porcine, compared with human, thyroid plasma membranes. The anti-idiotypes induce adenylate cyclase activation, iodide transport into dispersed thyrocytes and organization of these cells into follicular structures. The last two properties depend, at least in part, on the generation of cyclic AMP (Islam *et al.*, 1983b).

Furthermore, anti-idiotypic antibodies were found to interact with protein blots of thyroid plasma membranes, resolved under non-reducing conditions with a band at Mr $\approx 197\,000$ (Islam *et al.*, 1983a). This band corresponded to the TSH holoreceptor. The interaction was almost completely blocked by pre-incubation of nitrocellulose paper with bTSH (500 mU/ml) but not by insulin or human chorionic gonadotropin (figure 8).

These anti-TSH anti-idiotypes were, therefore, agonists which exhibited all the *in vitro* biological correlates of Graves's IgG (Farid *et al.*, 1983). The results also indicated that the antibody species accounting for the biological activity of the polyclonal Graves's IgG was that directed against the receptor and not against other membrane components close to the receptor. The results also suggested that, at least in some instances, Graves's IgG may indeed be an anti-idiotype (Farid *et al.*, 1983; Islam *et al.*, 1983b).

Anti-TSH Subunit Anti-idiotypes

The second class of anti-idiotypic antibodies was raised specifically to examine the mode of interaction of TSH with its receptor. As the dissociated α and β subunits of TSH are biologically inactive (Pierce and Parsons, 1981), it has not been possible to determine the relative contributions of the two subunits to the signals delivered by the hormone. It is generally assumed that signal specificity requires the β subunit, but its interaction with the receptor could be through anchoring or binding, while the α subunit delivers the hormone specific signal (figure 9).

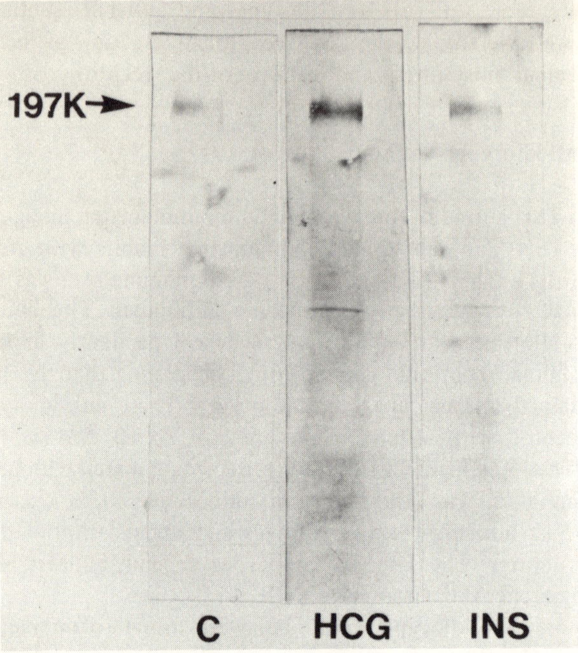

Figure 8 Binding of anti-TSH anti-idiotypes to the TSH holoreceptor ($Mr \approx 197\,000$). This binding is specific in that 500 mU/ml of human chorionic gonadotrophin (HCG) or insulin (INS) had no effect on binding.

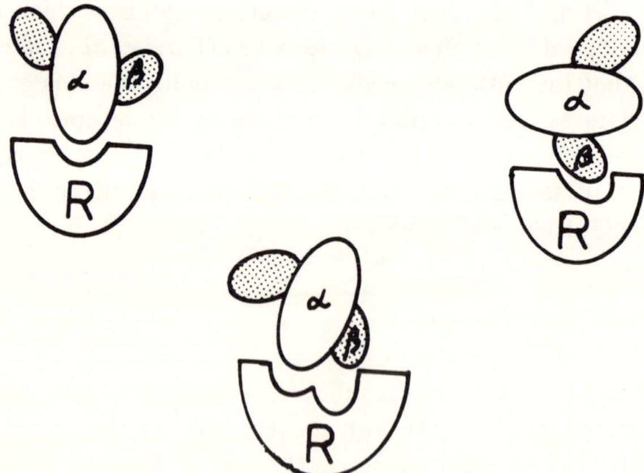

Figure 9 Potential ways in which the TSH α–β dimer interacts with the receptor: left, α subunits as binding moiety with β delivering hormone signal; right, β sub-unit is the binding moiety; centre, both subunits are involved in the signalling. In all probability, the model shown on the left is the most appropriate; it is, however, not certain whether TSH delivers two separate signals (not shown) or a conjoint single signal.

We raised monoclonal antibodies specific to the TSH α and β subunits which were then used to raise anti-monoclonal anti-idiotypes in rabbits (Briones-Urbina *et al.*, 1987). The characteristics of the monoclonal antibodies used are shown in table 1. The binding of ^{125}I human TSH to the anti-β subunit monoclonal antibody was inhibited by its complementary anti-idiotypes, in a dose-dependent manner, up to 48% at 500 mg IgG/ml. By contrast, ^{125}I-bTSH interaction with anti-α subunit monoclonal antibody was not influenced by the anti-α anti-idiotype. Therefore, whereas the anti-β subunit anti-idiotype is of the 'internal image' variety, the anti-α anti-idiotype is not (Farid and Lo, 1985; Farid, 1985;

Table 1   Anti-TSH subunit specific monoclonal antibodies

	Anti-α	Anti-β
Species	Rat	Rat
Ig isotype	IgM	IgG
Binding to ^{125}I-hTSH	+	+
Binding affinity K_D (10^{-10} M)	3.4	3.7
Displacement of bound ^{125}I-hTSH by bTSH	< 5%	< 3%
Glycoprotein hormone causing displacement of bound ^{125}I-hTSH	hTSH, hFSH, hLH, hCG	hTSH
Inhibition of membrane-bound ^{125}I-bTSH	−	+
Inhibition of adenylate cyclase activation	+	+

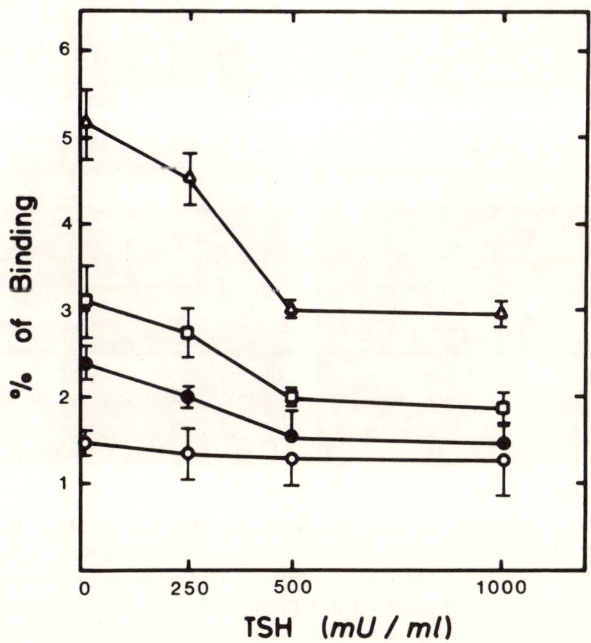

Figure 10   The binding of ^{125}I-anti-idiotypic antibodies to thyroid plasma membranes and their inhibition by TSH. Binding of anti-α + anti-β anti-idiotypes is additive and displaceable by TSH. Bars depict the SD.

Briones-Urbina *et al.*, 1987). It may be complementary to idiotypes in close proximity to the antigen binding site or may represent an 'epibody' (Farid, 1985). The anti-idiotypic antibody preparations were found to be without effect, alone or in combination, when tested for their ability to inhibit ^{125}I-bTSH binding to thyroid plasma membrane. This was in spite of the ability of iodinated anti-idiotypes to bind to thyroid plasma membranes (figure 10). The binding of the equimolar concentrations of radiolabelled anti-idiotype was additive. Some 40–65% of the bound anti-α and anti-β anti-idiotypes and their mixture was inhibited by 500 mU/ml of bTSH. In the case of the anti-α anti-idiotype and, particularly, with reference to the combination of anti-α and anti-β anti-idiotypes, residual binding was well above that of normal rabbit IgG. This was attributed to the stabilization of the receptor by these antibodies (Briones-Urbina *et al.*, 1987).

Each of the anti-α and anti-β anti-idiotypes has some stimulatory activity on basal thyroid plasma membrane adenylate cyclase, compared with normal rabbit IgG. The addition of equimolar quantities of the two anti-idiotypes resulted in a marked stimulation of adenylate cyclase when compared with that produced by 150 mU/ml of bTSH (figure 11). The more than additive influence of the two

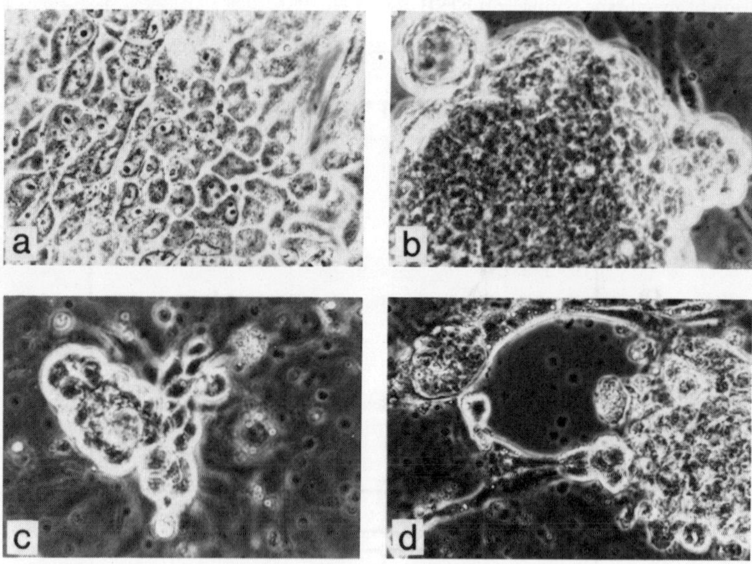

Figure 11   The influence of anti-idiotypes on the organization of thyrocytes into follicles. Photographs were taken on day 7 of culture with a phase contrast objective (25× –2×) through a green filter. (a) Anti-α anti-idiotypes are associated with elongated cells growing in a monolayer. (b) TSH 100 mU/ml. A large follicle is shown. (c) Anti-β results in a 'half-melon' appearance of follicles engaged in thyroglobulin synthesis. (d) Anti-β + anti-α anti-idiotypes follow the follicular type of structure of the cultured cells. (Normal rabbit IgG results in a monolayer similar to that of normal IgG and is not shown here.)

anti-idiotypes suggests co-operative interaction, i.e. the binding of one antibody to the thyroid plasma membrane increases the affinity of the other for the receptor. The combination of anti-α and anti-β anti-idiotypes was found to induce dispersed thyroid cells to organize into follicular structures (figure 11) and to promote the uptake of ^{131}I by these cells. The anti-β anti-idiotype alone had some effect on both assays, but the anti-α anti-idiotype had no influence on either. Finally, the capacity of these antibodies to bind to protein blots of thyroid plasma membrane under non-reducing conditions was tested. Neither of the two anti-idiotypes tested individually could be detected as interacting with the blotted peptide. However, when equimolar quantities of the two anti-idiotypes were tested, a clear band at $Mr \approx 200\,000$ was consistently observed (table 2). The seeming paradox between the finding that the radiolabelled anti-idiotypes bind to thyroid plasma membrane and the inability to demonstrate binding to the protein-blotted receptor can be resolved by noting that the protein blots are extensively washed in 200 mM NaCl in order to minimize non-specific binding. This procedure results in the removal of antibodies of low binding affinity and again emphasizes the co-operative interaction of the two anti-idiotypes in binding to the TSH receptor (Islam *et al.*, 1987).

Apparently, after binding to its receptor, TSH induces microaggregation of the receptor, which is necessary for adenylate cyclase activation. While it is conceivable that combination of the two anti-idiotypes acts through promoting receptor aggregation, we would need in addition, to invoke both specific interaction of each anti-idiotype with separate domains of the receptor and the bivalency of each of the two antibodies to account for the slight biological activity of the anti-β anti-idiotype and the co-operative influence of the two anti-idiotypes, particularly on protein-blotted receptor. The lack of an internal image anti-α idiotype does not allow for rigorous testing of the question of specificity (Farid, 1985; Briones-Urbina *et al.*, 1987).

In conclusion, the α and β subunits of the TSH receptor deliver two co-operative signals to the TSH receptor. The hormone specificity is indeed associated with the β subunit, the α subunit's contribution being to increase the affinity of the receptor for subsequent β subunit signalling (although it has not been possible for us to find out the order in which the two subunits interact

Table 2   Adenylate cyclase activation by anti-α and anti-β TSH subunit anti-idiotypes

	Normal rabbit IgG	Anti-idiotypes			TSH[b]
		Anti-α[a]	Anti-β[a]	Anti-α + anti-β[a]	
Percentage cyclase stimulation relative to buffer	-57 ± 2	-7.3 ± 3.1	-8.1 ± 0.9	87.3 ± 4.6	93 ± 6.8

[a] IgG was tested at a concentration of 250 μg/ml; thus, for the anti-idiotype mixture 125 μg/ml of each were used.
[b] 250 mU/ml crude bTSH (USV Laboratories, Mississauga, Ontario) were used.

with the receptor). This co-operative interaction is apparently crucial for receptor conformation requisite for the stimulation of adenylate cyclase systems. Studies comparing the interaction of free and receptor-bound bovine TSH with the monoclonal idiotypes also suggested that, after binding to the receptor, the bovine TSH molecule undergoes conformational changes such that new antigenic sites previously unrecognized by these monoclonal antibodies are exposed. The TSH receptor apparently comprises at least two functional domains, one of which is concerned with ^{125}I-bTSH binding and the second of which stimulates the cyclase system; this is a view consistent with work utilizing anti-TSH receptor monoclonal antibodies (Kohn *et al.*, 1985).

BIOSYNTHESIS AND TURNOVER OF THE TSH RECEPTOR

Data concerning the influence of TSH in regulating its own receptor are conflicting (see Farid *et al.* (1985) for review). Earlier studies variously suggested that pre-incubation of TSH with thyroid tissue either causes no change or increases the number of ^{125}I-bTSH binding sites. More recent *in vivo* and *in vitro* data, however, demonstrate down regulation of the receptor. All these studies enumerated receptors through their capacity to bind ^{125}I-bTSH. Many hormones, including TSH, have, however, been found to bind irreversibly to their receptors, thus making them unavailable for subsequent binding; hormone–receptor complexes are directed to intracellular destinations for further processing. The problem this implies may be circumvented by studying the receptors with specific antibodies. We utilized TSH subunit specific idiotypes to study the biosynthesis and turnover rates of the TSH receptor on thyroid cells (Briones-Urbina and Farid, 1987). Isolated porcine thyroid cells were cultured for 12–48 h in the presence or absence of bovine TSH; TSH was added in amounts varying from 50–500 mU/ml at different steps of the procedure. Thyrocytes were then endogenously labelled with [^{3}H]-leucine, for times ranging from 15 min to 6 h, to study the biosynthetic rate of the receptor. In other experiments, thyrocytes were labelled for 3 h (determined to be the optimal time for labelling) with [^{3}H]-leucine and chased with medium containing unlabelled leucine for periods varying from 2–96 h in order to determine the turnover rate of the receptor. At the end of the incubation period, cells were lysed, resolved in polyacrylamide gel and subjected to protein blotting. The holoreceptor, Mr $\approx$ 200 000 bands, and bands of reconstituted subunits as well as unrelated bands were identified by receptor-specific anti-idiotype, cut and counted (figure 12).

TSH was found to accelerate the biosynthesis of its receptor by very efficient incorporation of the receptor subunits into the holoreceptor Mr $\approx$ 200 000. The effect of TSH on new receptor synthesis was bimodal, both in terms of time and TSH dose (figures 13 and 14). After optimal receptor labelling, progressive decrement in the labelling rate was observed, whether or not thyroid cells were grown in the presence of TSH (figure 13). Similarly, TSH dosage above an optimum of 100 mU caused decrement of the senses of the rate of the receptor (figure 14).

In order to influence measurably receptor biosynthesis, TSH had to be left in a thyroid cell culture for several hours (more than 3 h but less than 12 h), suggesting that TSH action is mediated through transcription and/or mRNA stabilization (figure 15).

TSH was also found to reduce the half-life of its TSH receptor. The most dramatic effect of TSH on total thyroid cell receptor half-life occurred between 12 and 15 h of incubation with TSH. TSH receptor half-life decreased from

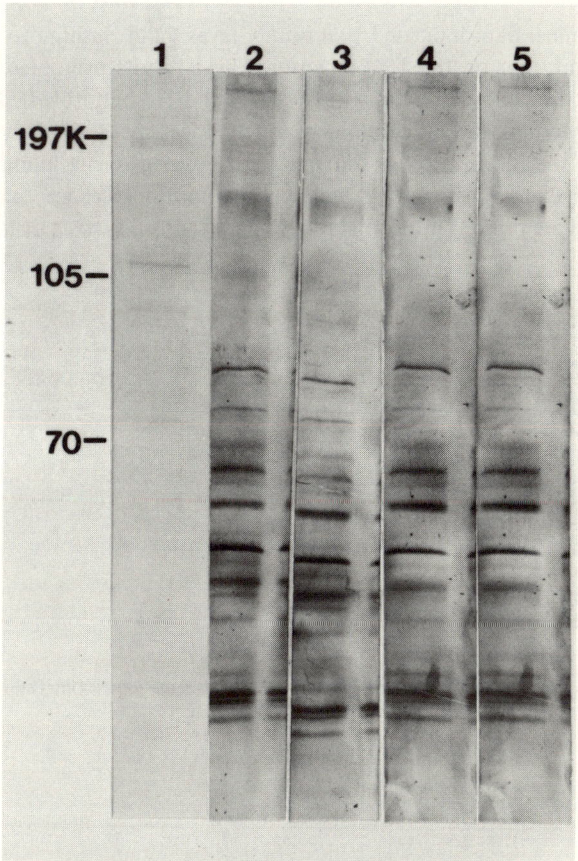

Figure 12   Interaction protein blots of thyroid whole cell lysate with receptor-specific anti-idiotypic antibodies. Lane 1, TSH binding identified with rabbit anti-bTSH. Lane 2, Mixture of anti-idiotypic antibodies. Lane 3, Blockage of the binding of anti-idiotypic antibodies by TSH to $M_r \approx 200\,000$ and $70\,000$ peptides. By contrast, porcine insulin (lane 4) (1 U/ml) failed to inhibit anti-idiotypic antibody binding to these bands and HCG (lane 5) (5 U/ml) brought about only partial inhibition of binding to the anti-idiotypes to the TSH receptor.

8.5 h to 3.3 h. Interestingly, this change coincided with replacement of the high affinity low capacity ^{125}I-bTSH binding site on thyroid plasma membranes by low affinity high capacity sites. The last observation points to a separate long-range mechanism of TSH-induced sensitization other than that involving the cyclase system, which is well documented. These *in vitro* experiments, pointing to positive regulation by TSH of its receptor, were recently confirmed by *in vivo* studies (Davies, 1985).

IMMUNOCYTOCHEMICAL STUDIES OF THE TSH RECEPTOR

Our biochemical data indicated that both Graves's and Hashimoto's IgG interact with different sites on the TSH receptor. These results prompted us to investigate the binding sites for TSH, Graves's IgG and Hashimoto's IgG at structural and ultrastructural level by immunocytochemical methods. Few studies have reported on the localization of antigens in thyrocytes using immunoassay technology. It has been shown by indirect immunofluorescence that microsomal autoantigens are present intracellularly, and on the cell surface of human thyroid

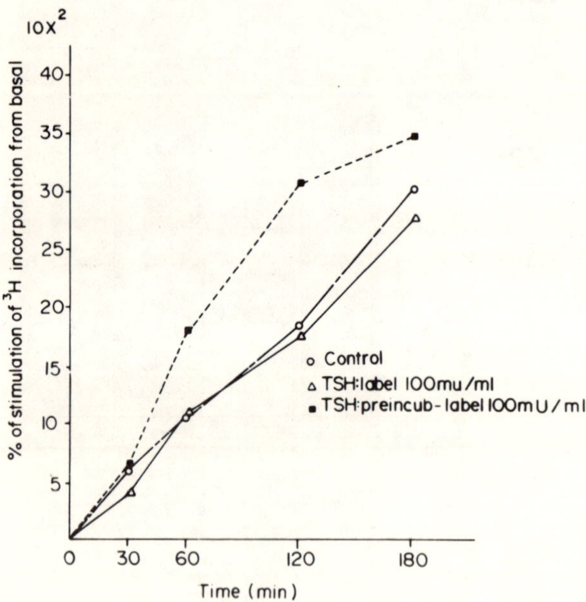

Figure 13   Effect of TSH on the synthesis rate of the Mr ≈ 200 000 polypeptide corresponding to the TSH receptor. Synthesis starts at 30 min in both groups. Maximal labelling is achieved by 3 h in TSH-stimulated cultures and at 6 h in TSH-untreated cultures. TSH, therefore, produces a shift to the left of the curve of the receptor synthesis rate.

cells maintained in monolayer cultures (Khoury *et al.*, 1981). Direct immuno-fluorescence studies indicate that the surface expression of these antigens on the thyroid cell epithelium is restricted to the apical border of the follicular cells (Khoury *et al.*, 1984).

The peroxidase-conjugated antibody method (Nakane and Pierce, 1967; Avrameas, 1969) appears to be convenient for the localization of tissue antigens and offers a useful alternative to the immunofluorescence technique (Petts and Roitt, 1971). We have used this method with porcine thyrocytes for the local-ization of bTSH and IgG from the sera of patients with Graves's (G-IgG) or Hashimoto's (H-IgG) disease (Farid *et al.*, 1985; Fahraeus-Van Ree and Farid, 1987a).

TSH AND THYROID AUTO-ANTIBODY BINDING SITES: LIGHT MICROSCOPY

Porcine thyroid fragments were fixed and prepared for immunoreaction or enzymatically dissociated in single cells (see legends to figures 16 and 17).

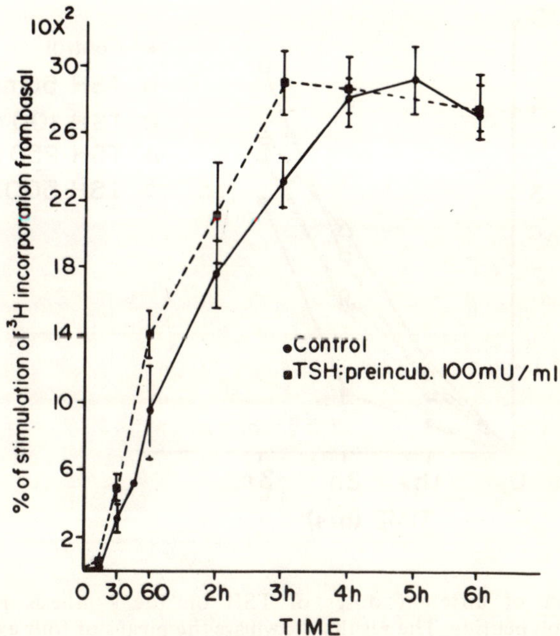

Figure 14   Effect of short term TSH stimulation compared with medium term stimulation on receptor synthesis. Incubation with TSH (100 mU/ml) medium term (15 h) accelerates the rate of synthesis of the TSH receptor, whereas short term incubation has no effect.

Cultivation of isolated porcine thyrocytes in bTSH-enriched medium leads to a monolayer with reconstructed three-dimensional follicles. The follicular cells in these monolayers and in the fragments contain a number of intracellular PAS-positive colloid droplets in the apical half of the cell. These cells are weakly immunostained with normal rabbit IgG (NR-IgG) and normal human IgG (NH-IgG) (figures 16-A, 17-1A and 17-2A), while anti-bTSH produces a weak-to-moderate immunoreaction (figures 16-B, 17-2B and 17-2C) and G-IgG and H-IgG a strong reaction (figures 17-2B–17-2D). Follicular cells which are in the process of forming follicles, and those which have already formed follicles, show the strongest immunoreactivity to these antibodies (figures 17-1C, 17-2B and 17-2D). This suggests a relationship between the number of antigenic sites identified and the functional activity of the follicular cells. Varying amounts of precipitate are found throughout the cytoplasm of all positive follicular cells. Some cells react strongly only in the perinuclear area, whereas others react in both perinuclear and nuclear areas. It has been found, using a fluorescence technique, that H-IgG antibodies are located at the cell surface and in the perinuclear area of human thyroid cells (Khoury *et al.*, 1981). This perinuclear compartment appears to be

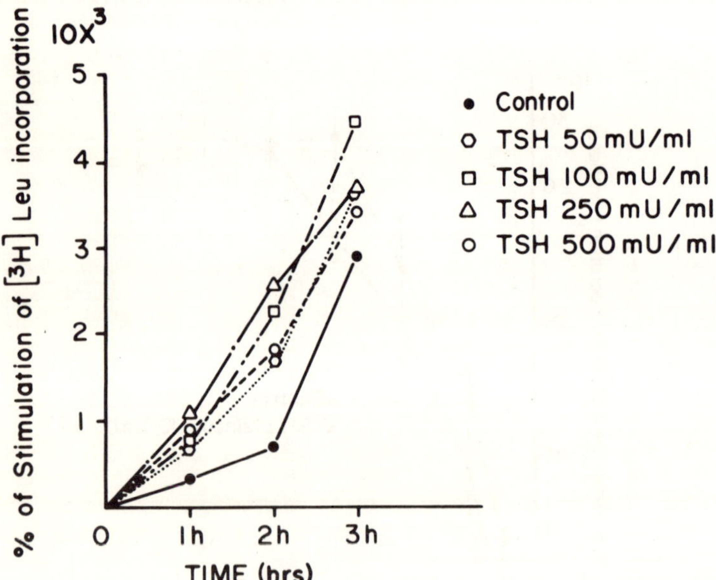

Figure 15   Effect of different doses of TSH on the synthesis rate of the $Mr \approx 200\,000$ polypeptide. The results shown are the means of four experiments. Standard deviations (which in no instance are $> 10\%$ of the mean) are not shown because of the proximity of the curves. [³H]-leucine incorporation into the receptor at 90 and 120 min was significantly different ($p < 0.05$) from that of the control at TSH doses of 50 and 100 mU/ml. Receptor labelling at these times was significantly lower at 500 mU/ml TSH than at 100 mU/ml TSH.

important for the transcellular transport of immunoglobulins (Rodewald, 1980; Hopkins, 1983). The fragments also show negative immunostained epithelial cells (figure 16-B), indicating non-reacting follicular cells and/or parafollicular cells.

Cells cultured in the absence of bTSH show minimal immunoreaction to anti-bTSH but moderate reaction to G-IgG and H-IgG. It has been suggested that the decline in antigenicity is caused by the functional de-differentiation of the thyroid cells in the absence of TSH (Khoury *et al.*, 1981; Bidey *et al.*, 1977). Apparently, the immunoreaction with anti-bTSH is specific, since pre-absorption

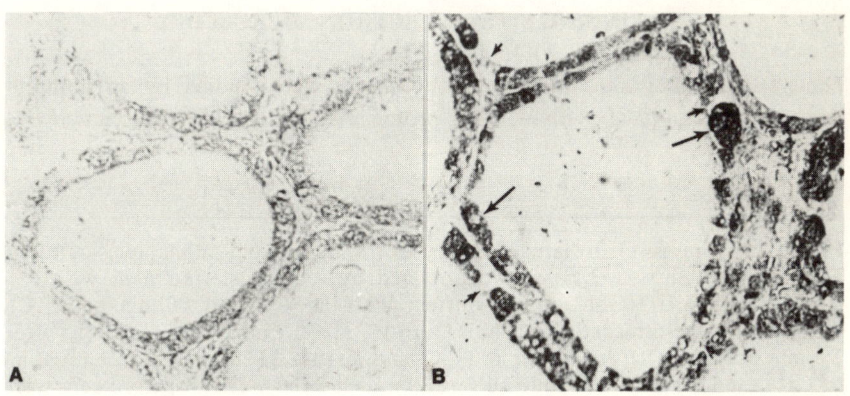

Figure 16   Immunostained consecutive sections of a porcine thyroid fragment, showing follicles with follicular cells reacting weakly to normal rabbit IgG (A) and strongly to anti-bTSH (B) as shown by the long arrows. Note the negative epithelial cells indicated by the short arrows in (B). (Magnification 350×.) Porcine thyroid fragments were fixed in 10% phosphate-buffered formalin, embedded in paraffin, sectioned at 5 μm, mounted on gelatin-coated slides, stained with periodic acid Schiff (PAS) and/or prepared for immunostaining. The indirect immunoperoxidase technique (Gartner *et al.*, 1985; Errick *et al.*, 1985) was applied, using as first antibody rabbit anti-bTSH (260 μg protein/ 100 μl) or G-IgG or H-IgG (200 μg protein/100 μl) diluted in binding buffer (BB) (20 mM Trizma hydrochloride and 25 mM sodium chloride, pH 7.6) containing 0.2% BSA (incubation times: 48 h at 4°C followed by 2 h at room temperature). The horseradish peroxidase labelled anti-rabbit IgG (1:100) or the enzyme-labelled anti-human IgG (1:200) was diluted in Tris buffer saline (TBS) (50 mM Trizma hydrochloride and 200 mM sodium chloride, pH 7.6) containing 0.2% BSA (incubation time: 2 h at room temperature). The staining solution consisted of 0.05% 3,3'-diaminobenzidine-4HCl in TBS buffer-containing 0.01% H_2O_2. Controls for specificity included (1) omission of the primary antibody, (2) replacement of the primary antibody with normal rabbit IgG (NR-IgG) or normal human IgG (NH-IgG), (3) pre-absorption of anti-bTSH and NR-IgG with bTSH (125, 250, 500 or 750 mU) and (4) exposure of sections of porcine liver fragments to the same immunochemical examination as the sections of thyroid tissue.

of anti-bTSH with bTSH (125 mU) results in complete disappearance of the immunoreaction. Pre-absorption of NR-IgG with bTSH from 125 to 750 mU does not abolish the immunoreaction. Moreover, porcine liver cells do not show any immunoreaction to NR-IgG, anti-bTSH, NH-IgG, G-IgG or H-IgG.

Pre-incubation of thyroid cell monolayer with bTSH leads to a strong reduction of the immunoreaction with G-IgG but does not affect the reaction with H-IgG (figure 17-3). These morphological results are in full agreement with our biochemical observations in that G-IgG interacts with the same cellular sites as does bTSH whereas H-IgG binds to a determinant on the TSH receptor separate from the one to which TSH and G-IgG bind.

TSH BINDING SITES: ELECTRON MICROSCOPY

The bTSH binding sites in porcine thyrocytes were studied by an immuno electron microscopical method, using protein A–colloid gold (pAg) complex as

---

Figure 17 (opposite) Isolated thyrocytes in 7 day old monolayer cultures. Thyroid fragments (2–3 g) were dissociated by sequential treatment with collagenase (2835 U/10 ml Tyrode buffer; 20 h at $4°$C and 20 min at $37°$C), ethylenediaminetetraacetic acid (EDTA) (10 ml of 2 mM Ca^{2+}- and Mg^{2+}-free Tyrode buffer; twice for 5 min at $37°$C) and dispase 2 (10 ml of 0.25% in 10 ml of Ca^{2+}- and Mg^{2+}-free Tyrode buffer; 30 min at $37°$C). The dispersed cells were plated in film-lined tissue culture dishes (Falcon 3006) and cultured in a hormone-free medium (Leibovitz-15 supplemented with 10% foetal calf serum and the antibiotics antimycotic and kanamycine) or in a medium with bTSH (150 mU/ml hormone-free medium) for 7 days. After the culture period, the cells were rinsed and fixed for 18–20 h at $4°$C in glutaraldehyde–picric acetic acid and washed successively in 80% and 70% ethanol and BB. The film liners were cut into small pieces, put in 24 multiwell plates and immunochemically stained in a manner identical to that used for the thyroid sections (see legend to figure 6) except for the use of different concentrations of antibodies (anti-bTSH, 65 μg protein/ 100 μl BB; g-IgG and H-IgG, 1.63 μg protein/100 μl BB). (1) Immunostained 7 day old porcine thyroid cell monolayer cultured in bTSH-enriched medium, showing cells with a weak immunoreaction to NR-IgG (A) and a strong reaction in cells and globular aggregates to anti-bTSH (B, C). (Magnification 365×.) (2) The same monolayer as in (1). The cells and globular aggregates show a weak reaction to NH-IgG (A), a strong reaction to Graves's IgG (B, C) and a very strong reaction to Hashimoto's IgG (D). Note the heavy precipitate around the nucleus shown by the arrow in C. (Magnification 365×.) (3) Immunostained 7 day old porcine thyroid cell monolayer cultured in control medium, showing cells reacting with G-IgG (A) and H-IgG (D). The reaction to G-IgG is strongly reduced by pre-incubation with bTSH (B), but the reaction to H-IgG is not affected by this pre-incubation (C). (Magnification 365×.) Some of the monolayers cultured in control medium were pretreated with NR-IgG or bTSH (100 μg protein/100 μl BB) for about 20 h at $4°$C and subsequently immunostained with NH-IgG, G-IgG or H-IgG as first antibody (see legend to figure 2 for concentrations used).

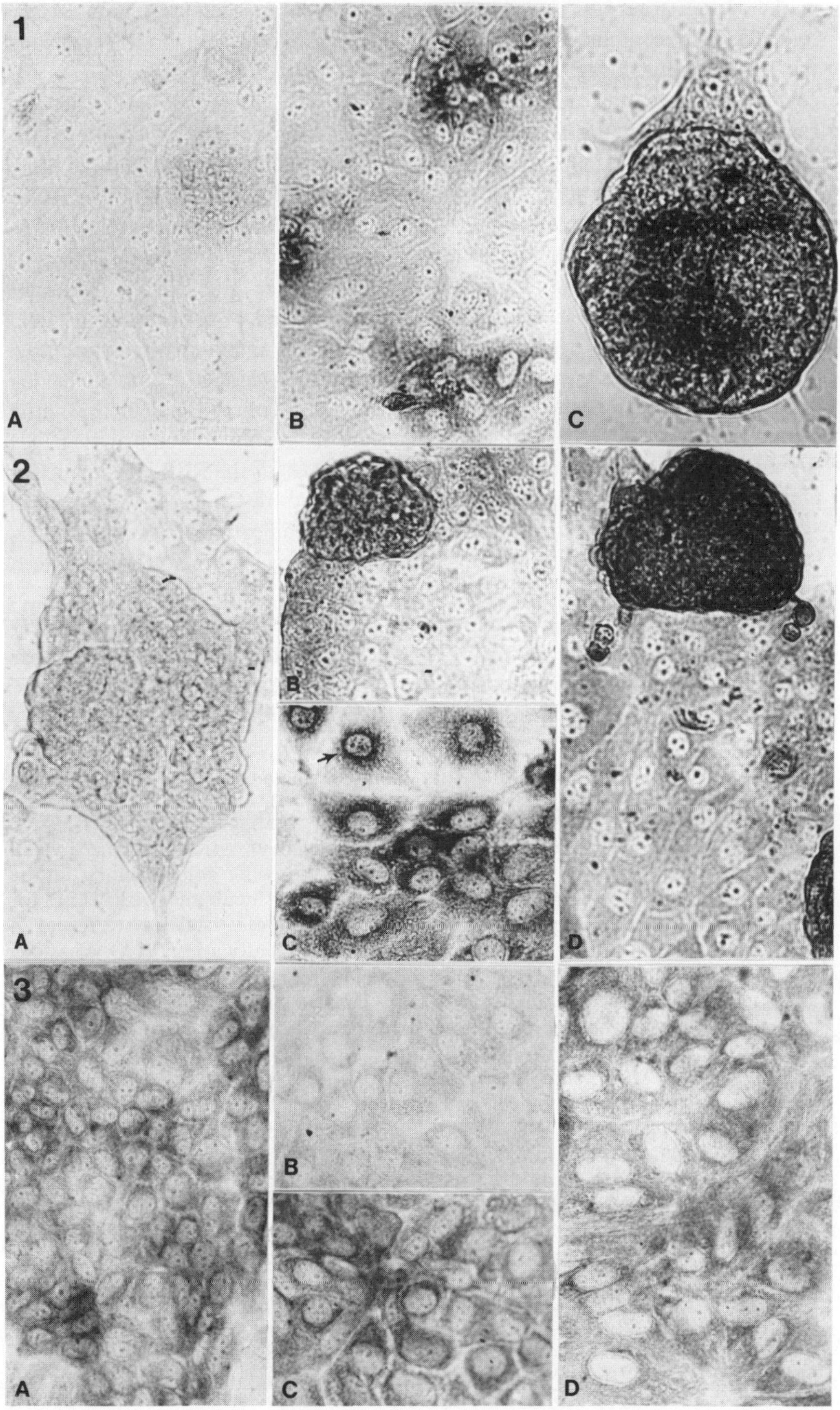

marker. In all groups of thyroid fragments studied (see legend to figure 18), the follicular cells contain prominent rough endoplasmic reticulum (RER) around the mitochondria, Golgi apparatus, lysosomes, microvilli and desmosomes, and coated vesicles in the apical parts of the cells. Two different stages of activity can be observed in the initial control fragments, one of these being well preserved with numerous phagosomes (intra-cellular colloid droplets), and the other poorly preserved with a condensed nucleus and almost no phagosomes. Fragments which are incubated for 20 h with bTSH show cellular debris in the follicular lumen. The follicular cells in these fragments show large dilations of RER and an abundant number of large droplets, often found in the basal part of the cell and against the nucleus (figures 18-B and 18-C). Almost no gold labelling is found on thyrocytes from initial control and control medium fragments while on thyrocytes incubated with bTSH for 60 min at 4°C gold labelling is found, especially at the basal membrane, in the collagen and in the blood capillaries (figure 18-A). Fragments which are incubated for 20 h with bTSH show groups of gold particles in droplets, in cisternae of the RER, at the nuclear membrane and within the nuclei (figures 18-B and 18-C). These results are in agreement with studies on bovine corpora lutea, indicating that several intra-cellular organelles, including the nucleus, contain gonadotropin, prostaglandin E and $F_{2\alpha}$ receptors (Rao and Chegini, 1983). It is difficult to determine the exact process of receptor-mediated endocytosis of TSH and the fate of the ligand-receptor complex inside the cell. This is due to the fact that intracellular organelles contain receptors and the internalized ligands bind to these organelles.

From our morphological results it can be concluded that porcine thyrocytes contain bTSH binding sites within the nuclei. This is in agreement with our *in vitro* biochemical data indicating that isolated nuclei and nuclear matrix of

---

Figure 18   (opposite) Electron micrographs of thyrocytes from porcine thyroid fragments. (A) Initial control fragment, clearly showing gold labelling at the basal membrane (BM) (arrowed). (B, C) A fragment incubated with bTSH for 60 min at 4°C and subsequently for 20 h at 37°C. Gold particles are found in large droplets (D) and within the nucleus (N). (Magnifications: (A) 45 500×; (B) 33 150×; (C) 29 250× (D) 45 500×.) Porcine fragments were fixed prior to, or after, incubation in a hormone-free medium (Liebovitz-15) or in a bTSH-enriched (100 mU/ml) hormone-free medium. Three incubation sequences were used for both of the incubated groups: (1) 60 min at 4°C; (2) 60 min at 4°C and subsequently at 37°C for 5 min or (3) for 20 h. The fixed tissue was prepared for immuno electron microscopical examination (Van Putten *et al.*, 1983) using anti-bTSH (65 μg protein/100 μl PBG comprising phosphate-buffered saline containing 0.15 M NaCl, 2.5 mM KCl and 0.01 M phosphate, pH 7.2, with added 0.2% gelatin and 0.5% bovine serum albumin) and anti-human TSH (anti-hTSH of dilution 1:30 000, 90 μg protein/100 μg PBG) as first antibody (incubation time: 2 h at room temperature) and pAg complex (Slot and Geuze, 1981) (gold particle size, 10 nm; dilution, 1:20 in PGB; incubation time, 1 h at room temperature) as a second reagent. Controls for specificity included (1) omission of the primary antibody and (2) replacement of the primary antibody with normal rabbit IgG.

BM
N
D
B
C
N
D
A

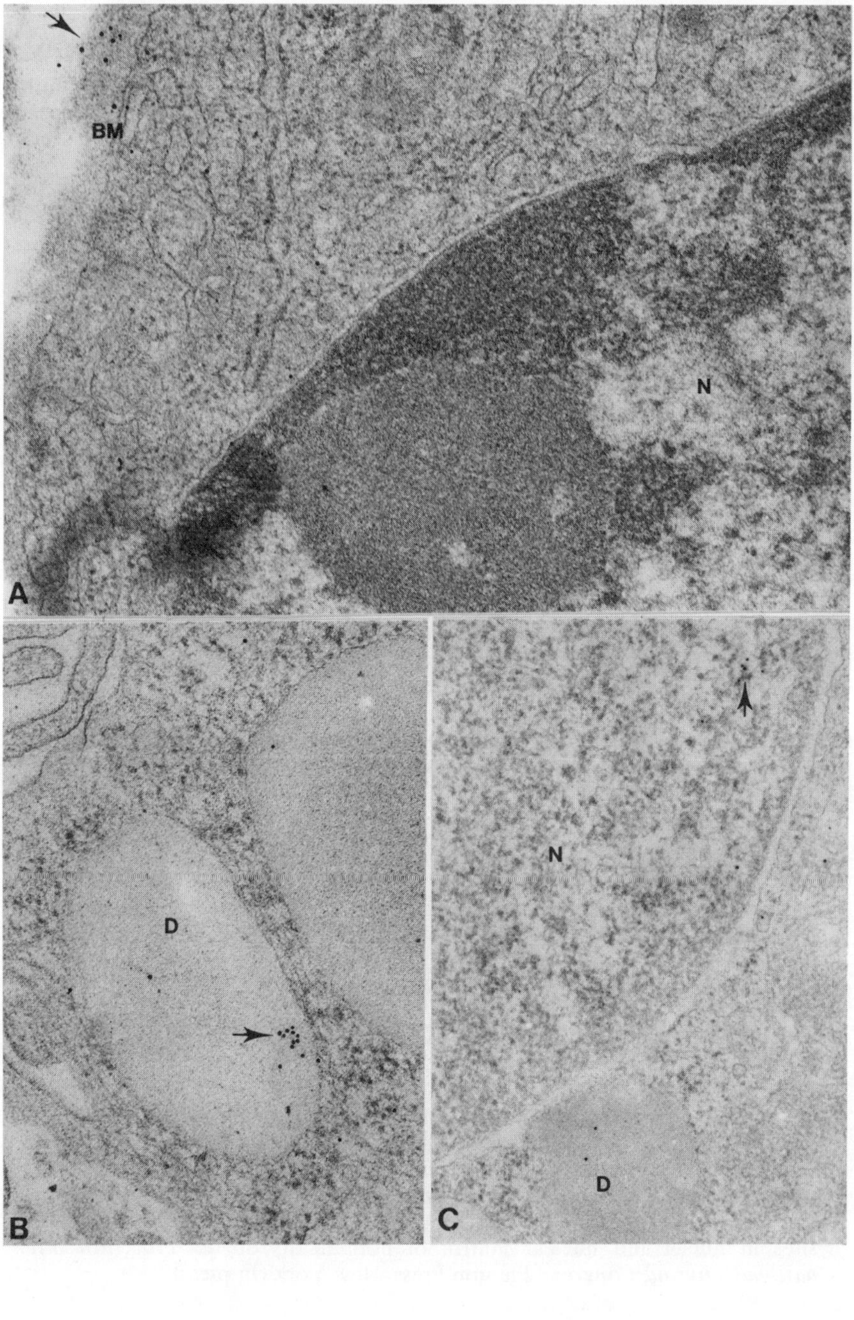

porcine thyrocytes have saturable and specific ^{125}I-bTSH binding sites (Fahraeus-Van Ree and Farid, 1987a,b). Some reports have already shown that protein and peptide hormones have a direct effect on the nuclei of target cells (Rao and Chegini, 1983).

These results provided the rationale for our present investigations on the potential role of nuclear receptors in mediating some of the physiological actions of TSH, e.g. stimulation of nuclear enzymes involved in ribonucleic acid synthesis.

ACKNOWLEDGEMENTS

This work was supported by grants from the Medical Research Council of Canada.

We are grateful to Dr. L. J. A. Van Putten for her support in carrying out the immuno electron microscopical study.

REFERENCES

Avrameas, S. (1969). Coupling of enzymes to proteins with glutaraldehyde. Use of the conjugates for the detection of antigens and antibodies. *Immunochemistry*, **6**, 43–52

Bako, G., Islam, M. N. and Farid, N. R. (1985). Photoaffinity labelling of the porcine thyrotropin receptor – effect of Graves' immunoglobulin G and anti-TSH anti-idiotypic antibodies. *Clin. Invest. Med.*, **8**, 152–159

Bidey, S. P., Marsden, P., Anderson, J., McKerron, C. G. and Berry, H. (1977). In-vitro studies of normal human thyroid cells: responses to thyrotrophin and dibutyryl cyclic AMP. *J. Endocrinol.*, **72**, 87–96

Briones-Urbina, R. and Farid, N. R. (1987). Control and biosynthesis and turnover of the thyrotropin receptor (submitted)

Briones-Urbina, R., Islam, M. N., Ivanyi, J. and Farid, N. R. (1987). Use of anti-idiotypic antibodies as probes for the interaction of TSH subunits with its receptor. *J. Cell. Biochem.* (in press)

Czarnocka, B., Ruf, J., Ferrand, M., Carayon, P. and Lissitzky, S. (1985). Purification of human thyroid peroxidase and its identification as the microsomal antigen involved in autoimmune thyroid disease. *FEBS Lett.*, **190**, 147–152

Davies, T. F. (1985). Positive regulation of the guinea pig thyrotropin receptor. *Endocrinology*, **117**, 201–207

Dumont, J. E. and Vassart, G. (1979). Thyroid gland metabolism and the action of TSH. In L. J. DeGroot, G. F., Cahill Jr., W. O. Odell, L. Martini, J. T. Potts Jr., D. H. Nelson, E. Steinberger and A. I. Winegard (eds.), *Endocrinology*, Vol. 1, Grune and Stratton, New York, 311–329

Errick, J. E., Eggo, M. C. and Burrow, G. N. (1985). Epidermal growth factor inhibits thyrotropin-mediated synthesis of tissue-specific proteins in cultured ovine thyroid cells. *Mol. Cell. Endocrinol.*, **43**, 51–59

Fahraeus-Van Ree, G. E. and Farid, N. R. (1987a). Bovine thyrotropin binding sites in nuclei and nuclear matrix of porcine thyrocytes. *Proc. 9th International Thyroid Congress*, Plenum Press, New York (in press)

Fahraeus-Van Ree, G. E. and Farid, N. R. (1987b). Immunocytochemical localization of bovine thyrotropin and thyroid auto-antibodies in porcine thyrocytes (submitted)

Farid, N. R. (1985). Anti-hormone anti-idiotypes are probes for receptor structure and function. *Immunol. Lett.*, **9**, 181–185

Farid, N. R., Briones-Urbina, R. and Bear, J. C. (1983). Graves' disease – the thyroid stimulating antibody and immunological networks. *Mol. Asp. Med.*, **6**, 355–457

Farid, N. R., Fahraeus-Van Ree, G. and Briones-Urbina, R. (1985). Structure, synthesis and cellular localization of the TSH receptor. In P. G. Walfish, J. R. Wall and R. Volpe (eds.) *Autoimmunity and the Thyroid*, Academic Press, Orlando, 249–271

Farid, N. R. and Lo, T. C. Y. (1985). Anti-idiotypic antibodies as probes for receptor structure and function. *Endocrine Reviews*, **6**, 1–23

Gartner, R., Greil, W., Demharter, R. and Horn, K. (1985). Involvement of cyclic AMP, iodide and metabolites of arachidemic acid in the regulation of cell proliferation of isolated porcine thyroid cells. *Mol. Cell. Endocrinol.*, **42**, 145–155

Heyma, P. and Harrison, L. C. (1984). Precipitation of thyrotropin receptor and identification of thyroid autoantigens using Graves' disease immunoglobulin. *J. Clin. Invest.*, **74**, 1090–1027

Hopkins, C. R. (1983). The importance of the endosome in intracellular traffic. *Nature*, **304**, 684–685

Iida, Y., Konishi, T., Kasagi, K., Endo, K., Misaki, T., Kuma, T. and Torizuka, K. (1983). Partial purification and properties of the TSH receptors from human thyroid plasma membranes. *Acta Endocrinologica*, **103**, 198–204

Islam, M. N., Briones-Urbina, R., Bako, G. and Farid, N. R. (1983a). Both TSH and thyroid stimulating antibody of Graves' disease bind to an Mr 197,000 holoreceptor. *Endocrinology*, **113**, 436–438

Islam, M. N. and Farid, N. R. (1985). Structure of the porcine thyrotropin receptor: a 200 kilodalton glycoprotein heterocomplex. *Experientia*, **41**, 18–23

Islam, M. N., Pepper, B. M., Briones-Urbina, R. and Farid, N. R. (1983b). Biological activity of anti-thyrotropin anti-idiotypic antibody. *Europ. J. Immunol.*, **13**, 57–63

Islam, M. N., Tuppal, R., Hawe, B. S., Briones-Urbina, R. and Farid, N. R. (1987). The thyroid "microsomal" antigen is an epitope on the thyrotropin receptor. *J. Cell. Biochem.* (in press).

Kajita, Y., Rickards, C. R., Buckland, P. R., Howells, R. D. and Smith, B. R. (1985). Analysis of thyrotropin receptors by photoaffinity labelling. Orientation of receptor subunits in the cell membrane. *Biochem. J.*, **227**, 413–420

Khoury, E. L., Hammond, L., Bottazzo, G. F. and Doniach, D. (1981). Presence of the organ-specific 'microsomal autoantigen on the surface of human thyroid cells in culture: its involvement in complement-mediated cytotoxicity. *Clin. Exp. Immunol.*, **55**, 995–998

Khoury, E. L., Bottazzo, G. F. and Roitt, I. M. (1984). The thyroid 'microsomal' antibody revisited. Its paradoxical binding in vivo to the apical surface of the follicular epithelium. *J. Exp. Med.*, **159**, 577–591

Kohn, L. D., Valente, W. A., Alvarez, F. V., Rotella, C. M., Marcocci, C., Toccafondi, R. S. and Grollman, E. F. (1985). New procedures for detecting Graves' immunoglobulins. In P. G. Walfish, J. R. Wall and R. Volpe (eds.) *Autoimmunity and the Thyroid*, Academic Press, Orlando, 217–247

Kohn, L. D., Valente, W. A., Lacetti, P., Cohen, J. L., Aloj, S. M. and Grollman, E. F. (1983). Multicomponent structure of the thyrotropin receptor: relationship to Graves' disease. *Life Sci.*, **32**, 15–30

Koizumi, Y., Zakarija, M. and McKenzie, J. M. (1982). Solubilization, purification and partial characterization of thyrotropin receptors from bovine and human thyroids. *Endocrinology*, **110**, 1381–1391

Lewinski, A., Bartke, A. and Smith, N. K. R. (1983). Compensatory thyroid hyperplasia in hemithyroidectomized snell dwarf mice. *Endocrinology*, **113**, 2317–2319

Martinez, A. C., Bernabe, R. R., de la Hera, A., Pereira, P., Cazenave, P.-A. and Coutinho, A. (1985). Establishment of idiotypic helper T-cell repertoires — early in life. *Nature*, **317**, 721–723

Nagakawa, H., Kotani, T., Ohtaki, S., Nakamura, M. and Yamazaki, I. (1985). Purification of thyroid peroxidase by monoclonal antibody-assisted immuno-affinity chromatography. *Biochem. Biophys. Res. Comm.*, **127**, 8–14

Nakane, P. K. and Pierce, Jr., G. B. (1967). Enzyme-labeled antibodies: preparation and application for the localization of antigens. *J. Histochem. Cytochem.*, **11**, 929–931

Nielsen, T. B., Totsuka, Y., Kempner, E. S. and Feilds, J. S. (1984). Structure of the thyrotropin receptor and thyroid adenylate cyclase system as determined by target analysis. *Biochemistry*, **23**, 6009–6016

Petts, V. and Roitt, I. M. (1971). Peroxidase conjugates for demonstration of tissue antibodies: evaluation of the technique. *Clin. Exp. Immunol.*, **9**, 407–418

Pierce, J. G. and Parsons, T. F. (1981). Glycoprotein hormones: structure and function. *Ann. Rev. Biochem.*, **50**, 465–497

Rao, C. V. and Chegini, N. (1983). Nuclear receptors for gonadotropins and prostaglandins. In R. A. Bradshaw and G. N. Gill (eds.), *Evolution of Hormone-Receptor Systems*, Alan R. Liss, New York, 413–423

Rodewald, R. (1980). Distribution of immunoglobulin G receptors in the small intestine of the young rat. *J. Cell Biol.*, **85**, 18–32

Sege, K. and Peterson, P. A. (1978). Use of anti-idiotype antibodies as cell-surface receptor probes. *Proc. Natl. Acad. Sci.*, **75**, 2443–2447

Slot, J. W. and Geuze, H. J. (1981). Sizing of protein A–colloidal gold probes for immunoelectron microscopy. *J. Cell Biol.*, **90**, 533–536

Valente, W. A., Vitti, P., Kohn, L. D., Brandi, M. L., Rotella, C. M., Toccafondi, R., Tramontano, D., Aloj, S. M. and Ambesi-Impiobato, F. S. (1983). Relationship of growth and adenylate cyclase activity in cultured thyroid cells: separate bioeffects of thyrotropin. *Endocrinology*, **112**, 71–79

Van Putten, L. J. A., Van Oordt, P. G. W. J., Terlou, M. and Peute, J. (1983). Histophysiological and immunocytochemical study on the nature of the thyrotrops in the pituitary of immature rainbow trout, *Salmo gairdneri*. *Cell Tissue Res.*, **231**, 185–198

Notes on Contributors

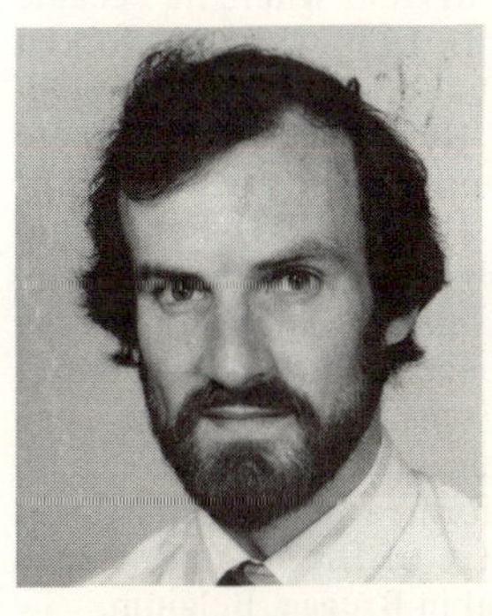

Robert Anthony, BSc, PhD, is a post-doctoral research assistant at the University of Glasgow. His research interests include immunology of liver disease and regulation of complement synthesis by hepatocytes.

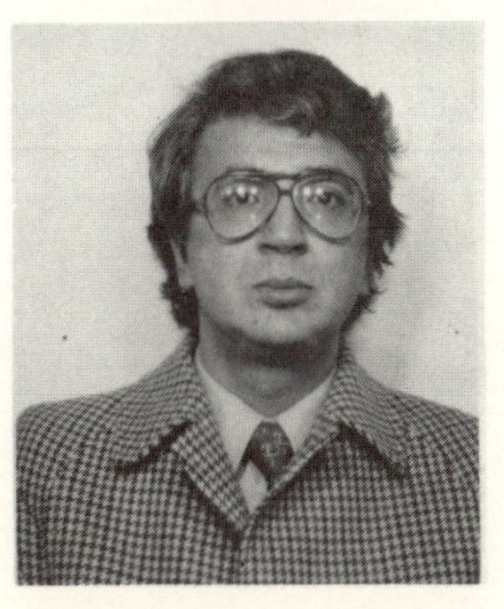

Francesco Bianco Bianchi was born in Brescia, Italy, on 20th January, 1939. He graduated in Medicine *cum laude* at the University of Bologna, Italy, on 12th November, 1963. He specialized in Internal Medicine in 1969 and in Gastro-enterology in 1970. He is now Associate Professor of Medicine at the University of Bologna and works at the Institute of Patologia Medica–Cattedra di Clinica Medica II.

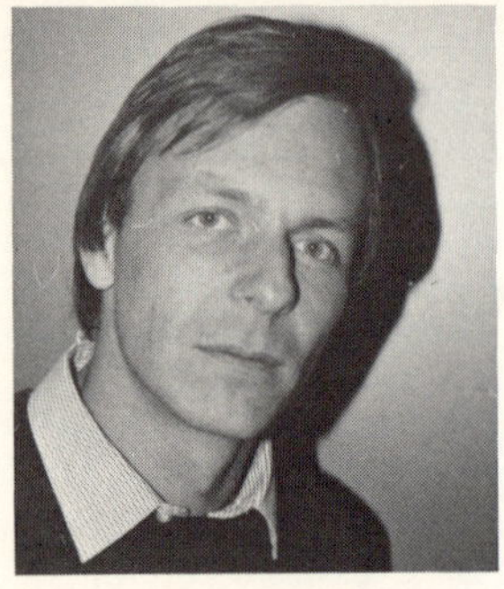

Professor R. Braun was born on March 24th, 1954 in Baden-Baden, Federal Republic of Germany, and grew up in Heidelberg, Stuttgart and Freiburg. After graduating from High School in 1973, he studied medicine at the Universities of Freiburg and Heidelberg and obtained his approbation and MD in 1979. During the period of his military service, he worked at the Ernst-Rodenwald Institute in Koblenz, Federal Republic of Germany, and subsequently held a post-doctoral position at the Institute for Virus Research, German Cancer Research Centre, Heidelberg. In 1985 he obtained a Habilitation in Virology, and was appointed Associate Professor at the Institute of Medical Virology at the University of Heidelberg in 1986. Professor Braun has received the Richtzenhain Award and the promotional award of the German Society for Hygiene and Microbiology.

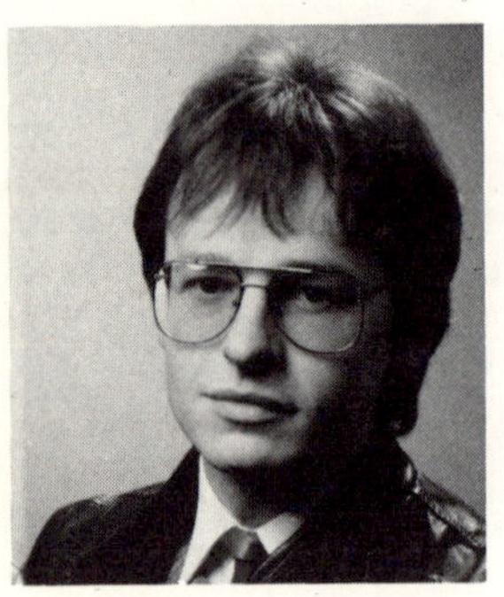

Dr. Jo B. J. Bury was born in Gent, Belgium, on 28th July, 1958. He started his studies in 1976 at the State University of Gent where he became a Pharmacist in 1981. In 1980–1981 he worked as an Assistant in the Laboratory of Toxicology of Professor Dr. A. Heydrickx at the State University of Gent. During the course of 1982–1985, he received an IWONL PhD–Fellowship to study the relationship between the structure and the function of plasma lipoproteins, for which the specific quantitation of the various apolipoproteins by a sensitive technique, such as ELISA, was a technical necessity. The experimental work was performed in the Department of Clinical Biochemistry of Dr. M. Y. Rosseneu in the St-Jan's Hospital in Brugge, Belgium.

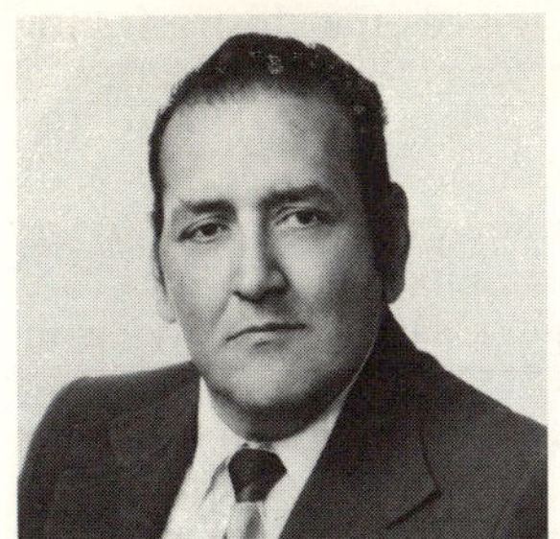

Dr. Albert Castro, PhD, MD, began his career in 1958 at the University of El Salvador, as Assistant Professor of Microbiology and Biochemistry; he became Professor and Head of the Dental Basic Sciences Department in 1965. In 1966 he was awarded a two-year NIH Postdoctoral Fellowship in diabetes and metabolism at the University of Oregon Medical School (UOMS), followed by a two-year NIH Senior Fellowship. His research concerned development of new hormone measurement techniques. This led to an Assistant Professorship in Pediatrics and co-Directorship of the Pediatric Metabolic Laboratory, UOMS, from 1969 to 1973. Dr. Castro moved to Miami, Florida, in 1973 to take up a post as a Senior Scientist and Associate Professor of Medicine at the Papanicolaou Cancer Research Institute; in 1975 he accepted a position in the Department of Pathology at the University of Miami (UM) School of Medicine; he was promoted to Professor in 1977, with secondary appointments in the Departments of Medicine, Microbiology and Immunology. During this time, he developed more than 40 immunoassays for steroids, hormones, drugs, etc. He is recognized as one of the original workers in immunochemistry and has more than 200 publications in scientific journals and 11 chapters in books. Dr. Castro serves as Research Director of the UM Latin-American Program, and as Co-ordinator of the Executive Program Committee, Inter-American International Technology Transfer and Training Program, and has served on the UM Senate. He is listed in numerous biographical publications including *Who's Who in America, 1984/1985, Who's Who in the World, 1984/1985* and *Who's Who in Frontier Science and Technology, 1984/1985.*

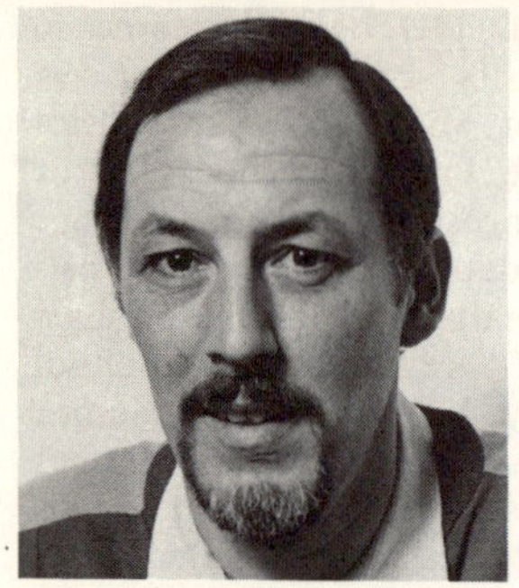

Co Coolen (1941) joined the Institute for Experimental Gerontology in 1975 after a career as a Research Assistant in Pathology. His main interest has been in the occurrence of spontaneous autoantibodies in *Praomys natalensis*. This animal (in appearance somewhere between a mouse and a rat — originally from southern Africa) defies the normal laws of immunology in that it carries high titres of autoantibodies from a very young age onwards. Notwithstanding these autoantibodies, the animal has a considerable life-span. *Praomys* has been advocated as a good animal model for age-related non-pathogenic autoantibodies encountered in man. Co Coolen specialized in immunohistological methods first, with emphasis on immunofluorescence, and later, on enzyme techniques.

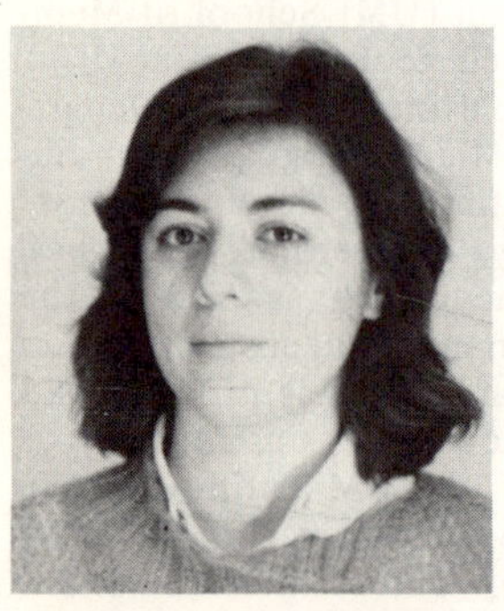

Cristina Crespi was born in Bologna, Italy on 17th February, 1958. She graduated in Medicine *cum laude* at the University of Bologna on 12th November, 1982. She is now specializing in Internal Medicine at the University of Bologna, and attending the Institute of Patologia Medica–Cattedra di Clinica Medica II.

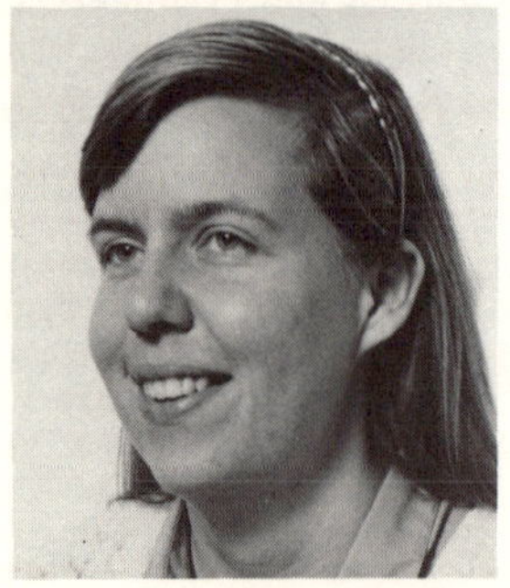

Carla Deen (1958) was trained in microbiological techniques. She joined the Institute for Experimental Gerontology in 1980 and has been working on monoclonal antibodies ever since. Her prime interest has been the epitopic structure of human immunoglobulins. She has shown that the epitopic structure may vary with assay conditions and has screened a large number of monoclonal antibodies for optimal performance. Selected mabs have been applied by her in immunogerontological research on the IgA system in man.

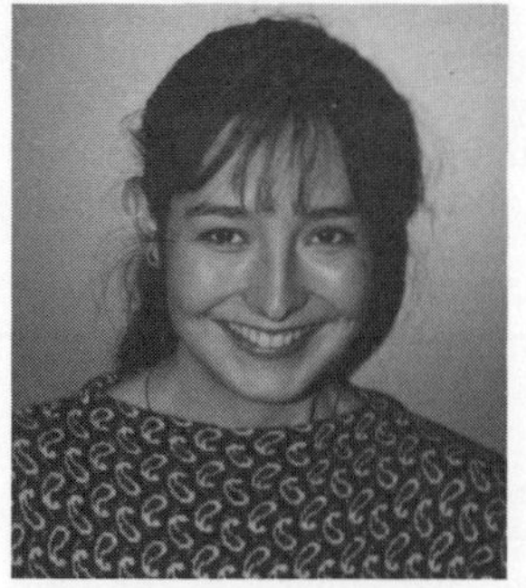

Gabi Dunkler was born on July 30th, 1960 in Esslingen, Federal Republic of Germany. She graduated from High School in 1979, and is now a student of medicine at the University of Heidelberg, in her final year. The subject of her thesis was the analysis of Herpes simplex virus antibodies by Western blots.

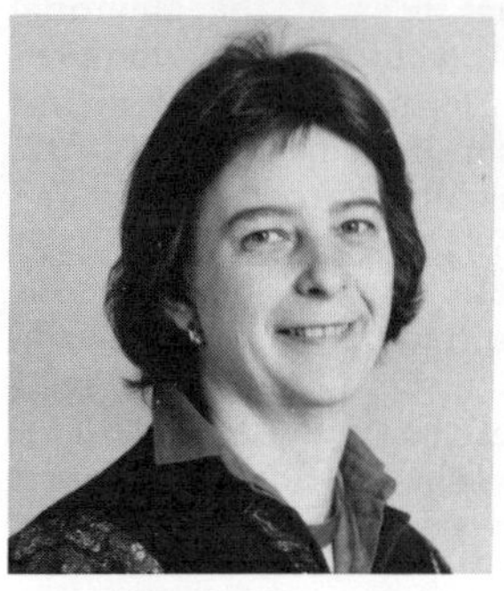

Goverdina E. Fahraeus-Van Ree is Dutch and was educated in the Netherlands. She graduated in Biology at the State University of Utrecht, the Netherlands, and completed her PhD thesis entitled 'In vivo and in vitro studies of the pituitary–ovary axis in the zebrafish (*Brachydanio rerio*, Ham. Buch.)' in 1977 at the same University in the Section for Comparative Endocrinology of the Zoological Laboratory. She worked in this research group from 1971 to 1982 as a Senior Research Scientist. Her research dealt with *in vivo* and *in vitro* studies of the pituitary–ovary axis of the zebrafish and the hormonal regulation of the gonadotropic cells in the pituitary of the juvenile rainbow trout. *Salmo gairdneri*. She was a visiting scholar for a year (in 1979) at the Marine Sciences Research Laboratory, Memorial University of Newfoundland, St John's, Newfoundland, Canada. She emigrated to Canada in late 1982, and is presently employed at the Thyroid Research Laboratory, Health Sciences Center, Memorial University of Newfoundland, St John's. Her special fields of interest are the kinetics of the interactions of hormones (TSH and insulin) and naturally occurring antibodies with the receptor (TSH and insulin) and their processing in the target cell.

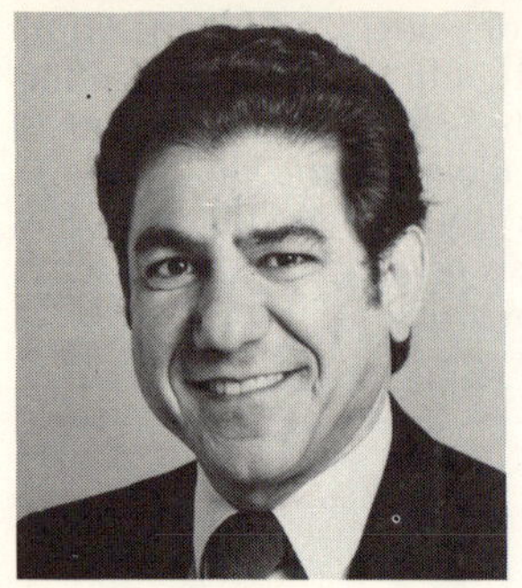

Dr. Nadir R. Farid is Professor of Medicine and Head of the Division of Endocrinology and Metabolism, Faculty of Medicine, Memorial University of Newfoundland, Canada. Dr. Farid, who is 42, received his education at Comboni College, Khartoum, and graduated from the Faculty of Medicine in 1967. He did his post-graduate training in Internal Medicine at the University of Khartoum in 1968–69, and at the University of Newcastle upon Tyne in 1969–1972. While at the University of Newcastle upon Tyne, he directed his interest towards clinical endocrinology, particularly in the field of thyroid work, and research. He took up a Research Fellowship with Dr. Robert Volpe at the University of Toronto in 1972–74, during which time he developed an interest in thyroid autoimmunity. He has been at the Memorial University since 1974, where he was appointed Assistant Professor, Department of Medicine. He has been a Professor of Medicine since 1983, and Chief of the Division of Endocrinology and Metabolism since 1981. Dr. Farid's interests include immunogenetic aspects of endocrine disease, the use of anti-idiotypic antibodies as probes for hormone receptors, and the structure and regulation of the synthesis of the TSH receptor. He has published 116 original papers on these subjects.

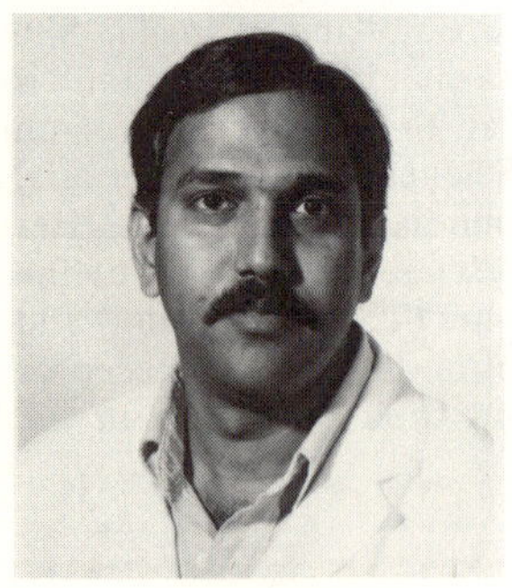

Shaik A. Gaffar was born in India and obtained his PhD in 1976 from the Indian Institute of Science, Bangalore, India. He received his post-doctoral training from the Laboratory of Immunodiagnosis, National Institutes of Health, Bethesda, Maryland, USA, from 1976 to 1979. Subsequently, he worked at the University of Kentucky, Lexington as a Senior Research Associate from 1979 to 1983. Since January 1984, he has been associated with Mark C Glassy as Postgraduate Researcher in the University of California Cancer Center, San Diego, California. Tumour immunology, immuno-chemistry of antigens as well as antibodies, radioimmunodetection of tumours, tumour metastasis and tumour-cell heterogeneity are some of his research interests.

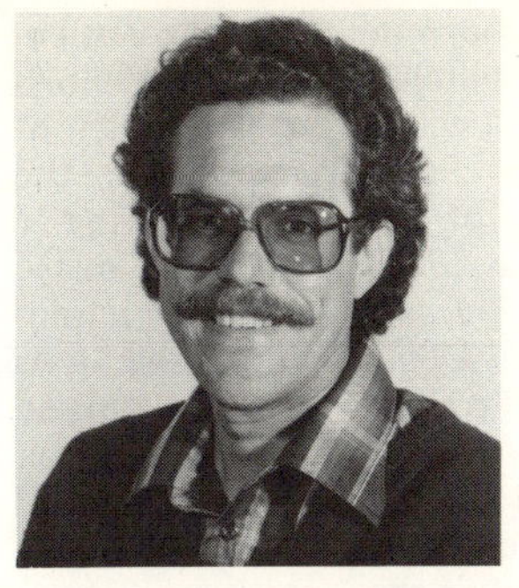

Mark C Glassy was born in the United States and received his BS degree in Biology from the University of San Francisco, California, in 1974. He was awarded a PhD in Biochemistry from the University of California, Riverside, in 1978. He then received his post-doctoral training in Molecular Immunology from Scripps Clinic and Research Foundation, from 1978 to 1980. In 1980 he joined the Department of Medicine, Division of Hematology/Oncology, University of California, San Diego as an Assistant Research Immunologist, and in 1981 became a member of the UCSD Cancer Center. Current research is focused on tumour antigens, mouse and human anti-cancer monoclonal antibodies, enzyme immunoassays, and other related aspects of tumour immunology.

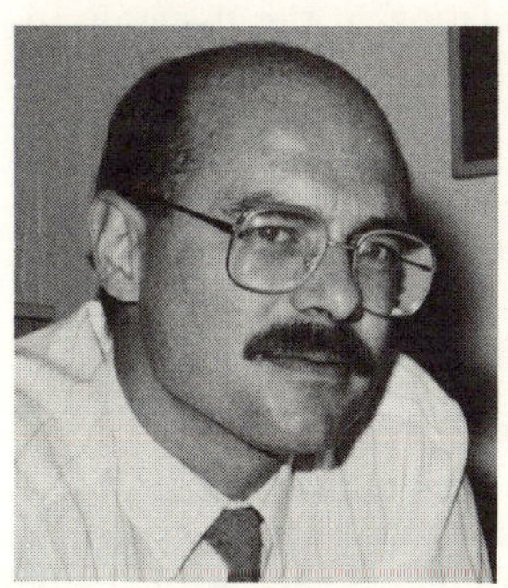

Dr. J. J. Haaijman (1947) received his MSc in Biology from the State University of Utrecht, The Netherlands. He joined the Dutch Organization for Applied Research (TNO) in 1972. His PhD degree was obtained for a thesis entitled 'Quantitative immunofluorescence, microscopy, methods and applications'. During sabbatical leave with Professor Dr. L. A. Herzenberg at Stanford University, Stanford, CA, USA he became acquainted with the technique of monoclonal antibody production. This was subsequently applied in studies of the human immunoglobulin system. Dr. Haaijman is author of numerous papers in the fields of immunology and gerontology. Recently, he was appointed Deputy-Director of the Medical Biological Laboratory of the Organization of Applied Research (TNO).

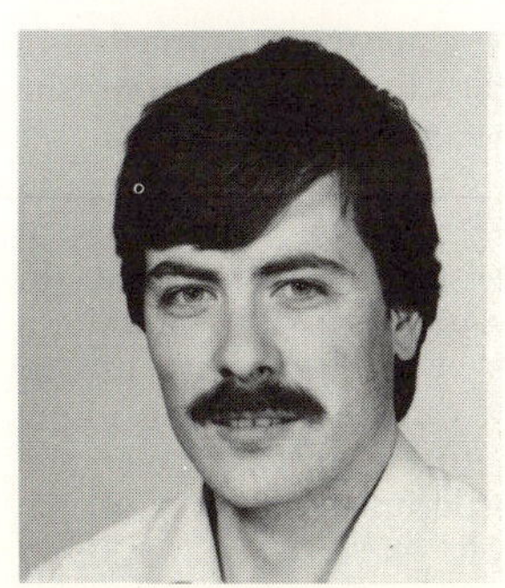

Allister O. Hamilton, BSc, is a Graduate Research Assistant at the University of Glasgow. His research interests include monocyte/macrophage differentiation, regulation of complement synthesis by mononuclear phagocytes and especially the role of interferons.

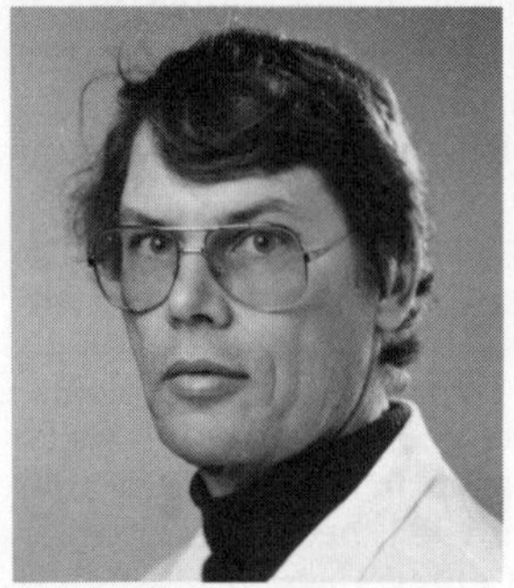

Dr. T. W. Jungi was born in 1945 near Zurich, Switzerland. After obtaining his Batchelor's degree he studied science at the University of Zurich, graduating in 1969, his major being the sensory physiology of insects. Following a period of teaching at high school and college level he took up a PhD programme in immunology at the Medical Department of the Swiss Research Institute, Davos. In 1974 he acquired his PhD degree at the University of Basel. Between 1975 and 1978 he was a Post-doctoral Fellow at the Trudeau Institute, Inc, Saranac Lake, New York, and at the Veterinary School of Medicine, Cornell University, Ithaca, New York. He investigated T-cell macrophage co-operation in a rat model of an infection with an intracellular pathogen, and continued these studies after returning to the Swiss Research Institute, Davos. His particular interest was devoted to the elucidation of the tissue disposition of long-lived memory T-cells and of the MHC restriction pattern imposed on protector T-cells in infection with *Listeria monocytogenes*. In 1982 he joined the Institute of Clinical and Experimental Cancer Research at the University of Berne, where he works in close collaboration with the Central Laboratory of the Swiss Red Cross Blood Transfusion Service. The major topic of his present work is the study of interactions of mononuclear phagocytes with other elements of defence, particularly with IgG antibodies and with blood platelets.

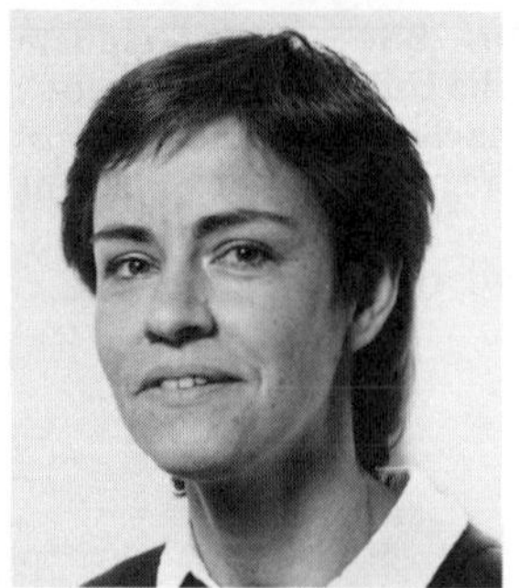

Tonny Kröse (1953) started her career as a Research Technician in Clinical Chemistry. She joined the Immunology Department of the Institute for Experimental Gerontology in 1975, where she first worked on age-related changes of the cytotoxic T-cell system. In 1980 her interest shifted to the immunoglobulin system and, notably, to the use of newly developed mabs directed against isotype-specific markers. Together with Co Coolen she analyzed the immunoglobulin (sub)class distribution of plasma cells in various lymphoid organs of man.

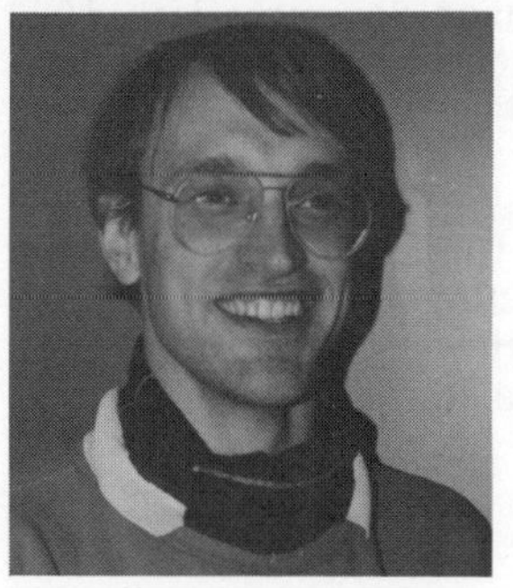

Joachim Kühn was born on November 11th, 1958 in Frankfurt am Main, Federal Republic of Germany. He studied medicine at the University of Saarland, Homburg-Saar, and obtained his approbation and MD in 1984. During the course of 1984 he worked at the Institute of Biochemistry in Homburg-Saar. Since 1985 he has been holding a post-doctoral position at the Institute of Medical Virology, University of Heidelberg.

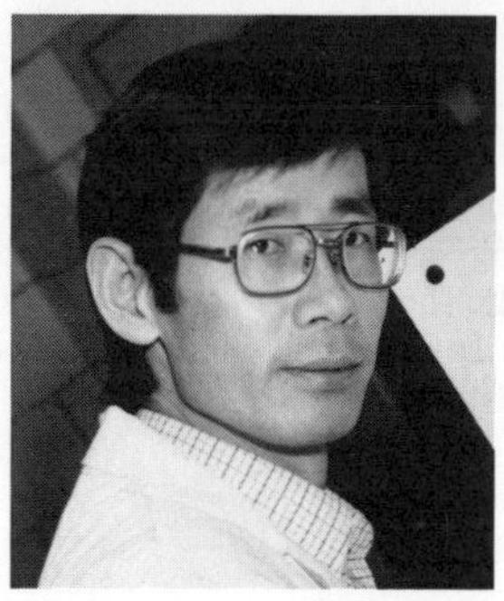

After obtaining his PhD in Biochemistry from Waksman Institute of Microbiology, Rutgers University, New Brunswick, New Jersey in 1975 in the area of microbial chemistry, **Dr. Nobuo Monji** spent one year at the Nippon Roche Research Center, Kamakura, Japan working in the area of drug pharmacodynamics and analytical methods, including the development of radio- and enzyme-immunoassays for small molecules. In order to obtain more extensive training in the development of enzyme-based immunoassay, he became a Post-doctoral Fellow, and later, a Research Assistant Professor at Professor Albert Castro's laboratory in the University of Miami School of Medicine, Miami, Florida. In 1980 he moved to the Medical Research Division of the American Cyanimid Company at Pearl River, New York, in order to pursue his industrial career. In 1984 he moved to the Genetic Systems Corporation, Seattle, Washington. He is currently working as a Program Manager in the development of polymer-based immunoassay for immunodiagnostics.

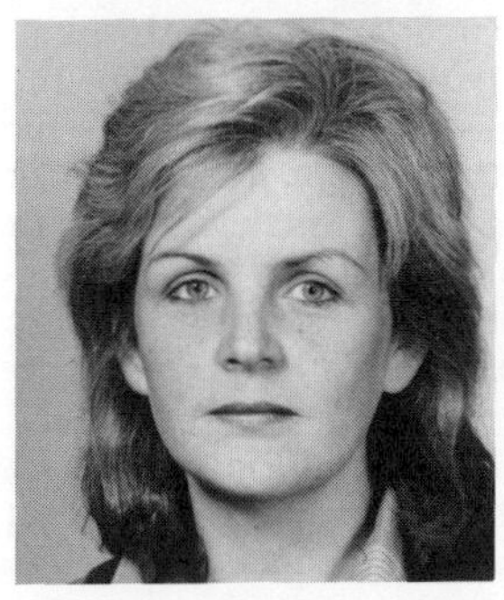

Lindsay Morrison, BSc, PhD, is a post-doctoral scientist working at the Western Infirmary, Glasgow. Her research interests include tumour immunology and the development of ELISA procedures for complement components and pathogenetic mechanisms of immune complex disease.

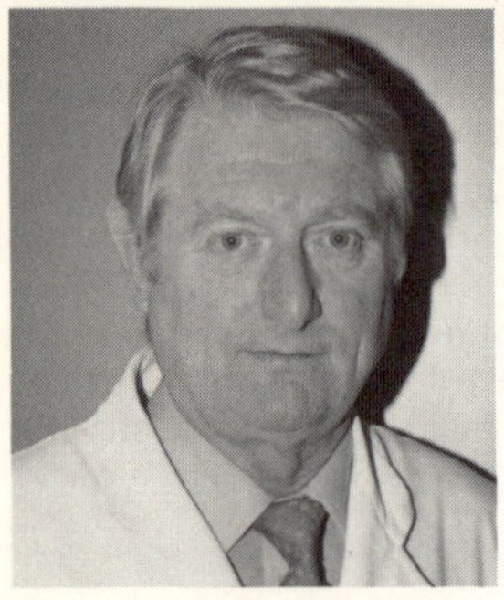

Klaus Munk was born on November 25th, 1922 in Berlin. He studied medicine at the University of Tübingen and obtained his approbation and MD in 1947. Since 1967 he has been Professor of Virology at the University of Heidelberg, Federal Republic of Germany. Professor Munk is Director of the Institute of Medical Virology at the University of Heidelberg, and Director of the Institute of Virus Research of the German Cancer Centre.

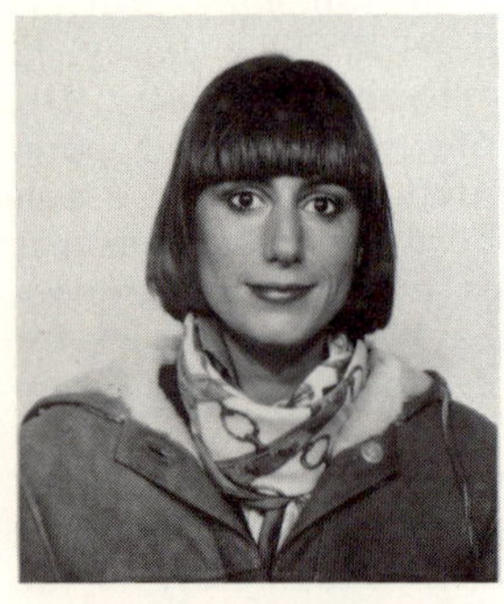

Monica Musiani was born in Bologna, Italy on 24th September, 1951. She graduated in Medicine *cum laude* at the University of Bologna in July 1975, specializing in virology in 1978 and in hygiene and public health in 1981. She is now Assistant at the Institute of Microbiology of the University of Bologna.

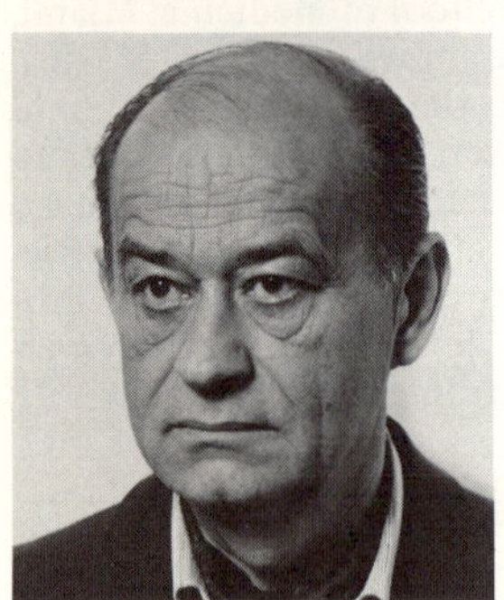

Jiri Radl (1930) obtained his MD in 1955 at Charles University, Prague, Czechoslovakia. He specialized in internal medicine and clinical laboratory techniques; his research work was devoted to serum proteins with special emphasis on immunoglobulins. His PhD thesis entitled 'Clinical and biochemical study of special forms of paraproteinaemias' was obtained in Prague in 1967. He came to the Netherlands in 1968, and worked with Dr. W. Hijmans at the Institute for Rheumatism Research, University Hospital, Leiden. During this period he worked on the setting up of standard fluorescent reagents for immunofluorescence microscopy to be used in the diagnosis of plasma cell malignancies. In 1971 he moved to the Institute for Experimental Gerontology of the Dutch Organization for Applied Research. Here, he studied age-related changes within the immune system and developed mouse models for multiple myeloma and benign monoclonal gammapathy. Dr. Radl is the author of 150 scientific papers.

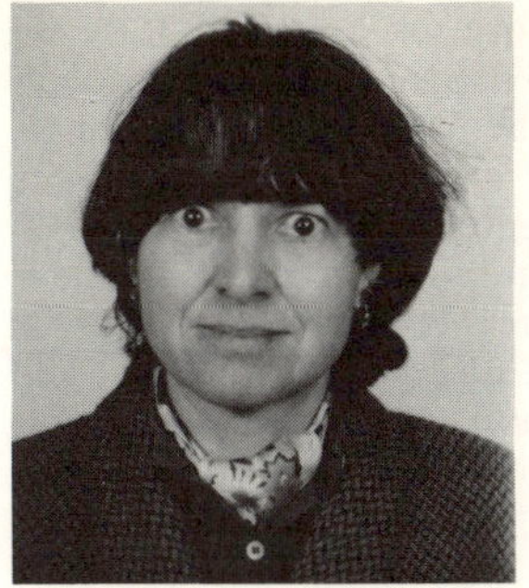

Maryvonne Rosseneu was born in France in 1944, and studied at the École Nationale Supérieure de Chimie in Paris, where she was awarded her degree as a Chemical Engineer in 1965. She obtained her PhD in 1972 at the University of Gent, Belgium, in Physical Chemistry, studying the dielectric properties of albumin, fatty-acid free and recombined with fatty acids. Her first interest in lipoproteins centred on the physicochemical properties of these macromolecules and especially on the phospholipid–apolipoprotein interactions. These *in vitro* studies, conducted mostly by microcalorimetry, required the immunological quantitation of specific apolipoproteins. This has led to her current interest in apolipoprotein fractionation and their application to compositional studies of lipoproteins, and to the characterization of normal and abnormal lipoproteins under pathological conditions.

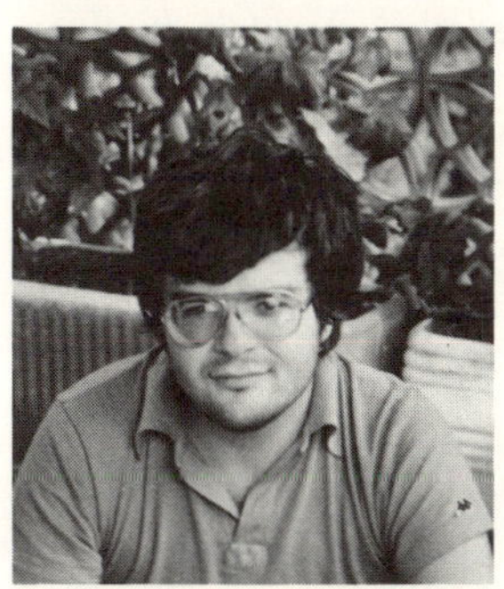

Pier Luigi Tazzari was born in Bologna, Italy on 15th February, 1956. He graduated in Medicine *cum laude* at the University of Bologna on 17th July, 1981, specializing in oncology in 1984. He is at present working at the 'L. & A. Seragnoli' Institute of Haematology of the University of Bologna.

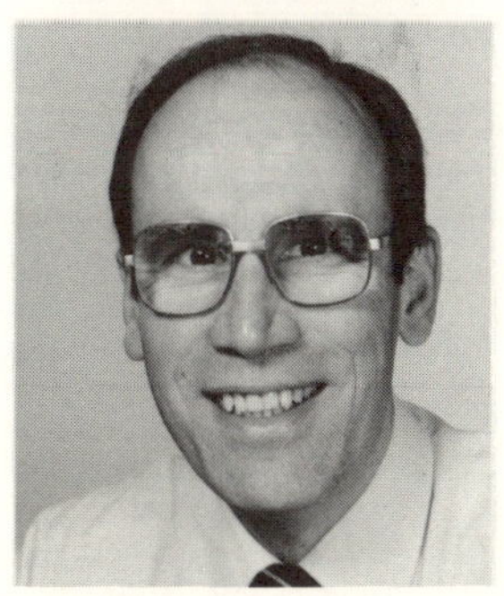

Professor Keith Whaley, MD, PhD, FRCP, FRCPath, is Professor and Honorary Consultant in Clinical Immunology at the University of Glasgow. His research interests include immunopathology of rheumatic and renal diseases, the role of complement in immune complex diseases and regulation of complement biosynthesis by mononuclear phagocytes and hepatocytes.

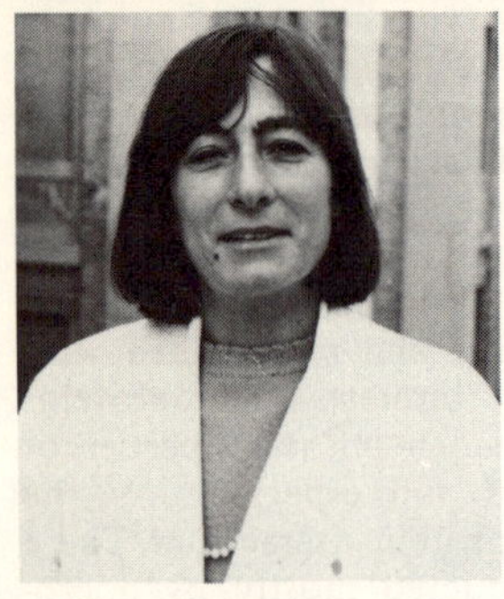

Daniela Zauli was born in Ravenna, Italy on 28th September, 1947. She graduated in Medicine *cum laude* at the University of Bologna, Italy, on 28th July, 1972, after which she specialized in gastroenterology in 1975, and in allergy and clinical immunology in 1979. She is at present Associate Professor of Clinical Immunology at the University of Bologna, and works at the Institute of Patologia Medica-Cattedra di Clinica Medica II.

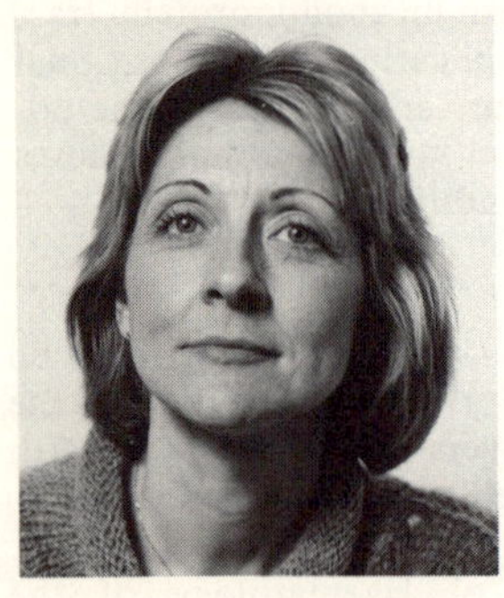

Jelly Zijlstra (1951) started out in T-cell immunology and joined the monoclonal group in 1980. Her interest has been directed towards the immunochemistry of mabs (purification strategies, conjugation with various reporter molecules) and the application of mabs in the tracing of phylogenetic relationships between Igs.

Index